ECSTASY

BB

ECSTASY:
THE COMPLETE GUIDE

A Comprehensive Look
at the Risks and
Benefits of MDMA

Edited by
JULIE HOLLAND, M.D.

Park Street Press
Rochester, Vermont

Park Street Press
One Park Street
Rochester, Vermont 05767
www.InnerTraditions.com

Park Street Press is a division of Inner Traditions International

Note to the reader: This book is intended as an informational guide. The approaches and techniques described herein should not be seen as an endorsement to use MDMA. They also should not be used to treat a serious ailment without prior consultation with a qualified healthcare professional.

Library of Congress Cataloging-in-Publication Data

Ecstasy : the complete guide : a comprehensive look at the risks and benefits of MDMA / edited by Julie Holland.
     p. ; cm.
Includes bibliographical references and index.
 ISBN 0-89281-857-3
 1. Ecstasy (Drug)
 [DNLM: 1. N-Methyl-3,4-methylenedioxyamphetamine—therapeutic use—Interview. 2. Nervous System—drug effects—Interview. 3. Risk Factors—Interview. QV 102 E194 2001] I. Title: Comprehensive look at the risks and benefits of MDMA. II. Holland, Julie, 1965-
 RM666.M35 E373 2001
 615'.785—dc21
                              2001002945

Printed and bound in the United States

10 9 8 7 6 5 4 3 2

Text design and layout by Priscilla Baker
This book was typeset in Janson with Morgan and Gill Sans as display faces

Using MDMA in Healing, Psychotherapy, and Spiritual Practice, originally published as "The Nature of the MDMA Experience and Its Role in Healing, Psychotherapy, and Spiritual Practice" by Ralph Metzner, Ph.D., and Sophia Adamson reprinted with the permission of the Helen Dwight Reid Educational Foundation. Published by Heldref Publications, 1319 Eighteenth St. NW, Washington, DC 20036–1802. Copyright © 1988.

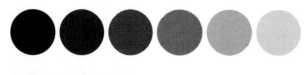

CONTENTS

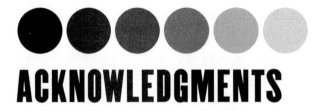

ACKNOWLEDGMENTS

I am indebted to Rowan Jacobsen and Lee Awbrey for their incisive and invaluable editorial assistance and to the diligent Dillon Euler for his role as a contributing editor. Marcia Means and Janet Jesso have done a thorough and exhaustive job as copy editors, which I truly appreciate. I'd like to thank Mark Kelly, my agent, and all the wonderful people at Inner Traditions International.

My sincere gratitude to Sasha Shulgin for patiently reviewing the finer points of all things chemical and historical, and to George Greer and Rick Doblin for providing details on the scheduling proceedings. Thanks also to Dave Nichols and James O'Callaghan for assisting me with some details of chemistry and neurotoxicity, respectively. Simon Reynolds, Harry Sumnall, and José Carlos Bouso taught me a thing or two about the history of the worldwide rave culture, and John Morgan filled me in on some details of the history of MDA. A special thank you to Jerome Beck for his help with the epidemiological statistics of MDMA use. I also appreciate Ilsa Jerome's help in summarizing Charles Grob's research, and Judy Ball's help with the statistics from SAMHSA. Thanks to Craig Bromberg and Joshua Wolf Shenk for their advice regarding the publishing industry and book publicity.

Jeremy Tarcher and R. E. L. Masters gave me assistance and encouragement early in the preparation of this project and I thank them for their belief in me and their advice. I also offer my humble gratitude to Dr. Carolyn Grey for her wisdom and guidance. MAPS and Rick Doblin have been a precious resource to me throughout the past fifteen years, and there is no doubt in my mind I would not be where I am today had Rick and I not met in the summer of 1985.

The following people were instrumental in helping me to assemble the chapter reviewing the MDMA laws throughout the world: Priya Narayanan, Brent Patterson, and Kiran Rao (India); Franco Landriscina, Livia and Alec Nicolescu (Italy); Jorge Gleser (Israel); Greg Duncan (Asia); Joanna Simon (Australia); Zephyros Kafkalides (Greece); Alex Mckay, Evan Rosen, and Adrienne Ward (United States); Harry Sumnall and John Henry (United Kingdom); Luc LeClair (Canada); and Tim Yuan (Brazil). Richard Glen Boire of alchemind.org was kind enough to offer eleventh-hour aid with the United States segment of that chapter.

Thanks also to the following people who donated their time to translate submissions from around the world: Sylvia Thyssen, Katrin Krollpfeiffer, and Chris Ryan.

I especially need to mention Joe Cosco, who originally gave me the idea of creating an MDMA book as a way to honor Nicholas Saunders, who died in 1998 and was an early and dedicated pioneer in espousing the therapeutic aspects of MDMA.

My friends, colleagues, and family have been attentive and supportive since this project began in the spring of 1998. A special thank you to my husband Jeremy, for his loving and playful care of our daughter while I was typing away.

Last, I wish to offer my heartfelt thanks to all the chapter authors, who donated their time and energy to make this book what it is. My biggest regret is that I could not include every submission that was requested, due to the publisher's concerns about this book's size. I humbly offer my apologies again to these authors, and have posted some of their chapters on my website for your perusal. I urge everyone to visit drholland.com to learn more, and also to make a donation to the Holland Fund for Therapeutic MDMA Research. All royalties from the sale of this book will go toward funding clinical MDMA research, and I thank you, the reader, for your contribution.

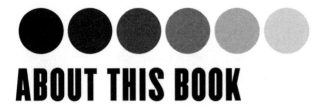

ABOUT THIS BOOK

This book is not about encouraging illicit drug use but rather about promoting mental health and physical safety. It is my belief that MDMA, when used as a prescription medicine in a therapeutic context, may have the potential to benefit various patient populations, and this warrants clinical research. My primary goal in organizing this book is to further that cause. However, I am also a firm believer in the harm reduction model. Because there are millions of people around the world using the drug Ecstasy in a dangerous manner, I feel obligated to educate them about how to reduce their risk of physical harm. Providing risk reduction information, which is a public health service, should not be interpreted as encouragement to abuse drugs.

Throughout this book I have tried to make the distinction when the authors are speaking of the known chemical MDMA versus the illegal, unknown substance called Ecstasy. All illegal substances are of unknown chemical makeup and purity. When a person buys Ecstasy at a rave, club, or from a dealer in any situation, there is no knowing what is being bought or ingested, thus increasing the risk of harm. There have been several reported deaths associated with PMA (paramethoxyamphetamine) sold in the guise of MDMA, and it is suspected that some cases of hyperthermia were due to dextromethorphan, alone or in combination with MDMA, as may occur with impure pills.

Due to the complex nature of MDMA several chapters in this book use fairly technical language—the treatment section in the chapter "Medical Risks Associated with MDMA Use" and the neurotoxicity review found in the chapter "Does MDMA Cause Brain Damage?" in particular. It is my hope that lay readers will have no trouble reading the rest of the book.

Proceeds from the sale of this book will go toward funding clinical research with MDMA. Donations to the Holland Fund for Therapeutic MDMA Research can also be made at the Web site Drholland.com, or by sending your tax deductible check to The Holland Fund c/o MAPS, 2105 Robinson Avenue, Sarasota, Florida 34232.

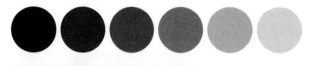

INTRODUCTION:
Medicine for a New Millennium

Julie Holland, M.D.

Every weekend around the world, nearly a million people are taking a drug they call Ecstasy. They hear from friends and the media that this "love drug" is an aphrodisiac, capable of creating feelings of love and empathy with others, or that it induces a "blissed-out" state, marketed as euphoria. The British government estimates that more than half a million hits of Ecstasy are sold every weekend in the United Kingdom, and authorities calculate that the use of Ecstasy increased by more than 4,000 percent between 1990 and 1995. In the United States, hundreds of thousands of doses of Ecstasy are consumed weekly; in the first five months of 2000, over four million hits of the drug were confiscated.

Although some will take Ecstasy in small social gatherings, the majority of people are trying this drug in a setting known as a rave. These are large, all-night dance parties in secret locations or in clubs, where techno music is typically played. The rave scene has been growing since the late 1980s in the United Kingdom and the United States—it has become a huge cultural phenomenon, eclipsing the LSD-inspired movement of the sixties in terms of the number of participants and the movement's longevity. In Spain, Germany, Israel, and Australia, weekly raves attract tens of thousands of revelers, and the majority of those in attendance are specifically seeking out Ecstasy. Even India is experiencing a significant increase in Ecstasy consumption, as the "new drug craze," now fifteen years old and still going strong, finally reaches that continent.

Almost everyone has heard of Ecstasy, the dance drug, but few know the whole story. Unknown to many, Ecstasy has a less recreational, more medicinal history. In the 1970s and 1980s, the chemical known as MDMA (methylenedioxymethamphetamine, or N-methyl-3,4-methylenedioxyphenylisopropylamine) was used secretly by a select group of psychiatrists and therapists in the United States and Europe. These private practitioners, some of whom called the drug Adam, had discovered a pharmacological tool that lowered their clients' defenses and allowed them to open up more completely to the psychotherapeutic process. In doses smaller than those typically used in the rave setting, MDMA would induce a gentle and subtle shift in consciousness, enabling its users to give themselves over to a frank and thorough self-analysis. A New York writer described his MDMA experience as being like a "year of therapy in two hours" (Adler 1985). The effects of MDMA fostered introspection and verbalization of profoundly meaningful aspects of personality and life history. Unlike earlier psychotherapy sessions in the 1950s and 1960s catalyzed by LSD, MDMA-supported therapy allowed patients to remain centered, focused, and able to think and speak clearly.

Painful and repressed memories typically are not accessible until years of therapy have uncovered them. Under the influence of MDMA, these psychic traumas often come to the foreground to be processed and analyzed in one intense session. The greatest difference, however, is that instead of feeling vulnerable and anxious during this experience, the patients remain relaxed, nearly fearless, and show a stronger sense of self and purpose. Feelings of depression and anxiety are replaced with a sense of ease and satiety. Therapists scattered throughout the United States and Switzerland were impressed by the consistent usefulness of this new drug and were giving it to their patients with remarkable results. Some therapists even conducted sessions with the terminally ill, assisting them to make peace with their families and themselves before death. An added and unexpected effect of MDMA is its potent pain-killing property. Terminal patients who had been in chronic pain found themselves pain-free for the duration of the MDMA session. Adam earned the reputation of being "penicillin for the soul" and a "psychic pain-reliever": it offered healing to all who partook.

The judicious, supervised, and infrequent use of single oral doses of MDMA as a psychiatric medicine may be a revolutionary tool to assist the fields of psychology and psychiatry. Dr. Mitchel Liester interviewed twenty psychiatrists who were personally familiar with the effects of MDMA. Roughly 85 percent of those surveyed said they thought that MDMA has substantial potential as an adjunct to the psychotherapy process. A large percentage of them spoke of psychological or spiritual benefits in their own lives that had resulted from MDMA use (Liester et al. 1992). The results of a survey of sixteen psychiatrists and therapists who had used MDMA in their practices were presented at a conference in Bern, Switzerland, in 1990. All of the twelve American and five Swiss clinicians felt that the general psychotherapeutic value of MDMA was "very positive." More than three fourths of these therapists stated that their patients had improved greatly in insight-based therapies and that the overall psychological value of MDMA was great (Harlow and Beck 1990).

Any psychiatric disorder that can be ameliorated by psychotherapy can be treated more quickly and more profoundly with MDMA-assisted psychotherapy. MDMA is also a useful tool in the field of medicine, helping those with chronic pain or psychosomatic illness and those who are dying. This medicine can help heal a person, and it also can strengthen the bonds between people. Many therapists have been impressed by the degree of empathy generated during an MDMA experience. This makes MDMA especially useful for couple's therapy and family therapy, in which patients need to have an understanding of what their loved ones are experiencing and of one another's emotions.

Like anesthesia given during surgery to allow for deeper incisions and removal of more malignant material, MDMA is a chemo-adjunct, given during therapy to allow for a more thorough examination of deeper layers of psychological material. In a field of medicine with no specialized equipment, anesthetics, or tools to help with the excavation required for successful treatment, a safe and versatile new medication had been discovered and added to the armamentarium. Therapists had found a way to make painful psychotherapy easier and faster.

MDMA had been used for over a decade as an adjunct to psychotherapy when, in 1985, the Drug Enforcement Administraton labeled it a Schedule I drug. In effect, the government was unilaterally stating that this drug had no medical utility and, like heroin and cocaine, it had a high potential for abuse. Overnight, what was once a medicine used by experienced clinicians became an illegal drug, its use punishable by a fine of up to $125,000 or fifteen years in prison. The reason for the DEA's ruling was that Adam, the therapeutic tool, had leaked out into the general community to become Ecstasy, the party drug. But because the drug was placed in Schedule I, no clinical work could move forward, and it became very difficult to obtain permission for human research studies. This action allowed illicit use to continue unabated but put a halt to any legitimate accumulation of knowledge about the drug. All hope for its clinical and therapeutic use evaporated. In response to the rapid scheduling of MDMA, a group of physicians banded together to educate the government about this special psychoactive substance and to fight for their clinical practices and for their patients. Some of those therapists are featured on the following pages.

This book is about the importance of bringing MDMA back into the fold of medicine. It is about reclaiming the legacy of MDMA and giving it back to the people who can benefit most from its judicious, supervised use. The contributors to this volume are people who have been involved with MDMA for many years and in some cases decades. They are scientists who perform MDMA research or psychiatrists who have administered MDMA to their patients. Members of the rave community, the clergy, and those navigating the regulatory waters in an attempt to make MDMA a prescription medicine also are represented. This book convenes multiple experts weighing in with facts and opinions concerning this controversial drug.

One purpose of this book is simple and can be summed up in two words: pain control. People have the potential to be hurt and helped by MDMA, and this book aims to educate both groups. Millions around the world are taking Ecstasy, and they need to be informed about the risks of their behavior and how to minimize any harm that may come from it. For instance, one of the greatest risks from unsupervised use of Ecstasy and dancing in overheated environments is heatstroke. For millions of ravers worldwide, this should be taken as a strong recommendation to stay cool at a rave, take plenty of breaks, and drink a moderate amount of water. Clinical research and human studies are essential in helping us learn more about minimizing the dangers of illicit Ecstasy use.

When the forbidden cookie jar is placed on a high shelf out of reach, a child is more determined than ever to get to it. When a drug is scheduled, it goes underground. It becomes inaccessible to researchers but readily available on the black market. People then buy illicitly made substances that are unregulated and use them in a clandestine environment where they are unsupervised and miseducated. When millions of people take a legal drug every week (for example, alcohol), the medical community typically sponsors thorough research and public education. This is not true with MDMA. Instead of scientific evidence about the actual effects of MDMA, we get rumors, innuendo, and good copy. The government itself loses credibility as it overstates the dangers of drug use. The amount of misinformation being disseminated about Ecstasy via the media and the Internet is irresponsible and alarming. An important aim of this book is to educate the average Ecstasy user about MDMA—to offer reliable information from legitimate sources and professionals who are familiar with the complex risk/benefit analysis of this drug.

The second purpose of this book is to present the idea that we can do better than simply minimizing the harm associated with illicit Ecstasy use. We can offer MDMA as a beneficial medicine. We can remind everyone of Ecstasy's earlier incarnation as a drug once known as Adam, and we can stress the importance of future clinical research into the therapeutic uses of MDMA. This book delineates the possible therapeutic advantages to be gained by guided MDMA experiences and emphasizes the need for further clinical research. All proceeds from the sale of this book will go toward funding future studies.

Like any other medicine, MDMA has indications and contraindications—situations where its use would be helpful and other instances where its use is ill advised. Like any other potent medicine, there is a therapeutic index that needs to be respected—a safe dose and a dangerous dose, a recommended frequency of dosing, and many guidelines to prevent misuse. As with chemotherapy for cancer or lithium for manic-depression, this strong medicine needs to be carefully administered and monitored. Like any powerful tool, it should be used by people who are properly trained, educated, and supervised. And like any power tool, it should come with an instruction manual. This book, I hope, will serve as that manual.

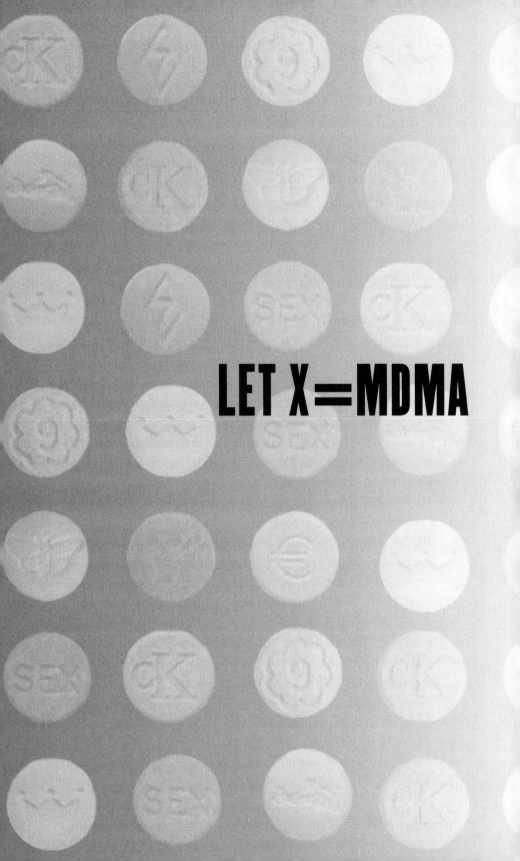

LET X=MDMA

Introduction

MDMA, also known as Ecstasy (X, XTC, E, Rolls), is a semi-synthetic drug, since it is related to many chemicals found in nature. The tree that gives us nutmeg and mace *(Myristica fragrans)*, as well as its essential oil safrole, is the most commonly known relative of MDMA, but the sassafras root is, in fact, a much more potent source of safrole. Safrole is the major natural precursor in the synthesis of MDMA. Other natural elements that have chemical similarities to MDMA are parsley, dill, and the calamus root (Shulgin and Shulgin 1991).

MDMA is chemically related to the amphetamine group of drugs, which includes methamphetamine (speed) and MDA (3,4-methylenedioxy-amphetamine, an analog, or chemical cousin, and metabolite, or breakdown product of MDMA). It belongs to the family of phenethylamines, as does mescaline. MDMA shares some chemical properties with mescaline, but MDMA is not a hallucinogen. As a matter of fact, its subjective effects are not like any other drug. Unlike alcohol or anti-anxiety drugs, there is no clouding of consciousness or sedation, and unlike cocaine or methamphetamine, there is no agitation or paranoia. Its effects are more easily controlled and predictable than LSD or psilocybin. The chemical effects of MDMA more closely resemble an immediately acting antidepressant such as fluoxetine (Prozac), but the euphoria and calm are more profound. So distinct is MDMA that most chemists and psychopharmacologists believe that it deserves its own classification. The two proposed class names are "empathogen," meaning "to create an empathic state," and "entactogen," meaning "to create a touching within."

When administered by a trained psychiatrist to a properly prepared patient, MDMA produces a consistently reliable response in nearly all users. In the context of a therapeutic session, the feeling of a low dose of MDMA can best be compared to taking a deep, cleansing breath. If you try this, you will notice a very mild change in how you feel. In a therapeutic situation without many distractions, the feeling from a low dose of MDMA is similarly subtle and mild. Dr. Lester Grinspoon dubbed it a "gentle invitation to insight" (Klein 1985). It is a slight shift in perception—you may feel a little calmer and more centered, or you may feel that you have all that you need.

8

At higher doses of MDMA, that feeling of satiety becomes a fortified self-image, a sense of enhanced capacity and strength. Taking that effect a step further, it becomes euphoria, intense self-love and self-acceptance. This is why experiences with MDMA can be so curative. Having feelings of confidence and self-worth can be invaluable during psychotherapy, allowing for the exploration of painful material. Lessening anxiety to explore core issues or repressed memories, and feeling calm in the face of what would typically be considered threatening, help accomplish a great deal in therapy. Experiencing these feelings of self-love and acceptance, sometimes for the first time in years, can be therapeutic all on its own.

Depression, anxiety, and feeling uncomfortable in your body and in your life stem in large part from self-hatred. Self-loathing is universal; it is hidden, and it is malignant. It manifests in self-destructive, addictive patterns of drug use, compulsive eating, or escapist behaviors, such as numbing yourself with television. These sabotaging behaviors impede progress toward life's goals. MDMA increases the ratio of love to fear. The capacity to love yourself and love others triumphs over the anxiety about doing just that. Allowing yourself to see and accept all that you are opens the path toward healing. People are scarred, and they are scared. MDMA often allows them, for the first time, to accept themselves fully and to feel a love for themselves that they may never have experienced. A major marker of successful psychotherapy is understanding, accepting, and loving yourself and your place in the world. Good psychotherapy often works, but it takes years. MDMA markedly accelerates and intensifies the process.

A fringe benefit of the MDMA-assisted psychotherapy session is a fortified bond with the therapist. The feelings of self-love tend to flow outward, growing into acceptance and love of the people around you, and in this way the therapeutic alliance is solidified. A sense of trust, that the therapist cares about the patient and is trying to help, carries over into subsequent sessions without the drug, strengthening the entire psychotherapy process.

Other subjective effects of MDMA include feeling less hopeless and more socially connected, which are two crucial issues in the context of working with people who are depressed or suicidal. Because there is a renewed sense of strength and a belief in the capacity to deal with life's problems, the typical feelings of hopelessness that arise during an episode of depression are quieted.

When people are suicidal, they often are lonely, with few social connections, but the MDMA experience can provide a sense of belonging to a bigger whole, of being connected to all of humankind and nature. MDMA can effectively interrupt feelings of depression, hopelessness, and isolation.

Optimally, a session with MDMA should include experiencing courage and hope, seeing your goals, and sensing your purpose. Your life makes sense; you, as a person, make sense—these are the components of the ecstatic experience. The beauty of this experience is that you come to know and feel the result of successful therapy in advance; MDMA points out the proper direction and provides the incentive to pursue it. At the peak, you are transported to your goal; you get a guided tour of your ultimate self-realized destination. Dr. Claudio Naranjo, a therapist who has worked with MDMA, referred to the peak as a "brief, fleeting moment of sanity." You gain a clearer understanding of what it will take to arrive at this place of peace in the future, and you see that you could get there on your own, over time, without the drug. With a good guide and careful integration of what you have gleaned from the experience, you understand the changes that are necessary in your life for you to return to that place of love and acceptance.

THE HISTORY OF MDMA

Julie Holland, M.D.

Although MDMA (methylenedioxymethamphetamine) has been in the public spotlight only since the mid-1980s, its history extends back to the beginning of the twentieth century. MDMA was synthesized some time before 1912. The German pharmaceutical giant Merck was attempting to create a new medication to stop bleeding when it stumbled across MDMA as an intermediate step in the synthesis. On Christmas Eve in 1912, Merck filed the patent for this styptic medication, called hydrastinin; MDMA was included in the patent application as an intermediate chemical only (Beck, 1997). The patent was received in 1914 and has long since expired. For this reason, MDMA no longer can be patented. Contrary to the stories of most reporters and even some scientists, there was no use mentioned for MDMA in Merck's patent application. MDMA was never marketed as an appetite suppressant, nor was it used in any way during World War I. Its chemical cousin, MDA (methylenedioxyamphetamine, an analog and metabolite of MDMA), however, was patented by Smith Kline French and tested as an appetite suppressant in humans in 1958. It was then abandoned because of its psychoactive properties; this is likely the cause of the confusion.

Between 1912 and 1953, MDMA appears twice in the scientific literature. Both times it is cited as a side product of chemical reactions, news that was published and received with very little fanfare. In 1953, the Army Chemical Center funded secret testing of various psychotropic chemicals, including MDMA, for their potential as espionage or "brainwashing" weapons. These toxicity and behavioral studies, which were declassified in 1969, were performed at the University of Michigan using animals; no human studies were conducted at that time. MDMA was given the code name EA 1475. Some people mistakenly believe that the EA stands for "experimental agent," but it really abbreviates Edgewood Arsenal, where the chemicals were synthesized. Eight psychotropic drugs were studied (mescaline, DMPEA, MDPEA, MDA, BDB, DMA, TMA, and MDMA) in rats, mice, guinea pigs, dogs, and monkeys (Hartman et al. 1973). In late 1952, human studies using MDA were conducted at the New York State Psychiatric Institute, where a volunteer was inadvertently given an overdose of the drug by the researchers and died. MDA became popular before MDMA, in the mid-1960s in the hippie subculture of the Haight Ashbury area in San Francisco (Beck and Rosenbaum 1994). Nicknamed the love drug and the mellow drug of America, MDA was reputed to impart a high that was described as a sensual euphoria that lasted for six to eight hours. Psychotherapeutic studies of MDA reported facilitation of insight and heightened empathy (Naranjo et al. 1967; Naranjo 1973), but the drug was declared illegal in the United States by the Controlled Substances Act of 1970.

Although MDMA did not become popular until the early 1980s, a sample was obtained in Chicago in 1970; it was finally analyzed, and the results published in 1972 verified it was indeed MDMA (Gaston and Rasmussen 1972). Sasha Shulgin, the chemist who often is credited erroneously for creating MDMA, did not synthesize MDMA until September 8, 1976. The first published human study of MDMA appeared in 1978. In this article Dr. Shulgin and another chemist, Dave Nichols, described its subjective effects as "an easily controlled altered state of consciousness with emotional and sensual overtones" (Shulgin and Nichols 1978). Shulgin, who lived in California and had many friends in the scientific community, some of whom were therapists, introduced MDMA to a few of his colleagues. He had had experiences with many psychedelics by that time and felt that this substance in particular could be useful to the psychotherapeutic process. One therapist, referred to as Jacob in Myron Stolaroff's book *The Secret Chief*, was so impressed with the effects of MDMA that he came out of retirement and began to introduce other therapists to the drug. This led to a slow spread of underground psychotherapeutic work in the late seventies and early eighties. Psychotherapist Ann Shulgin estimates that as many as four thousand therapists were introduced to MDMA during Jacob's tenure.

In March of 1985 Deborah Harlow, Rick Doblin, and Alise Agar, who referred to their group as Earth Metabolic Design Laboratories, sponsored a meeting on MDMA at the Esalen Institute in Big Sur, California. Several therapists who used MDMA in their practices and other psychiatrists who used various other psychedelics were invited to attend. According to an article by George Greer (1985), who attended the conference, "The combined clinical experience in using MDMA during the past several years totaled over a thousand sessions." Because of what had happened with LSD, which many researchers thought was a valuable tool but which was outlawed once too many people had gotten wind of it, most MDMA enthusiasts agreed to keep quiet. The media was discouraged from spreading the word, and very little was published about MDMA until a story broke in the *San Francisco Chronicle* in June 1984.

The name the therapists had given to MDMA was Adam, signifying "the condition of primal innocence and unity with all life" described in the Bible's account of the Garden of Eden (Metzner and Adamson 1988). But MDMA acquired a new name among recreational users of the drug. It is widely accepted that the name Ecstasy was chosen simply for marketing reasons. It is a powerful, intriguing name to attach to a psychoactive substance. The person who named the drug, an alleged dealer who wishes to remain anonymous, had this to say: "Ecstasy was chosen for obvious reasons, because it would sell better than calling it Empathy. Empathy would be more appropriate, but how many people know what it means?" (Eisner 1989).

By the early 1980s, recreational use of MDMA had begun in earnest. A group of entrepreneurs in Texas, known to most as the "Texas group," started to produce and distribute MDMA in small brown bottles under the brand name Sassyfras, a nod to the naturally occurring essential oil of sassafras that is a chemical precursor to MDMA (Eisner 1989; Collin and Godfrey 1997). Because MDMA was not yet a scheduled, or illegal, drug, people could order it by calling a toll-free number and paying for it with their credit cards. It also was available at certain nightclubs in Dallas and Fort Worth, Texas, where over-the-counter sales at the bars were subject to tax. All of this MDMA-fueled nightlife got the attention of Texas Democratic senator Lloyd Bentsen, who sat on the Senate Judiciary Committee and urged the Drug Enforcement Administration (DEA) to make the drug illegal. When the Texas group heard about impending legislation, they stepped up production, from estimates of thirty thousand tablets a month to as much as eight thousand tablets a day. In the few months before MDMA became illegal, it is possible that the Texas group made as many as two million tablets of Ecstasy (Eisner 1989; Collin and Godfrey 1997).

The DEA published their intention to declare MDMA a Schedule I drug on July 27, 1984, in the Federal Register. A Schedule I drug is prohibited for every application, has no recognized medical use, and cannot be prescribed by a physician. In response to the DEA's proposal, a group of psychiatrists, psychotherapists, and researchers (Thomas Roberts, George Greer, Lester Grinspoon, and James Bakalar), together with their lawyer, Richard Cotton, filed a letter within the thirty-day period allotted by law to the DEA administrator, Francis Mullen, requesting a hearing. The request was granted, and the DEA scheduled hearings in Los Angeles, Kansas City, and Washington, D.C.

On May 31, 1985, the DEA announced that it would not wait for the hearings to be completed before acting, because their recent data indicated that the drug was being abused in twenty-eight states. On an emergency basis, the DEA "scheduled" MDMA, taking advantage of a law passed in October 1984 that allows drugs to be scheduled for one year, without hearings, if there is enough concern for public safety. MDMA is the only drug that has been scheduled in this manner. The ban took effect July 1, 1985. The emergency action was an interim measure to curb Ecstasy abuse until the longer administrative process could be completed. The DEA also initiated efforts to criminalize all aspects of MDMA internationally. An expert committee of the World Health Organization recommended that MDMA be placed in Schedule I but urged countries to "facilitate research in this interesting substance"(World Health Organization 1985). The chairman of this group voted against scheduling MDMA and felt that the decision should be deferred while awaiting data on the substance's therapeutic usefulness. MDMA was placed in Schedule I internationally on February 11, 1986.

The DEA hearings took place in February, June, and July of 1985. Many psychiatrists, research scientists, psychotherapists, and, of course, lawyers took part. People who had experience giving MDMA to patients testified as to the unique utility of MDMA to catalyze the therapeutic process, to enhance insight and communication between spouses, family members, and therapist and patient. Speaking on behalf of the DEA were those who felt that MDMA caused brain damage. Dr. Lewis Seiden of the University of Chicago presented data from animal studies of MDA, demonstrating changes in the axon terminals of rodents given injections of large amounts of that substance. Humans do not take MDMA by injection, but ingest it orally. Moreover, these two drugs are very different in terms of their effects and how long they last, and they have opposite active optical isomers [see "The Chemistry of MDMA" for more details]. Nonetheless, the MDA neurotoxicity data seemed to make an impact for the prosecution's side.

To meet the criteria for Schedule I, the DEA had to prove that MDMA had no accepted medical use and a high potential for abuse. Unfortunately, the fact that no scientists had performed double-blind, placebo-controlled studies examining the clinical efficacy of MDMA hurt those challenging the DEA's move to schedule the drug. There simply was no proof, beyond the anecdotal, that MDMA did what the therapists said it did. Based on the weight of all of the evidence presented at the three hearings, thirty-four witnesses in all, Judge Francis Young, handed down an opinion on May 22, 1986. Because he felt that there was an accepted medical use for MDMA, he recommended to the DEA that MDMA be placed in Schedule III. This would allow clinical work and research to proceed unhindered and would permit physicians to prescribe MDMA.

The DEA's administrator, John C. Lawn, was not convinced, and Judge Young's recommendation was ignored. During the course of an appeal by Dr. Lester Grinspoon, (from December 22, 1987, to March 22, 1988, a period of time referred to affectionately as the "Grinspoon window"), MDMA was again unscheduled. Grinspoon won his case—the first circuit court of appeals in Boston ruled that the DEA could not use the fact that MDMA did not have Food and Drug Administration (FDA) approval as the basis for their argument that it had no medically accepted use. There were other points at issue. Congress gave the U.S. Attorney General, not the DEA, the power to schedule drugs on an emergency basis. The Attorney General was authorized to delegate that authority to the DEA, but the DEA acted against MDMA before the Attorney General had formally delegated that power. This intriguing loophole was used successfully by several attorneys to argue for overturning the convictions of their clients for MDMA possession and trafficking, convictions that took place before the permanent scheduling of the drug. At the end of all the trials and appeal, John Lawn and the DEA permanently placed MDMA in Schedule I on March 23, 1988.

As a result of the trials, the media got wind of the situation—"Miracle Medicine/Party Drug Goes on Trial" ran the headlines. Many questions began to be posed. Was MDMA an amazing therapeutic tool, as proposed by the West Coast shrinks? Was it a killer drug that causes brain damage, as promulgated by the DEA? Every magazine article and every television news story was free publicity for the drug Ecstasy. The so-called hug drug or love drug was a hot story in the summer of 1985. Indeed, that was when I first heard of MDMA. I remember feeling sorry for the psychiatrists who had based their practices on MDMA-assisted psychotherapy. How hard it must be for them when they had seen the benefits of its proper use. Many of these practitioners, not willing to risk their licenses and livelihoods to administer an illegal drug, ceased using it. But some continued, becoming "underground" therapists. As Ann Shulgin described it, "MDMA is penicillin for the soul; you don't give up penicillin when you see what it can do" (Shulgin and Shulgin 1991).

Some time in the early 1980s, a group of intravenous heroin users in northern California made national news when they inadvertently injected themselves with MPTP (1-methyl-4-phenyl-1,2,5,6-tetrahydropyridine), the unfortunate product of a botched attempt to concoct a synthetic opiate. [See "MDMA Myths and Rumors Dispelled" for more details.] In at least seven of these individuals, a severe form of parkinsonism developed, with shaking tremors and impressive episodes of near paralysis (Ballard et al. 1985). This made for amazing copy, and many television talk shows aired images of these patients on the same shows that were explaining the other popular drug of that time, MDMA. Because of this synchronicity many people became confused and assumed that MDMA caused Parkinson's disease. MPTP has been shown to be toxic to dopamine-producing neurons and is now used as a chemical model for mimicking Parkinson's disease. MDMA has never been shown to damage dopamine-producing neurons or cause parkinsonian symptoms.

With the increased media coverage of Ecstasy during the mid-1980s came growing recreational use of the drug. Several surveys of college campuses reflected this trend—anywhere from 8 percent to 39 percent of those surveyed admitted using the drug [see appendices]. In the early eighties, Ecstasy use in the gay club scene of New York, specifically at Studio 54 and Paradise Garage, enhanced its cachet. British disc jockeys and such performers as Soft Cell and Boy George returned to England from trips to New York City extolling the virtues of the drug. Couriers began smuggling Ecstasy into England from America. There are rumors that the followers of Bhagwan Shree Rajneesh, an Indian guru based in the Pacific Northwest, were proponents of MDMA and may have helped lay the foundation for its international distribution, particularly into the Netherlands, where MDMA remained legal until 1988 (Collin and Godfrey 1997).

Some researchers place the beginning of the rave movement on the Spanish island of Ibiza, where two tablets of Ecstasy were confiscated by police in 1986 (Capdevilla 1995; Gamella and Roldán 1999). Certain DJs from London started "spinning" at the nightclubs there in the summers of 1985 and 1986. The summer of 1987 was huge on Ibiza, with large gatherings at the *discotecas* fueled by Ecstasy and an eclectic mix of music. Paul Oakenfold, an English DJ, tried to import that sound and vibe back to London during the winter of 1987, at the Project Club (Reynolds 1998). Afterward, large all-night dance parties, called raves, began to be held in underground locations or in clubs, with a growing number of attendees taking Ecstasy. What followed thereafter, in 1988, was Britain's "Summer of Love," when the raves were held outdoors with thousands in attendance. Unfortunately, that summer also brought the United Kingdom's first Ecstasy-related death: twenty-one-year-old Ian Larcombe, who was alleged to have taken eighteen Ecstasy tablets at once.

The rave phenomenon sweeping the United Kingdom, which was considered the largest youth movement in Britain's history (Collin and Godfrey 1997), was soon exported back to the United States. New York's Frankie Bones, a DJ and producer, brought the rave to the United States after visiting England in 1989. His "STORMraves" began in warehouses in the outer boroughs of New York and eventually took place monthly throughout 1992, the so-called Second Summer of Love. NASA (Nocturnal Audio and Sound Awakening), a popular rave at the Manhattan club Shelter, kicked off in July 1992, and one of the first large U.S. raves in San Francisco, Toon Town, debuted in 1991 (Reynolds 1998). Raves are still going strong in the San Francisco Bay Area, and Oakland's version, called massives, bring anywhere from five thousand to thirty thousand attendees.

Throughout the nineties, both rave scenes—in the United States and the United Kingdom—fed off each other and grew to become a substantial part of the youth culture in each country. Worldwide consumption of Ecstasy continued to grow exponentially, and raves of thousands of people became increasingly common, spreading throughout Europe, Australia, Israel, and India. At times the Ecstasy supply in the United States and the United Kingdom was sporadic; occasionally, there seemed to be an abundance of methamphetamine compared with MDMA, but at other times, the European market seemed to be flooded with Ecstasy. The sources were underground labs and possibly even abandoned pharmaceutical companies, in Eastern European (former Iron Curtain) countries (Saunders 1993, 1995). The DEA also regularly cited Amsterdam as being a major relay point for Ecstasy manufacture or distribution. Many significant Ecstasy seizures in Amsterdam, Los Angeles, and Newark, New Jersey, airports have been well publicized in the past several years. Russian and Israeli organized crime rings have been implicated in the drug's current distribution network, as have Hassidic Jewish couriers.

By the late nineties, government seizures of Ecstasy in the United States had increased by 450 percent. Congress held hearings in June 2000 and reported that Ecstasy seizures by the United States Customs Service had risen from less than five hundred thousand tablets during 1997 to more than four million tablets in the first five months of 2000. Also in 2000, the mobster Sammy "the Bull" Gravano was collared for distributing Ecstasy and admitted to financing sales of twenty-five thousand tablets a week. A dealer in Miami claimed that he could unload one hundred thousand tablets in forty-eight hours.

The Monitoring the Future Study, a yearly survey of eighth-, tenth-, and twelfth-graders in the United States, shows a steady increase in the percentage of students who say they have tried Ecstasy. In 1996, just over 6 percent of twelfth-graders reported using the drug. In 1999 the number jumped to 8 percent, and in 2000, 11 percent of students reported taking Ecstasy. Emergency room visits attributed to Ecstasy and reported through the DAWN (Drug Abuse Warning Network) surveying system also have risen, from 319 in 1996 to 2,850 in 1999.

In May 2000, Representative Judy Biggert of Illinois introduced bill HR 4553, the Club Drug Anti-Proliferation Act, to combat club drug trafficking, distribution, and abuse in the United States. This bill was meant to include a group of drugs that are known to be used at raves—MDMA, ketamine (an anesthetic), Rohypnol and GHB (sedative hypnotics), and LSD (a hallucinogen)—according to the National Institute on Drug Abuse (NIDA). The bill called for the U.S. Sentencing Commission to amend the federal sentencing guidelines to provide for higher penalties for the manufacture, distribution, and use of Ecstasy. Further, the bill asked for five million dollars in funding to the Public Health Service for school- and community-based abuse and addiction prevention programs aimed at Ecstasy, PMA (paramethoxyamphetamine, a dangerous and potent ingredient in certain "bogus" Ecstasy tablets), and related club drugs.

The club drug provisions were attached to the Children's Health Act of 2000, which passed in the House and Senate in September 2000. The sentencing provision that would have equated MDMA penalties with those of methamphetamine was removed. Also removed was a particularly alarming provision that would make it a crime to distribute information about the manufacture, acquisition, or use of a controlled substance. Specifically, the word "teaching" had appeared in the original draft of HR 4553, which would have made the publication of this book a criminal offense.

At a July 2000 DEA conference on club drugs, it was estimated that two million hits of Ecstasy were coming into the United States every week. These rising statistics, in addition to several deaths due to PMA, caused the government to crack down on club drugs. A website was set up by NIDA specifically to educate America's youth on the dangers of these drugs. Supporting the claims that Ecstasy is a dangerous drug is the NIDA-funded research of the Johns Hopkins University neurologist George Ricaurte, who has made a career out of giving large doses of MDMA to laboratory animals and publicizing the axonal changes he has documented. [For more information, see "Does MDMA Cause Brain Damage?"]

A fascinating consequence of the government's crackdown on club drugs is the media coverage of Ecstasy and its effect on our nation's teens. The Monitoring the Future study statistics for 2000, a survey of fifty thousand students, reflected the largest one-year percentage point increase among twelfth-graders for any drug class in the twenty-six-year history of the study. Eleven percent of high school seniors in the year 2000 had tried Ecstasy at some time in their lives.

But NIDA has chosen to demonize the drug instead of offering guidelines for safer use or publicizing the specific behaviors that endanger the user. It is well known that overheating and dehydration are real risks encountered at a rave, but the government has opted to ignore these issues in favor of scare tactics and slogans. Contrast that with the British legislation enacted shortly after Dr. John Henry reported the first cases of Ecstasy-associated overheating at raves in 1992. In January 1993 the Safer Dancing Campaign was launched in Manchester, with joint backing from Lifeline (a harm reduction group) and the Manchester city council. This ensured that clubs would be monitored for temperature, air quality, and the availability of "chill out" areas, water, and harm reduction information.

Also distressing is the lack of clinical research of MDMA in the United States and around the world. Because MDMA was made illegal in 1985, sanctioned MDMA-assisted psychotherapy completely ceased in the United States, and little published research beyond anecdotal reports of cases has made its way into the literature. One research group in Switzerland did obtain permission from the government to conduct research on what they called "psycholytic psychotherapy," and they conducted MDMA-assisted sessions from 1988 until 1993. No clinical research on MDMA was being done in the United States at all until the FDA finally agreed, in the summer of 1992, to allow Dr. Charles Grob to conduct human studies of MDMA, using people who had taken the drug before. His study commenced in May 1994.

Since that time two more research groups in the United States have obtained permission to give MDMA to human subjects, but no therapeutic studies have been undertaken in this country yet. At a MAPS-sponsored (Multidisciplinary Association of Psychedelic Studies) conference held in Israel in August 1999, clinical researchers from around the world met for the first time to share their findings, their assessments of where we stand with respect to research, and future plans in the exploration of this invaluable medicine. There is a ray of hope to round out this history. On November 9, 2000, in Spain, a doctoral candidate, José Carlos Bouso, administered the first dose of MDMA in a research protocol designed to test the efficacy of the drug to treat post-traumatic stress disorder. "The four-hour session went very well, and the patient seemed to have gotten to a deeper, more therapeutic level." I hope that this is the first in a long line of treatment studies.

WHAT DOES MDMA FEEL LIKE?

Gary L. Bravo, M.D.

Why do people take MDMA? Among the terms used to describe the experience are empathy, acceptance, closeness, insight, lack of defensiveness, peace, oneness—"ECSTASY." These terms for the state of consciousness associated with MDMA are common in first-person accounts and so-called anecdotal reports in the scientific literature.

Although MDMA was one of the more intensely studied novel chemical compounds in the 1980s and 1990s, the focus of interest for most of the hundreds of published reports was its alleged toxicity to serotonin neurons, with a secondary focus on adverse reactions among users. Because of these emphases and the 1985 scheduling of MDMA as part of the most restricted class of regulated drugs (those with "no accepted medical use" and a "high potential for abuse"), clinical research into the nature of the MDMA experience has been meager. Amid the furor about the dangers of MDMA abuse have been the claims of psychotherapists and medicinal chemists that MDMA ingestion results in a unique and useful state of consciousness.

What is this state of consciousness? How is MDMA different from other psychoactive or psychedelic drugs? This chapter focuses on what the scientific literature tells us about the subjective experience of people under the influence of MDMA and related phenethylamines. In addition, mention is made of the acute and less severe side effects of MDMA use, which contribute to the subjective experience.

As with the traditional psychedelics (and all psychoactive drugs, to some extent), the MDMA experience seems to be greatly dependent on "set and setting." "Set" refers to the intentions, preparation, and mental and physical capacities of the user, and "setting" refers to the user's physical and interpersonal environment. The experience of a person who takes MDMA in the context of psychotherapy or for spiritual exploration is bound to be different from that of a person using the drug in a recreational setting, or in a rave, or in an experimental laboratory setting. Nevertheless, there seems to be a unique MDMA profile that is reliably common to all contexts and distinguishes MDMA from other mind-altering drugs. This profile is characteristic of a group of methoxylated phenethylamines, which have chemical structures related to both amphetamines and mescaline-type psychedelics. The chemicals in this class are so uniquely different from other psychoactive drugs that they have been proposed to constitute a new class of drugs—the "entactogens," which means "to touch within" (Nichols 1986). Another proposed term is "empathogen," stemming from their empathy-producing effects. MDMA is the prototype and most studied of these compounds. Closely related are 3,4-methylenedioxyethylamphetamine (MDE or Eve) and 3-methoxy-4,5-methylenedioxyamphetamine (MMDA).

Another drug known since the 1950s, MDA, has been considered to have empathogenic effects at low doses and psychedelic effects at high doses. An early published description of the qualities of the MDA experience could be used as a generalized prototype of the entactogenic experience (Turek et al. 1974). Ten subjects who were given MDA reported the following effects, as measured by the Psychedelic Experience Questionnaire: "feelings of peace and tranquillity, feelings of tenderness and gentleness, increase in the beauty and significance of music, feelings of emotional closeness with the companion, increased awareness of the importance of interpersonal relationships, feelings of joy, experience of oneness in relation to an inner world within, sense of being at a spiritual height, experience of pure being and pure awareness, gain of insightful knowledge experienced at an intuitive level, feeling that the state of consciousness experienced during part of the session was more real than normal awareness of everyday reality, and loss of the usual sense of time."

How has the MDMA state been characterized? Greer and Tolbert (1990) summarize from their experience their interpretation of how MDMA works: "In the right circumstances, MDMA reduces or sometimes eliminates the neurophysiological fear response to a perceived threat to one's emotional integrity. . . . With this barrier of fear removed, a loving and forgiving awareness seemed to occur quite naturally and spontaneously."

Another characterization of the effects of MDMA is that of powerful empathy with others. Empathy is defined in the psychiatric literature as the "capacity to understand what another person is experiencing from within the other's frame of reference (standing in the other's shoes). In empathy one feels as the other person does, but recognizes that other feelings are possible; there is no fusion or identification with the patient" (Ayd 1995). Unfortunately, the subjective experience of empathy is difficult to quantify, and there is a paucity of research on this purported quality of the empathogens. MDMA differs from the traditional psychedelics by rarely producing ego disorganization and disintegration, leaving reality testing relatively intact. "As compared with the more familiar psychedelic drugs, it [MDMA] evokes a gentler, subtler, highly controllable experience which invites rather than compels intensification of feelings and self-exploration. The user is not forced onto any mental or emotional path that is frightening or even uncomfortable" (Grinspoon and Bakalar 1986).

The first mention of MDMA's psychological effects was in a report by Shulgin and Nichols (1978), who pointed out the rapid onset of effects, usually within half an hour, and the diminishment of the effects after another two hours. Early attempts at quantifying the MDMA experience, which took place before the DEA scheduling of the drug, were small, uncontrolled case studies of MDMA sessions that focused on healing specific problems or on psychospiritual exploration. Greer and Tolbert (1986) published a summary of the subjective effects of MDMA in twenty-nine subjects; all reported positive changes in their attitudes or feelings during the session and increased feelings of closeness and intimacy with anyone present. Twenty-two subjects cited some cognitive benefit, such as an expanded mental perspective, insight into personal patterns or problems, or improved self-examination. Common undesirable effects during and after the sessions were jaw tension, teeth clenching, insomnia, fatigue, and decreased appetite.

In another pioneering study of MDMA's acute effects, Downing (1986) looked at physiological parameters of twenty-one subjects in a group MDMA session and found that all of them showed elevations in blood pressure, pulse rate, and pupillary dilatation. Appetite was generally suppressed, and deep tendon reflexes were enhanced. Some subjects had ataxia (difficulty walking), and more than half had jaw clenching. Subjects experienced euphoria, increased physical and emotional energy, and heightened sensual awareness; three reported sexual arousal.

For many years after the scheduling of MDMA in 1985, before the FDA approved research, studies of the MDMA experience were limited to surveys. In one of the more notable studies (Peroutka et al. 1988), Stanford undergraduates were asked about their MDMA use; 40 percent of the students reported having tried it. The most common acute effect was a sense of closeness with other people, experienced by 90 percent of the respondents. The term "closeness" is not defined in the report; it is stated only that "the subjects thought that they were more verbal during this time and were able to interact better with other people." Other acute effects documented in this report, which emphasized adverse effects, were jaw tension (75 percent), rapid heartbeat (72 percent), teeth grinding (65 percent), dry mouth (61 percent), and increased alertness (50 percent). Other effects, experienced by 20 percent to 42 percent of the subjects, were "luminescence of objects," tremor, palpitations, sweating, difficulty concentrating, tingling, insomnia, hot or cold flashes, increased sensitivity to cold, dizziness or vertigo, visual hallucinations, and blurred vision. Less acute effects of MDMA experienced by users (in the 24 to 48 hours after ingestion) included drowsiness (36 percent), muscle aches or fatigability (32 percent), lingering sense of closeness (22 percent), depression (21 percent), tight jaw muscles (21 percent), difficulty concentrating (21 percent), and headache (17 percent).

A more detailed structured interview was done by Liester and colleagues (1992), who surveyed twenty psychiatrists who each had used MDMA from one to twenty-five times. The most common acute effects were altered time perception (90 percent), enhanced ability to interact with or be open with others (85 percent), decreased defensiveness (80 percent), decreased fear (65 percent), and changes in visual perception (55 percent). Half of these subjects reported heightened awareness of emotions and less aggression. The most common adverse effects (not necessarily experienced as adverse by the subjects) were diminished desire to perform mental or physical tasks (70 percent), decreased appetite (65 percent), jaw tension (50 percent), diminished libido (45 percent), higher levels of restlessness/agitation (35 percent), teeth grinding (30 percent), and increased anxiety (25 percent). A later study

(Davison and Parrott 1997) of the subjective effects of MDMA used questionnaires, interviews, and a standardized test of psychoactive drug effects, the Profile of Mood States (POMS), to assess retrospective self-reports of twenty recreational Ecstasy users in England. On the POMS, subjects reported feeling energetic, elated, agreeable, and confused. The "composure vs. anxiety" scale and the "confidence vs. uncertainty" scale were surprisingly unchanged from baseline. Physiological changes described were faster heart rate, higher body temperature, sweating and dehydration, dilated pupils, and tight jaw. Psychological effects were feelings of happiness, exhilaration and energy, warmth and friendliness, calmness and relaxation, and heightened perception of sound, color, and touch.

A sociological study of one hundred Ecstasy users in Australia (Solowij 1992) attempted to provide data that characterized the unique MDMA state of consciousness. In this survey, the following terms distinguished the MDMA experience from that of amphetamines and hallucinogens: happy, easygoing, accepting, sensual, and euphoric. The other common adjectives that were used to describe the experience were talkative, open-minded, confident, and carefree.

Grob undertook the first federally approved study of the acute effects of MDMA in the United States (1996, 1998). Eighteen subjects with previous Ecstasy experience were given placebo, medium-dose, or high-dose MDMA, and physiological and psychological parameters were measured. Both the POMS and the State Trait Anxiety Inventory were administered during the period of acute intoxication but "proved to be of mixed value," since they revealed only a "lack of negative symptomatology during the experimental drug sessions." However, the Altered States Graphic Profile showed significant increases on the hedonic and arousal continuum for both the medium- and high-dose ranges. Subjects tended to have mild elevations in body temperature and modest increases in heart rate and blood pressure (though two subjects had significantly elevated blood pressures).

A unique double-blind, placebo-controlled laboratory study conducted by Hermle and coworkers (1993) in Germany reported the results of MDE given to fourteen volunteers. On several psychological and cognitive tests there were no significant differences in cognitive functions between subjects and controls. The researchers concluded that MDE "produced a partially controllable state of enhanced insight, empathy, and peaceful feelings," and that "the major effects of MDE were a reduction of anxiety, an increased drive with pronounced partly euphoric and partly depressed mood, and an improved responsiveness in, and openness to, communication. . . . Unlike hallucinogenic drugs, MDE neither disturbed perception, nor formal thought processes, nor memory, and did not produce psychotic symptoms such as hallucinations, with the exception of one case." That case was of a volunteer who showed signs of toxic psychosis with paranoia and auditory and visual hallucinations (Gouzoulis et al. 1993). Another subject had an unpleasant reaction characterized by anxiety.

Later, Vollenweider and colleagues (1998a) conducted a double-blind, placebo-controlled study of thirteen volunteers using a typical recreational dose of MDMA (1.7 mg MDMA per kg body weight). Using the Adjective Mood Rating Scale and the Altered State of Consciousness rating scale, they found that during the peak effects of MDMA, subjects evidenced enhanced mood and well-being, associated with moderate derealization and depersonalization (feeling that they, or their surroundings, were not real), thought disorder, and anxiety. The rating of increased anxiety was on a particular subset of the anxiety scale related to "thoughtfulness-contemplativeness," and subjects said that they felt no increase in subjective anxiety. Subjects also reported experiencing increased responsiveness to emotions, heightened openness, and a sense of closeness to other people. Most subjects became more verbal, although a few desired to withdraw. The investigators found that the MDMA group did not differ from the placebo group in the results of the Stroop test, a measure of selective attention. These results are consistent with those of earlier prospective and retrospective reports on the psychological effects of MDMA.

Tolerance to the Subjective Effects of MDMA

Does MDMA lose its effectiveness with repeated administration? Early studies of the psychotherapeutic use of MDMA report the effects of a "booster" dose of approximately half the original dose taken two to three hours after the first, to extend the peak effects (Greer and Tolbert 1986). Most users report that repeated doses do not extend or increase the desired empathogenic effect but that the unpleasant "amphetamine-like" side effects are more pronounced in proportion to the dose. In addition, a tolerance to the desired effects extends for as long as twenty-four to thirty-six hours. One of the more interesting features of the MDMA experience is that repeated administrations tend to lead to decreasing desired effects, regardless of the amount of time that elapses between doses. Beck and Rosenbaum's in-depth interviews of one hundred MDMA users (1994) found this "cumulative tolerance" to be a common phenomenon, though not universal. Reasons given by users for decreased use of MDMA were the following: (1) They "get the message," in other words, they feel that after they use MDMA a few times there is no more learning to be done, the novelty has worn off, and the new state of consciousness is more readily available. (2) They enjoy the high less and less. (3) They have more negative after effects, such as fatigue, malaise, and headaches. One study compared subjects who took Ecstasy at a weekend dance club with those who took alcohol and found that the Ecstasy users were significantly more depressed five days after taking the drug (Curran and Travill 1997). Another report compared subjects who took Ecstasy at a weekend dance club with those who did not take the drug at the same club. Results showed that all subjects reported positive moods while they were at the club, but when they were assessed again after two days, the Ecstasy users felt "significantly more depressed, abnormal, unsociable, unpleasant and less good tempered" than controls (Parrott and Lasky 1998).

Spiritual Effects

MDMA experiences are often described in spiritual terms, and so far these data elude scientific analysis. MDMA frequently is labeled as a "heart-opening" drug. Those who work with subtle and esoteric energies believe that MDMA opens the "heart chakra," a term that comes from Hindu spiritual beliefs. It refers to those energies that make up the psychospiritual body, which is located in the heart region; they emanate unconditional acceptance of and strong connection to others. The way in which MDMA accomplishes this is unknown, but this seems to be a unique effect of the empathogens. Other psychedelic drugs can produce the same effect in a somewhat more unpredictable way.

The MDMA condition also has been likened to a state of advanced meditation, a state of peace and subtle bliss in which distracting thoughts are minimal or nonexistent. One Zen teacher had this to say: "Ecstasy is a wonderful tool for teaching. For example, I had a very keen student who never succeeded in meditation until Ecstasy removed the block caused by his effort when trying to meditate" (Saunders 1995). A Benedictine monk stated that "the drug facilitates the 'awakened attitude' all monks seek" (Eisner 1989). The utility of the MDMA experience for spiritual purposes awaits a true science of experimental mysticism.

Conclusion

How do we generalize and characterize the MDMA state of consciousness? The results of the studies described here validate the classification of MDMA as the prototype of a new and unique class of psychoactive drugs—the entactogens or empathogens—that reliably imbue the user with a sense of interpersonal closeness, acceptance of self and others, feelings of "oneness," and a potent sense of well-being. Enough claims have been made for the usefulness of the effects of MDMA to medicine, psychiatry, and the science of consciousness that it deserves to be investigated thoroughly. In addition, the short- and long-term risks of MDMA use in medicine or psychotherapy and the effects of its nonmedical use also demand careful investigation. Only prospective studies of MDMA in human populations, using creative and interdisciplinary research protocols, will begin to provide some understanding of this unique psychoactive chemical.

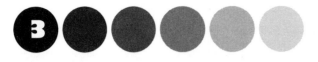

HOW MDMA WORKS IN THE BRAIN

Jessica E. Malberg, Ph.D., and Katherine R. Bonson, Ph.D.

The pharmacology of MDMA primarily involves two brain chemicals: serotonin and dopamine. These neurotransmitters help nerve cells communicate with each other (as described below) and each of them have their own complex neural systems and behavioral responses. MDMA acts in the brain through three main neurochemical mechanisms: blockade of serotonin reuptake, induction of serotonin release, and induction of dopamine release. With these actions, MDMA is essentially a combination of the effects of fluoxetine (Prozac), the serotonin reuptake inhibitor and antidepressant; fenfluramine (Pondamin), the serotonin releaser (and the "fen" in "fen-phen"); and amphetamine, a dopamine releaser. Additionally, MDMA can directly interact with receptors in a variety of neurotransmitter systems and can act as a monoamine oxidase (MAO) inhibitor. This chapter will explain how each of these different mechanisms function at the cellular level with an eye toward how these actions can ultimately affect behavior and mood.

How Neurotransmitter Systems Function in the Brain

Before we attempt a complicated discussion of the neurochemical effects of MDMA, readers may benefit from a basic orientation to the way that the nervous system functions in the brain. Nerves communicate with each other by electrical and chemical means. When an electrical signal reaches the end of one neuron, there is a gap before the start of the next neuron. This space is known as a synapse. A synapse cannot be bridged with an electrical signal;

communication between neurons continues with the release of a chemical from the presynaptic neuron. This chemical, called a neurotransmitter, is synthesized and stored in this presynaptic space. Once released, the neurotransmitter floats across the synapse and can bind postsynaptically on the next neuron to protein structures known as receptors. When the receptor is occupied with the chemical, it causes the induction of a new electrical signal, and nerve cell communication continues. Neurotransmitters also can bind to presynaptic receptors, which function in a negative feedback mode to reduce the release of more neurotransmitter.

The normal functions of the presynaptic neurotransmitter cell are storage, release, and reuptake of its neurochemical. We can explain this concept using the example of serotonin (5-hydroxytryptamine, or 5-HT) neurons. Storage simply means that 5-HT is stored inside the cell, in one of two forms. Single molecules of 5-HT floating in the cytoplasm (the fluid in the cell) are characterized as either free-floating or cytoplasmic. 5-HT also can be found sequestered within the cell in storage packages called vesicles. Release of 5-HT occurs when a neuron is activated, causing the presynaptic terminal to release stored 5-HT into the synapse. The released serotonin then can bind to any of fourteen currently known serotonin receptor subtypes. These receptors are located both postsynaptically and presynaptically and are concentrated by subtype in particular regions of the brain. For instance, the 5-HT2 receptor, which is stimulated by hallucinogenic drugs, is found in high concentrations in the frontal cortex, an area of the brain responsible for higher cognitive processing.

After a certain amount of time, 5-HT will stop binding to the receptor and will become free again in the synapse. At this point, 5-HT can do one of three things: (1) It can be recycled into the presynaptic neuron through a reuptake mechanism (transporter) so that it can be stored for future release. (2) It can be degraded by an enzyme such as monoamine oxidase subtype A (MAO-A), which metabolizes 5-HT into 5-HIAA (5-hydroxyindoleacetic acid). (3) It can diffuse away out of the synapse. All of these actions terminate the effect of the neurotransmitter.

The serotonin reuptake mechanism is sometimes called the transporter protein. The 5-HT transporter is located on the outside membrane of the presynaptic cell, facing the synapse. Reuptake begins when the 5-HT in the synapse binds to the 5-HT transporter. Once a molecule of 5-HT is bound to the transporter, the transporter changes shape (or configuration) and moves the 5-HT to the inside of the cell, where the 5-HT "falls off" and is released into the cytoplasm of the cell. The transporter then reorients itself toward the outside surface of the presynaptic membrane to continue its uptake function for the next molecule of 5-HT. The net effect of the action of the 5-HT transporter is removal of 5-HT from the synapse. There are many transporters on presynaptic serotonin membranes throughout the brain, so the reuptake mechanism does not rely on a single site at a time, working to recycle serotonin molecules. Drugs that "block" the reuptake mechanism occupy the site that would normally be occupied by 5-HT. This prevents 5-HT from binding to the transporter, so it is left out in the synapse, where it can reattach to a postsynaptic receptor. Thus, a drug that causes reuptake inhibition essentially prolongs the effect of any released serotonin. This is the mechanism of action of many antidepressants known as selective serotonin reuptake inhibitors (SSRIs).

MDMA and the 5-HT Transporter

How does MDMA fit into the function that we have just described? Although we have previously discussed the two mechanisms of 5-HT release and blockade of uptake separately, MDMA is unusual pharmacologically, because it can produce both of these effects at the same time. MDMA functions similarly to the antidepressant fluoxetine in that both drugs occupy the 5-HT transporter site and prevent 5-HT from binding to the transporter. In contrast to fluoxetine, MDMA also is taken up by the transporter after it is bound and is deposited into the presynaptic cell. This action does not occur with fluoxetine because of its relatively large size, which allows it to occupy the 5-HT transporter site but prevents its entry into the presynaptic cell. MDMA is closer in size to 5-HT than fluoxetine and therefore is able to enter the cell as if it were 5-HT.

Once inside the presynaptic cell, MDMA induces the release of 5-HT into the synapse. This is a four-step process:

1. MDMA is released from the transporter into the cell when the transporter undergoes a change in "configuration" (shape) and the MDMA falls off.

2. The transporter then has the correct configuration to bind cytoplasmic 5-HT (the serotonin in the neuron, not the synapse).

3. The bound 5-HT is transported out of the presynaptic cell, and when the transporter changes configuration again, the 5-HT falls off into the synapse.

4. The transporter is then in the correct configuration to bind more MDMA that is available in the synapse and repeat the process.

[For diagrams to help explain this process, please refer to the Ecstasy slide show on the Web site www.dancesafe.org]

MDMA's ability to induce 5-HT release is common to all substituted amphetamines, including methamphetamine and fenfluramine. Under normal circumstances, 5-HT is not released in large amounts but is tightly regulated in the brain. Thus, the main effects of MDMA—inhibition of 5-HT reuptake and release of 5-HT from the presynaptic neuron—flood the synapse with atypically large amounts of 5-HT. Within three to six hours after MDMA administration, so much 5-HT has been released that there is a temporary depletion of 5-HT in the presynaptic cell. Additionally, MDMA inactivates the enzyme (tryptophan hydroxylase) that is necessary for synthesis of new 5-HT, so that cells cannot make enough 5-HT to reach baseline levels. Since low levels of serotonin are associated with depression, this may account for the transient mood swings that follow MDMA use in humans. Within twenty-four hours, however, new serotonin can be synthesized, and 5-HT levels return to normal (Schmidt 1987). Longer-lasting depletions of 5-HT have been seen only when high doses of MDMA are given repeatedly for long periods of time. Similar depletions of 5-HT also are seen with long-term administration of fenfluramine [see "Does MDMA Cause Brain Damage?"].

Scientists have created a mouse that does not have the 5-HT transporter in its brain—this is known as a "transgenic mouse" or "knockout mouse," because the genes that are responsible for the transporter have been knocked out of the genetic makeup of the mouse. This mouse is useful scientifically to test how the absence of a transporter affects a living biological system, especially when it is challenged with drugs. In regular mice, MDMA will produce an increase in the amount of movement that mice make around a cage. But when 5-HT transporter knockout mice were given MDMA, there was no increase in their locomotion (Bengel 1998). This suggests that without a 5-HT transporter, MDMA could not get into the cell and cause its various effects. In contrast, when amphetamine was given to regular and knockout mice, both groups showed an increase in locomotion (this is thought to be because of increased dopamine). Thus, it was concluded that the 5-HT transporter is required for MDMA to exert its effects.

MDMA and Dopamine

MDMA also causes the release of dopamine (DA), but to a lesser extent than release of 5-HT. The release of DA appears to rely on the previous release of 5-HT, since blockade of the 5-HT transporter with fluoxetine suppresses the increase in DA after MDMA administration (Nash and Brodkin 1991). This principle also has been borne out in genetically altered mice that lack a 5-HT transporter, in whom MDMA does not cause hyperactivity (a measure of dopamine action). Conversely, giving drugs that increase 5-HT synthesis before the administration of MDMA causes an even greater increase in DA release (Gudelsky and Nash 1996). It should be noted that the effect of 5-HT on DA release involves the DA transporter as well, since inhibition of the DA reuptake mechanism also will prevent DA release in response to MDMA.

This effect of 5-HT on DA release may occur through the 5-HT2 receptor, since activation of this site in the absence of MDMA is known to increase DA release. To test whether the 5-HT2 receptor is involved in MDMA-induced DA release, 5-HT2 antagonists were given before administration of MDMA. These antagonists were found to block the increase in DA from MDMA, but they did not affect the resting levels of DA before MDMA (Schmidt et al. 1991). Given the connection between MDMA neurotoxicity and DA release [see "Does MDMA Cause Brain Damage?"], 5-HT2 antagonists might be useful in the prevention of any possible damage from high-dose MDMA.

MDMA and 5-HT Receptors

Although the primary effects of MDMA are on the transporter sites in 5-HT and DA systems, there is evidence of direct interactions between MDMA and other receptors. The most intriguing work in this area has shown that MDMA has a slight affinity for the 5-HT2 receptor. This is interesting, because the hallucinogenic response from the classic psychedelics (such as LSD) has been correlated to activation of the 5-HT2 site.

MDMA often is characterized by users as having some psychedelic properties (despite the lack of hallucinations); it is therefore not surprising that the site associated with the psychedelic experience is activated to a small degree by MDMA. However, when rats are trained in drug discrimination studies to identify when they have received MDMA by pressing a certain lever, they do not press that lever when LSD is given to them instead. This suggests that the internal experience of classic hallucinogens is different from that of MDMA, in agreement with results from studies of human beings, which report a distinction between these drugs.

Additionally, the increased body temperature that is seen after MDMA ingestion may be the result of 5-HT2 activation, since stimulation of this receptor with other drugs is known to cause hyperthermia. This conclusion is strengthened by the fact that pretreatment with fluoxetine does not block MDMA-induced hyperthermia, suggesting that preventing 5-HT release by occupying the reuptake sites is not sufficient to inhibit the body temperature effects of MDMA.

Another receptor that may play a role in the action of MDMA in the brain is the $5-HT1_B$ site. This receptor is thought to be important in producing feelings of calmness, and drugs that activate this site are known in psychiatric research as "serenics." Exploration of this receptor with MDMA has shown that there is a similar pattern of increased locomotion in rats when MDMA or $5-HT1_B$ agonists are given. In contrast, the pattern of locomotion with $5-HT1_A$ or 5-HT2 agonists is not similar to that from MDMA.

When rats are given repeated doses of MDMA and become tolerant (that is, they do not respond behaviorally to a dose of MDMA at the same level as they did before drug administration), they also fail to respond to the effects of a $5-HT1_B$ agonist—this is known as cross-tolerance. Cross-tolerance also happens when rats are made tolerant to repeated administration of the 5-HT1_B agonist and are subsequently given MDMA. This suggests that MDMA shares a common mechanism of action with 5-HT1_B agonists. Finally, drug discrimination studies have shown that rats trained to identify MDMA will press the MDMA lever when they are given trifluromethylphenylpiperazine (TFMPP), a drug with 5-HT1_B properties. TFMPP has been promoted on underground drug information Web sites as being similar to MDMA when combined with a stimulant.

MDMA and Interactions with Other Drugs

Selective Serotonin Reuptake Inhibitors (SSRIs)

It has been shown that people who have taken fluoxetine or other SSRIs, like paroxetine (Paxil) or sertraline (Zoloft), for at least three to four weeks for depression have a reduced response to LSD and other hallucinogens (Bonson 1996a, 1996b). Our new research has found that a similar effect exists with MDMA. Most (but not all) people who take SSRIs for a long period of time report a reduced or completely eliminated response to MDMA. This decrease in response to MDMA in people who have taken SSRIs occurs because SSRIs occupy the same site on the 5-HT transporter that MDMA uses. Because an SSRI was there first, MDMA has nowhere to bind on the transporter and cannot be taken up into the presynaptic serotonin cell. Since all the SSRIs that are used as antidepressants have extremely long durations of action, MDMA simply diffuses away out of the synapse without ever having any psychoactive effect.

People who are not under treatment for depression also take fluoxetine in single doses before ingestion of MDMA. This practice is based on familiarity with neurotoxicological studies using rodents and monkeys that suggest that fluoxetine can blunt the serotonin-damaging effects from repeated high doses of MDMA when it is taken either before or three to four hours after MDMA. As expected, when fluoxetine is taken immediately before (in one dose) or concurrently with MDMA, it can decrease the MDMA response in humans. But since the effects of MDMA have dissipated by four hours after ingestion, taking fluoxetine after the effects of MDMA have worn off will not interfere with the response to MDMA and may still produce the desired protective effects.

Dextromethorphan (DXM)

It has recently been reported that what is sold as Ecstasy can sometimes contain only dextromethorphan (DXM), instead of MDMA (Baggott et al. 2000). When users discover that these tablets do not produce the desired MDMA effect, they might be inclined to purchase Ecstasy from another dealer in hopes of obtaining real MDMA. In a situation where a person ingests both DXM and MDMA, it is possible that this drug combination could produce what is known as the serotonin syndrome. This behavioral condition is characterized by muscle spasms, gastrointestinal problems and diarrhea, confusion, agitation, incoordination, shivering, fever, and sweating.

The serotonin syndrome can be brought on by any combination of drugs that increase serotonin availability in the brain. It seems to be especially likely with combination of SSRIs from different sources. Although DXM is primarily thought to be an NMDA (N-methyl-D-Aspartate) antagonist, it also has SSRI properties. This means that there can be an extra increase in serotonin when MDMA is also in the body. It is noteworthy that the liver enzyme that metabolizes MDMA (cytochrome P450 isozyme 2D6, or CYP2D6) can be inhibited by the continued presence of MDMA. Since DXM also relies on CYP2D6 for its metabolism, if this enzyme is not functioning, both MDMA and DXM may continue to act in the brain for extended periods and increase the risk of serotonin syndrome.

MAO Inhibitors

It is well known that the combination of a MAO inhibitor and an amphetamine can induce a dangerous increase in blood pressure known as hypertensive crisis. During this hypertensive reaction, the heart will race at life-threatening levels, and if medical attention is not sought immediately, unconsciousness and death are possible outcomes. Since MDMA is an amphetamine, it should never be taken by someone who is taking an MAO inhibitor. The medical literature has reported severe reactions to MDMA in persons taking MAO inhibitors since 1987, and several people have died. It should be noted that there are two types of MAO inhibitors—those that block the A form and those that block the B form of MAO. MAO-A inhibitors are typically antidepressant agents, such as phenelzine (Nardil), tranylcypromine (Parnate), and isocarboxazid (Marplan). It is these drugs that are dangerous in combination with MDMA, leading to the excessive increase in blood pressure.

Many hallucinogen enthusiasts are also familiar with natural forms of MAO-A inhibitors, such as those found in the plants Syrian rue or pegnalum *(Peganum harmala)*. It is important, however, to appreciate that no MAO-A inhibitor, natural or synthetic, should ever be taken with MDMA because of the risk of hypertensive crisis.

There are also MAO-B inhibitors—selegiline (deprenyl) is the most commonly known. These drugs are not thought to have the same risk factors as MAO-A inhibitors when combined with other drugs or certain foods. However, to be on the safe side, it is advisable not to take MAO-B inhibitors with MDMA.

Hallucinogens

The practice of combining MDMA with LSD is known as "candy flipping." Although some people take both drugs simultaneously, others take them at separate times. When the drugs are taken at different times, it is more common for LSD to be ingested first, since it has a longer duration of action (eight to twelve hours) than MDMA (two to four hours). MDMA is ingested after the LSD has begun to take effect. The candy-flipping experience has been described as "mellowing out the effects of tripping on acid," without eliminating the experience of LSD. Taking MDMA after LSD-induced hallucinations have subsided has been reported to bring back hallucinatory effects. The interpersonal "entactogen" qualities of MDMA can merge with the colorful aspects of LSD to create what has been described as "psychedelic brandy." A related experience is reported when MDMA is combined with hallucinogenic mushrooms—this interaction is known as an MX missile. There are currently no reports in the medical literature or in the underground press of adverse physical or psychological effects of combining MDMA with LSD or mushrooms. Caution is advised, though, since each person's biological and psychological makeup is different and some people may be predisposed to untoward effects after certain drug combinations.

Summary

It is unclear at this stage in scientific research just how the distinct psychoactive effects of MDMA relate to the various pharmacological mechanisms of action. Since drugs that mimic the individual actions of MDMA (such as fluoxetine at the transporter, fenfluramine in releasing serotonin, amphetamines in releasing dopamine, LSD at the 5-HT2 receptor and 5-HT1$_B$ agonists) do not produce the full MDMA response by themselves, it can be concluded that each of these actions must occur simultaneously for the unique effects of MDMA to emerge.

THE CHEMISTRY OF MDMA

David Nichols, Ph.D.

When I asked Dr. Holland what she wanted me to present in this chapter, she replied, "Explain the molecule to the masses. . . . Keep it elementary." That is a somewhat daunting task, because for many people who attended college or university, organic chemistry is a subject that is best forgotten. Those of you who have never had the experience of a basic organic chemistry course may still have heard horror stories about the subject or you are at least aware that it instills a kind of instinctive fear into most non-chemistry majors. In my opinion, chemistry itself is beautiful, and legendary accounts of its difficulty are greatly exaggerated. I hope to prove that here and even to instill a basic understanding of chemistry into those formerly thought to be immune to such attempts.

Acids and Bases

Where to start? Our discussion probably should begin with acids and bases. Most people are familiar with these terms. For example, the acid in most car batteries is a solution of sulfuric acid. It will burn the skin, eat through cotton clothing, and dissolve many kinds of metals that are placed into it. Acid rain is rainfall that has absorbed diluted sulfuric acid vapors from polluted air. It would have the same effect as battery acid if it were it to be concentrated to the same strength. Sulfuric acid, as well as hydrochloric acid and nitric acid, are known as inorganic, or mineral, acids, because they lack the presence of carbon atoms, and things containing carbon atoms are generally referred to as "organic" molecules. There are, however, a great many organic acids. Perhaps one of the most common is ordinary vinegar. Vinegar is a dilute (about 3%) solution of acetic acid. There are a number of other common acids that the reader will recognize. For example, aspirin is acetylsalicylic acid, and vitamin C is ascorbic acid. Although these are much weaker acids than mineral acids, they nevertheless have the same essential property—that is, they give off hydrogen ions, or protons (positively charged atoms), and it is these protons that lead to the unique chemistry of acids.

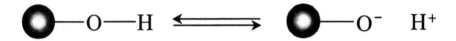

Figure 1. Ionization of a prototypical acid by loss of a proton (H⁺).
Lines indicate chemical bonds.

At the left of figure 1 is shown an idealized acid, where the sphere can represent any sort of organic molecule or a group of inorganic atoms. On the right is shown the loss of the proton from the acid, with a positive charge on the hydrogen atom (H^+) and a balancing negative charge on the oxygen atom (O^-) of the acid molecule. Each chemical bond consists of two electrons, and normally one electron is contributed to the bond by each of the bonding partners. When the proton left the acid, however, it left both electrons with the oxygen atom. It is therefore one electron short of being electrically neutral (and hence has a positive charge, +). The oxygen atom is one electron in excess of neutrality and hence carries a negative electric charge (–). This process of the proton leaving the acid, because it creates charges in the groups involved, is called ionization.

For the purposes of this discussion, we are not really as interested in acids as we are in their chemical counterparts, bases, because many drug substances, including MDMA, are organic bases. Bases have the property of being attracted to protons, the H^+ shown in figure 1. Since acids give off H^+ and bases are attracted to, and interact with, H^+, when the two are mixed together there is an "acid-base" reaction. If the proportions of the two species are exactly equivalent, we say that "neutralization" has occurred. That is, we have neutralized the acid with the base or vice versa.

There are very strong and caustic inorganic bases, such as sodium hydroxide (lye), employed commonly in a drain cleaner marketed as Drano, which has the ability to chemically react with and dissolve greases and fats. More relevant to our interests, however, are the weaker organic bases, which are ultimately chemically related to ammonia. The gas ammonia has a structure where a nitrogen atom (N) is attached (bonded) to three hydrogen atoms. Everyone has no doubt smelled a bottle of household ammonia. That product is, in fact, a weak solution of ammonia gas dissolved in water, but the smell of ammonia gas is quite pungent.

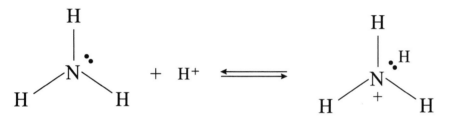

Figure 2. *Ammonia accepts a proton to become an ammonium ion. Lines indicate chemical bonds. The two dots between the N and H also denote a completely equivalent bond, which is indicated this way only to show that the two electrons in one of the bonds both came from the nitrogen atom.*

Figure 2 illustrates ammonia reacting with a proton (from an acid) in a neutralization reaction to become an ammonium ion, or ammonium salt. This reaction occurs because organic bases (amines) have a pair of electrons that are not normally involved in the formation of a chemical bond. These electrons are represented in figure 2 as the pair of black dots adjacent to the central nitrogen (N) atom. There is a strong attraction between the negative character of these electrons and the proton, which bears a positive electronic charge (+) because it does not possess enough electrons to make it electrically neutral. After the neutralization reaction, the central nitrogen atom has four hydrogen atoms attached to it as well as the positive charge brought by the proton, shown as the + sign. Organic molecules that bear a positive charge are often given names ending in "onium." Because this new product was derived from ammonia, it is called ammonium. Thus, if the proton came from sulfuric acid, the final compound would be called ammonium sulfate. If the proton came from acetic acid, the product would be called ammonium acetate.

If one replaces the H atoms of ammonia with small organic groups (units that contain carbon atoms), these resulting molecules are called organic bases, or amines. The low-molecular-weight amines have an ammonia-like, or fishy, smell. In fact, the smell of fish is due to the formation of very small amounts of these amines as the fish slowly decomposes. Amines behave much like ammonia in that they react with protons to form salts. Salts of organic bases are most often white crystalline substances, which possess a bitter taste and are usually water-soluble. Salts of amines with complex structures are typically named after the amine itself, followed by the name of the acid that was used to prepare the salt. That is, while the neutralization of ammonia with hydrochloric acid gives ammonium chloride, neutralization of a more complex base, such as amphetamine, would give a salt with the name amphetamine hydrochloride.

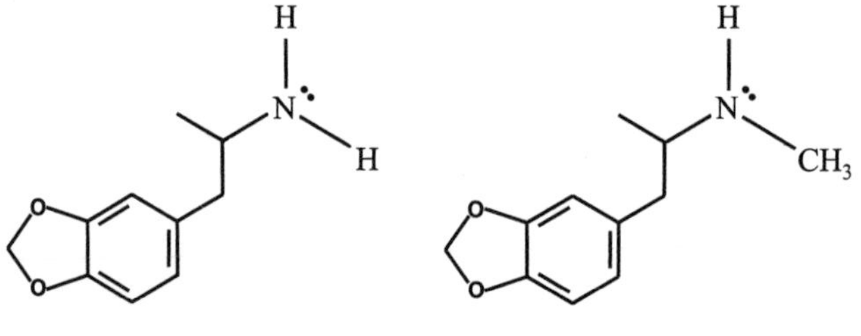

Figure 3. Methylenedioxyamphetamine (MDA) on the left and methylenedioxymethamphetamine (MDMA) on the right. Relative molecular sizes are exaggerated to emphasize the basic amine portion of the molecule. The letter O represents an oxygen atom. The straight lines represent chemical bonds, and the vertex of each angle between the bonds represents a carbon atom. Hydrogen atoms have been omitted from these structures except at the nitrogen atom, for greater clarity.

By now the reader may be wondering, "Where is this going, and what has it got to do with MDMA?" The structures of MDA and MDMA are illustrated in figure 3, and I hope that this figure will provide the beginning of an answer to that question. We see here, on the left, the chemical relationship between ammonia and MDA as one where a hydrogen atom attached to ammonia has been replaced by the lightened structure on the left with two joined rings and extra chemical bonds. The basic properties of the nitrogen atom (N), however, are not substantially changed. It will still attract the proton from an acid, will become "neutralized," and will form a bitter, water-soluble salt. Similarly, MDMA, on the right, is simply a modification of MDA, where the hydrogen atom pointing toward the lower right has been replaced by a CH_3, a methyl group. This is the origin of the "meth" part of "methamphetamine." It is still an organic base and will behave quite a bit like both MDA and the prototypical base, ammonia.

You may now be thinking, "Okay. I see that MDA and MDMA are organic bases, but where did all that molecular stuff on the left come from that is attached to the N atom?" The history of organic chemistry really begins with natural products: molecules that are produced by living things. In particular, there are many plants that have characteristic smells and tastes, many of which have been used for millennia as herbs, spices, and perfumes. For example, figure 4 illustrates the structures of several natural molecules that come from plants you will recognize. In most cases, these substances are oils that make a major contribution to the flavor or aroma of the natural product. Because these plants have characteristic flavors and aromas, chemists seek the active principles, or "essential oils," from them to make natural products. These substances then serve as starting materials for a variety of different kinds of organic chemical products. One could obtain the oil and carry out chemical reactions that change atoms, or replace bonds, to lead to new organic compounds. The structure of the naturally occurring material thus may be viewed as a sort of scaffold, or template, upon which new structures can be built.

The molecule safrole (seen in figure 4) was used for many years as a

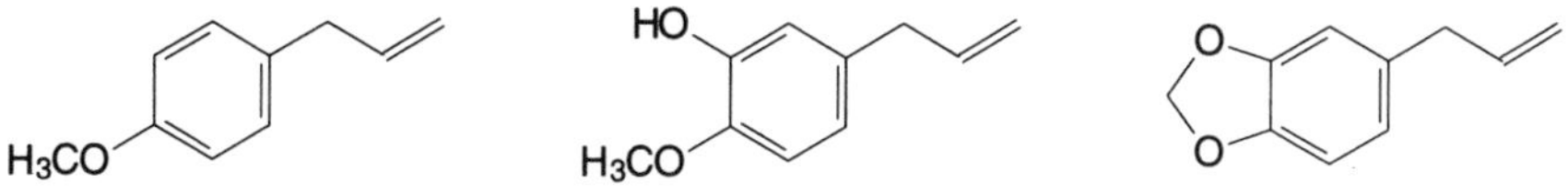

Figure 4. Molecular structures of a few common, naturally occurring odor and flavor molecules: anethole (from anise) eugenol (from cloves) safrole (from sassafras) (cited from left to right).

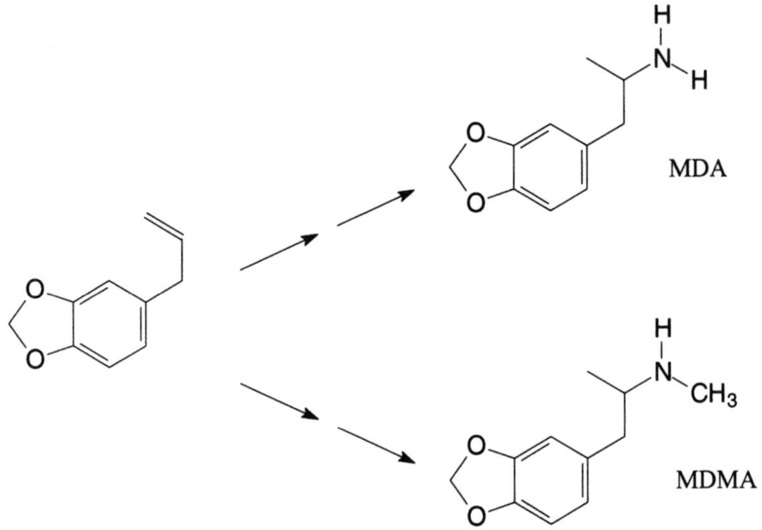

Figure 5. Safrole as the origin of MDA and MDMA.

flavoring agent in root beer and is the major flavor component of sassafras root bark, from which one makes sassafras tea. After safrole was found to produce liver tumors in rats, it was no longer available for commercial flavoring. Nevertheless, many organic molecules are still made using materials derived from sassafras oil and safrole. It is perhaps not too surprising that chemical and pharmaceutical companies made many derivatives of safrole; it was a cheap and plentiful starting material. Without trying to describe the intricate details of the actual chemistry involved, figure 5 will suffice to show in a general sense the way in which safrole evolved into MDA and MDMA. At this point, the reader should keep two facts firmly in mind. First, MDA and MDMA are organic bases and react with acids to form water-soluble salts, and, second, the greater portion of the structure of these molecules is derived from safrole, which comes from sassafras root.

There is one other issue with which we now need to deal. It concerns a property called stereochemistry. While we have been drawing chemical structures as sets of lines, polygons, and letters on a page, in fact, these molecules are three-dimensional, occupying specific shapes in space. Figure 6 illustrates a stereo-pair view of MDMA. That is, this figure can be viewed to give the reader a three-dimensional representation of MDMA. To achieve this

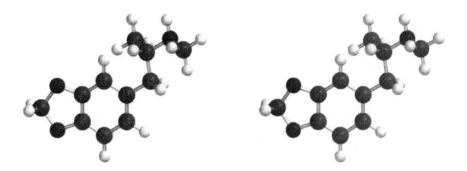

Figure 6. A three-dimensional, stereo-pair representation of (+)-MDMA. This orientation is the same one illustrated in figure 7 as the original molecule rotated about the axis below the mirror image. The atoms in this figure are not scaled to size, so as to show the individual bonds more clearly.

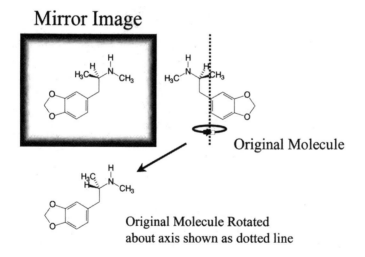

Mirror Image

Original Molecule

Original Molecule Rotated
about axis shown as dotted line

Figure 7. The concept of organic molecules that are mirror images. The original molecule at the top right is shown reflected in a mirror on the left, so that the upper-left image is a mirror image of the original molecule. One may rotate the original molecule around an imaginary axis (shown as the vertical dotted line) to obtain the molecule on the lower left. A comparison of the upper mirror image with the rotated original molecule below it shows that the two molecules are not identical in their three-dimensional structure.

result, one must look at the figure while crossing your eyes. When your eyes are crossed, you will see more than two images. Let your eyes relax so that the images slowly drift back together until there are only three images, then focus on the central image. If you are able to do this, you should see a three-dimensional image of the MDMA molecule.

One other complicating feature of MDMA that we need to discuss is the fact that there are really *two* types of MDMA molecules. Because chemical bonds cannot easily break, the arrangement of groups connected to a carbon atom with four bonds can be represented in two ways, which prove to be mirror images. Figure 7 shows these mirror images. Now compare the two images on the left, the one in the panel under "mirror image" and the one directly below it. They are not the same. In the mirror image, the H atom is attached with a dashed line, meaning that it projects back behind the plane of the paper, while the CH_3 is attached by a dark, wedge-shaped bond, to show that it projects above the plane of the paper. In the image below that, however, the two groups are reversed. Thus, the spatial arrangement of the groups attached to the carbon atom next to the N atom is different, and the groups are different in that they are mirror images. There are two specific names that are used interchangeably for mirror image organic molecules: "optical isomers" and "enantiomers."

Although the chemical properties of mirror image molecules, or enantiomers, are identical (for example, they have the same boiling point, their salts have the same melting point, and they have the same water solubility and the same affinity for protons), they do have one unique property. If one prepares a solution of the salts of mirror image molecules and then shines a beam of plane-polarized light through the solution, it turns out that the two enantiomers will cause the light beam to rotate in opposite directions and by the same amount. Optical isomers are sometimes called (+) or (–) isomers, depending on whether they rotate plane-polarized light to the right or to the left, respectively. Thus, MDMA exists either as (+)-MDMA or as (–)-MDMA. The importance of optical isomers does not lie in their simple chemistry, however, but in their interactions with living systems, because all living systems are made largely of building blocks that are optical isomers. Some of the most important constituents of mammalian species, of which we are an example, are proteins that are constructed of amino acids of only one type.

These are called L-amino acids (L for levo, or left), and they have core structural features that are identical in all of them; they have the same three-dimensional framework. Indeed, the proteins of nearly every living thing on this earth are made up exclusively of L-amino acids.

The consequences of this are profound for the actions of drugs and other molecules that affect our biological systems. Imagine for a moment a world where people only have right hands—not a right hand and a left hand but only right hands. Now suppose that we build a factory to produce gloves to keep all those hands warm. But somewhere in the design department a mistake is made. When the factory starts up, it produces gloves that fit only left hands. Even though we know that right hands are the mirror images of left hands, these left-handed gloves do not fit the hands of the people in that right-handed world.

Organic chemists often use this analogy between hands to explain mirror image molecules, and it is apt. If one can generalize this concept to the idea that all molecules made of L-amino acids have a sort of "handedness," one can appreciate the fact that when molecules have mirror images, only one of them will interact well with proteins in the body. Let me extend this analogy, to be absolutely sure that this point is clear. Imagine that there are important proteins in the body that have cavities shaped like very small left-handed gloves. Let's call these places "receptors" because they receive, or provide a reception for, certain important messenger molecules. If we administer a drug that is made of mirror image molecules that somehow resemble small hands (meaning that we have a mixture of molecules that resemble small left hands and small right hands), it is only the molecules resembling the shape of left hands that will fit into these receptors, just as left-handed gloves fit only left hands and right-handed gloves fit only right hands. The mirror image molecules shaped like small right hands will not fit into these particular receptors. That does not mean, however, that the molecules shaped like little right hands always have no effect at all. Indeed, there may be another place in the body where there are receptors shaped like right-handed gloves, where molecules shaped like left hands will not fit. In some cases both mirror image molecules may have significant effects in the body, but they are almost always different effects, occurring in different systems, governed by different kinds of receptors.

Finally, one more thing to remember is that most times when an organic chemist synthesizes a new organic molecule with a carbon atom to which four different groups are attached, the product is a 50:50 mixture of mirror images. Half of the molecules rotate plane-polarized light to the left (–), and half rotate it to the right (+). In a 50:50 mixture, these rotations exactly cancel each other out, and no rotation is observed. This mixture of half "left" and half "right" molecules is called a racemic mixture, or a racemate. If you have managed to stay awake through this discussion, you should now have the basic knowledge to understand the MDA and MDMA molecules well enough to proceed to a very introductory discussion of how they interact with the body.

In about 1967, the molecule known as 3,4-methylenedioxyamphetamine (MDA) gained popularity as a recreational substance. It was known as the "love drug," because it seemed to produce in users a feeling of emotional closeness, of loving and of being loved. MDA is a racemic mixture and therefore contains a 50:50 mixture of mirror image molecules. While mirror image molecules interact differently with certain receptors in the body, it is not always the case that only one mirror image molecule is active and the other inactive. It was discovered about ten years ago that MDA is an example where both mirror image molecules of MDA have different effects that contribute to the effect of racemic MDA. The enantiomer of MDA that rotates plane-polarized light to the left, (–)-MDA, was found to have long-lasting effects that resemble those of LSD and other classical hallucinogens. That action is believed to be due to activation of a type of brain serotonin receptor called the 5-HT2$_A$ receptor. On the other hand, the enantiomer of MDA that rotates plane-polarized light to the right, (+)-MDA, was found to be shorter in duration of action and not to have much of an LSD-like effect. It is more of a stimulant. Its actions seem to be related to its ability to be taken up into brain neurons that release the brain chemicals, or neurotransmitters, called serotonin and dopamine and somehow to cause the neurons to spill out their stores of both these neurotransmitters. The mechanism of action through which that occurs is not yet completely clear. But the neurons have specialized proteins called "reuptake pumps," and it is currently believed that drugs like (+)-MDA are carried into the neurons by this uptake pump. Furthermore, it is thought that the ability to be pumped into the neuron is an important part of the process whereby the neuron begins to release its stored neurotransmitter.

About ten years later, someone decided to prepare and sample some 3,4-methylenedioxymethamphetamine, or MDMA, and found that it had unusual and unique effects on the human psyche. A comparison of MDA and MDMA is shown in figure 3. The only difference is the presence of the methyl group, which is attached to the nitrogen atom. This methyl group does not profoundly change the chemical properties or the base strength of MDMA when compared with MDA. It does have consequences in terms of the biological effects, however. First, adding a methyl group to the nitrogen atom makes the molecule more lipid (fat) soluble. This means that because the brain is made largely of lipids, MDMA has a greater solubility in brain tissues. In general, drugs that have greater solubility in lipids and an action in the brain also have a faster onset of action but a shorter duration of action. Based only on this observation, one could predict that MDMA should products its effects faster than MDA but have a shorter action than MDA. This is in fact what is observed.

The different times to onset and duration of action for MDA and MDMA is confounded somewhat by the fact that the N-CH$_3$ has a second important effect: it makes the molecule too large to fit comfortably into the brain serotonin 5-HT2$_A$ receptor that is responsible for LSD-like actions. That receptor is only minimally activated by MDMA; hence MDMA lacks significant LSD-like effects. The N-methyl group does not affect the ability of the reuptake pump to transport MDMA into neurons that utilize serotonin and dopamine, however. It is nearly as potent as MDA in that regard. Recalling that (–)-MDA has effects resembling LSD but that (+)-MDA has more of a stimulant effect, we can see that (–)-MDMA lacks LSD-like effects but that (+)-MDMA retains the ability to cause neurons to release their stores of dopamine and serotonin. Remember, too, that these drugs, as used on the street, have equal mixtures of their mirror image molecules. That is, street MDA is an equal mixture of (+)-MDA and (–)-MDA, and the effects in humans are the result of the two different actions of MDA, the LSD-like actions of (–)-MDA and the neurotransmitter-releasing actions of (+)-MDA. Likewise, street MDMA is an equal mixture of (+)-MDMA and (–)-MDMA, where the LSD-like effects of (–)-MDMA essentially have been destroyed by the N-CH$_3$ group, but the neurotransmitter-releasing effects of (+)-MDMA are still intact.

Based on this discussion, we can conclude that if one ingests a dose of MDA, the resulting effect is long lasting and has elements of LSD-like actions, due to the (–)-MDA. It also has the neurotransmitter-releasing effects that make one feel stimulated and probably lead to the unique emotional enhancement that is characteristic of MDA. By contrast, the effects of MDMA should be faster in onset and shorter acting; the LSD-like effects should be much less intense or completely absent, due to the inactivity of (–)-MDMA; while the stimulant effect and the mood-enhancing effects due to release of neurotransmitter should remain. What that means in practical terms is that (–)-MDMA has almost no effect at ordinary doses, whereas (+)-MDMA produces effects that are nearly identical to racemic MDMA, but at only one-half of the dose required for the racemate. That is, (+)-MDMA is about twice as potent as racemic MDMA, and the effect of ordinary clandestinely produced MDMA mostly resembles the experience one would obtain if one took pure (+)-MDMA.

And what about the "neurotoxicity" that is reported in rodents and monkeys after administration of MDA or MDMA? This toxic effect is related in some way to the ability of these molecules to cause neurons to release their stored neurotransmitters, dopamine and serotonin. As we might predict from the preceding discussion, because it is the (+)-isomers of both MDA and MDMA that affect the uptake pump and cause release of neurotransmitter, it is these (+)-isomers that are also more "toxic" to the neuron axons and terminals. [See "Does MDMA Cause Brain Damage?" for more details about MDMA neurotoxicity.]

It may be germane at this point to discuss one other point that is sometimes brought up—the fact that the original emergency scheduling of MDMA as a controlled substance was based on data that had been collected for MDA. Looking again at figure 3, we see that the two molecules differ only in the presence of the CH_3 unit attached to the N atom of MDMA. At the time of the scheduling, MDA had for some years been in Schedule I of the Controlled Substances Act and was classified as a hallucinogen. Reports by users of MDMA suggested that MDMA was a rather benign substance, with much milder effects and a shorter duration of action than MDA. Thus, proponents of MDMA argued that MDA was very different from MDMA and that the neurotoxicity data produced by studies of MDA could not be applied to the

effects of MDMA to justify scheduling MDMA. From a chemical and pharmacological standpoint, however, those arguments are difficult to defend.
While it is true that adding an N-CH$_3$ to amphetamine to give methamphetamine produces subtle changes in the effects on humans, the two structures
have generally similar pharmacologic characteristics.

As we have seen from the earlier discussion, a similar transformation from
MDA to N-CH$_3$-MDA, or MDMA, abolishes the hallucinogenic effects that
are possessed by the (–)-isomer within racemic MDA. It does not, however,
markedly change the ability of the substances to cause the release of neurotransmitters from brain neurons, which is due to their (+)-isomers. As you
will discover from reading other chapters in this book, the neurotransmitter-
releasing properties of MDMA are at the heart of its ability to produce the
reported serotonin neurotoxicity. Therefore, we can see that an extrapolation from the toxic effects of MDA to a prediction that the same effects
would occur with MDMA was justified. Sometimes small changes in molecular structure cause dramatic changes in their actions on biological systems, but in other cases, like this one, a change may be largely inconsequen-
tial in terms of a particular property.

It has often been said that MDMA is a sort of hybrid between mescaline
and amphetamine. Now that the reader has some facility in understanding
the structural elements of MDMA, it may be useful to consider what such a
statement means. Clearly, MDMA has the same backbone, or framework,
that is seen in methamphetamine. This similarity is evident in figure 8, which
illustrates the structures of (+)-methamphetamine on the left, (+)-MDMA in
the middle, and mescaline, on the right.

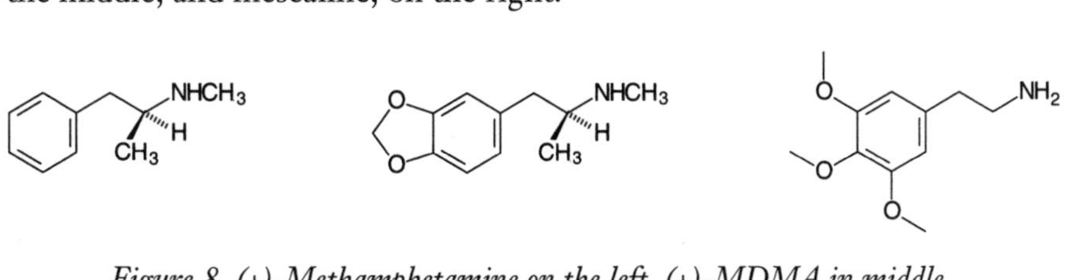

*Figure 8. (+)-Methamphetamine on the left, (+)-MDMA in middle,
and mescaline on the right.*

(+)-Methamphetamine is also a molecule that causes neurons to release
their stored transmitters. It is quite potent compared with MDMA, having a

typical therapeutic dose of 5–10 mg, given orally. Typical doses of MDMA range from perhaps 75 mg to more than 150 mg. Methamphetamine is a stimulant of the central nervous system and produces increased motor activity, decreased appetite, and a sense of well-being or even euphoria at higher doses. It is generally believed that its effects are mostly due to its ability to release the neurotransmitter dopamine from dopamine-containing neurons in the brain. This is a property that it shares with other stimulants, such as amphetamine and cocaine. It is widely believed that drugs that produce feelings of well-being and euphoria produce elevated levels of brain dopamine. In that sense, one might view MDMA in a similar way. It also has the ability to cause the release of dopamine from neurons, although it is much less potent in its ability to do so than methamphetamine. Because MDMA can produce feelings of well-being and euphoria, one might imagine that those effects also are related to its actions on dopamine systems.

Methamphetamine can bring about the release of other neurotransmitters from their neurons, including both norepinephrine and serotonin. There is little appreciation of the importance of either of these actions to the overall effects of that substance on humans. MDMA also possesses the ability to release both norepinephrine and serotonin. Its effects on norepinephrine systems are less potent than the effects of methamphetamine, and there is no recognition at present that this aspect of its mechanism of action is important to the overall effect. On the other hand, the ability of MDMA to induce the release of the stored neurotransmitter serotonin is enhanced over that of methamphetamine. This feature of the action of MDMA has been the focus of much of the research into the pharmacology of MDMA. Indeed, investigators have looked so intensely at the serotonin-releasing actions of MDMA that they have largely ignored the important role that dopamine release probably plays in its actions.

What is the relationship between MDMA and mescaline? Both molecules contain a phenyl ring (a ring of carbons) two carbons away from the amino group, so they are both phenethylamines (as is methamphetamine). And they both contain oxygen atoms attached to the phenyl rings. Beyond those features, there is not much else the two molecules have in common. My own opinion is that the comparison between MDMA and mescaline is not a good one. MDMA is really just a methamphetamine structure with oxygen atoms on the ring. While it is true that these oxygen atoms are largely responsible for the ability of MDMA to induce the release of neuronal serotonin, there is no evidence that mescaline has the same effect. Thus, the oxygen atoms on the mescaline ring do not have the same biological consequences as they have in the MDMA structure.

It is hoped that the reader now has a general appreciation of the basic chemical properties of MDMA. Although we have not discussed the detailed chemistry, it also should be apparent why sassafras oil, or its major component, safrole, are of concern to drug enforcement authorities. In addition, the comparisons between MDMA, amphetamine, methamphetamine, and mescaline should help provide a framework for appreciating some of the published discussions concerning how molecular structure affects biological action. This chapter is by no means intended to be comprehensive. Many people are interested in MDMA, from a variety of perspectives, and lack significant knowledge of organic chemistry. What I have tried to do is provide rudimentary knowledge upon which further understanding of these or similar substances can be based.

MDMA MYTHS AND RUMORS DISPELLED

Julie Holland, M.D.

Ecstasy Drains Your Spinal Fluid

The only way to remove spinal fluid from the body is with a surgical intervention called a lumbar puncture, better known as a spinal tap. In the mid-1980s, ongoing research required spinal taps on Ecstasy users. It is possible that this rumor began because of this practice. MDMA research may drain your spinal fluid, but recreational Ecstasy use does not.

Ecstasy Causes Parkinson's Disease

Parkinson's disease is a neurological illness that affects one's ability to move fluidly and causes a tremor when a person is sitting still. Its cause is unknown, but its effects are damaged dopamine neurons in a part of the brain known as the substantia nigra. MDMA does not damage dopamine neurons in any part of the brain, and Ecstasy use does not cause Parkinson's disease. In 1983, intravenous drug users, believing they were purchasing a form of heroin called China White, inadvertently injected MPTP (1-methyl-4-phenyl-1,2,5,6-tetrahydropyridine) into their veins.

Designer meperidine (Demerol) is sold as MPPP (1-methyl-4-phenyl-4-propionpiperidine). Specific conditions are required for the chemical reaction to produce MPPP. In the event of incorrect synthesis, where the pH is too low or the temperature is too high, a contaminant, MPTP, is formed. MPTP damages dopamine neurons. These intravenous drug users were left with a severe Parkinson's-like syndrome. Because MPTP and Ecstasy were popular in the media at the same time (the summer of 1985), many TV programs ran shows on so-called designer drugs that featured videos of the immobilized MPTP victims as well as segments about Ecstasy. These two stories became forever linked in the minds of many Americans.

A Single Dose of Ecstasy Causes Irreversible Brain Damage

Like all potent medicines, MDMA has a recommended dose and a toxic dose. No evidence exists that a single therapeutic dose of MDMA (roughly 125 mg) causes any damage to the nervous system. The widely publicized animal studies concerning brain damage involved repeated high-dose injections, given twice daily for four days. The changes reported do not involve the cell body but rather the tail, or axon terminals, of the nerves. Giving MDMA to test animals at lower temperatures has been shown to minimize these changes. Animal studies show that single oral doses, 2.5 mg/kg body weight, given every two weeks on four occasions to squirrel monkeys yielded no adverse effects on brain structure. One study that used a single oral dose of 5 mg/kg did cause some axonal damage in baboons. The equivalent dose in humans would be much larger than the therapeutic dose used for psychotherapy.

MDMA Was Initially Marketed as an Appetite Suppressant

MDMA was created in a laboratory in the early 1900s; a patent application was filed by Merck in 1912 and granted in 1914. Merck stumbled across MDMA when the company tried to synthesize hydrastinin, a vasoconstrictive and styptic medicine. MDMA was merely an unplanned by-product of this synthesis. The entire synthesis was patented, including intermediary products. No mention is made in the patent of using MDMA as an appetite suppressant (Beck 1997). No clinical trials were performed at that time, and MDMA was never marketed. Also, it is reasonable to assume that there was little need for an appetite suppressant in the early 1900s. The source of the confusion is clear: MDA, the analog and metabolite of MDMA, was patented by Smith Kline French and tested in 1958 on 180 human subjects as an anorectic. The medicine was abandoned due to its psychoactive side effects.

Ecstasy Is an Aphrodisiac

While MDMA can enhance communication and feelings of closeness between lovers, its physical effects tend to make erections and orgasm more difficult to achieve in most users. Some users do find that MDMA can enhance their appreciation of touch and movement, called kinesthetic awareness. This may be one reason why Ecstasy use is so popular in dance clubs and has earned the nickname the "hug drug."

Ecstasy Is a Date Rape Drug

The American media has a habit of labeling most new drugs as "date rape" drugs, perhaps to instill fear in the minds of news watchers. A date rape drug is one that renders the drug taker unconscious and therefore vulnerable to attack. Although some people may lose their inhibitions with MDMA or may feel a novel closeness to another person, MDMA does not cause a clouding of consciousness; it is not a sedative. In therapeutic doses, MDMA enhances attention and concentration. There is typically full retention of the events experienced under the influence of MDMA.

There Is Heroin in Ecstasy Pills

Because MDMA is illegal and there is no government-regulated quality control, tablets sold as Ecstasy vary tremendously in content. Many street sample analyses have been performed by harm reduction groups, results of which are often available on the Internet [see www.DanceSafe.org]. While it is common for some pills to contain methamphetamine (speed) or MDE (methylenedioxyethylamphetamine [Eve, a chemical cousin to MDMA]), the impurities more often are caffeine, dextromethorphan (cough suppressant), or decongestants. No survey has ever yielded heroin as an adulterant in an Ecstasy pill. It would not be cost-effective for pill manufacturers to use heroin in their pills, nor would the effects of heroin mimic the effects of MDMA as closely as the other additives.

Ecstasy Puts Holes in Your Brain

MTV ran a story of a woman with manic-depressive illness who had a history of polydrug abuse. During the program, they showed a three-dimensional image of her SPECT scan (single positron emission computed tomography), which is a measurement of blood flow in the brain. The areas of lower blood flow were displayed as blank spaces, while the areas of normal blood flow were shown as brain tissue. This method of displaying SPECT results is misleading, because the areas of low flow look like patches of missing tissue. MDMA does not destroy large areas of brain tissue. It does not cause neuronal cell death. Charles Grob has shown, via SPECT scans, that single doses of MDMA do cause decreased brain blood flow in certain areas, but this was not shown to be permanent [see "Clinical MDMA Research: A Worldwide Review" for more detail].

Ecstasy Turns Your Brain into Cartilage

There is simply no scientific basis for this rumor. Cartilage does not grow in the brain under any circumstance. I have been unable to discover the source of this rumor.

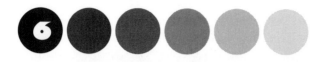

THE GODPARENTS OF MDMA
An Interview with Ann
and Sasha Shulgin

Julie Holland, M.D.

JH: What do you two think about MDMA as a medicine, versus its use as Ecstasy in the rave culture?

AS: It should be pretty well known by now, by anyone who knows anything about the subject, that MDMA was first discovered as a psychotherapeutic agent. It didn't become a street drug until sometime after it had been used in therapy. It is an insight drug. That's its main use. The effect of MDMA, for most people, is that it allows insight without fear. There isn't the usual defense against feelings of self-rejection and guilt. You can explore your shadow self, your dark side. It takes away the feelings of self-hatred and condemnation, which are the biggest obstacles to insight. That's what makes ordinary psychotherapy take so very long. It takes a long time for the therapist to get patients just to look at what's there, at what they're doing to themselves, and to try to do so without negative judgment and blame. For reasons we don't understand, MDMA allows people to do this, typically in one session.

SS: There's another aspect that ties this together a little bit with the rave scene. It seems that MDMA allows most people to accept other people. In the case of therapy, it's a matter of accepting yourself and therefore being able to speak to a therapist with a fair amount of honesty and less reserve. You can explain where you are and why you're there, and, of course, that's the whole art of therapy, to get people to acknowledge that and be able to accept themselves. There is also the acceptance of others—that is one of the reasons the drug is so successful at raves. There is no paranoia about revealing anything about yourself. You do it openly and honestly and with recall. You open yourself up to yourself and to others.

AS: As Sasha says, there is complete recall; there is no amnesia for the event. Also, there is never any loss of control, which is probably the main unconscious fear that most people have in taking any drug that affects the mental processes. With a lot of psychedelics, especially at high doses, there can be a feeling that you don't have any control, and that is never present with MDMA.

MDMA is also great for marital therapy. It enables two people to step out of the negative patterns that they might set up between themselves so that they can't communicate openly anymore. They've gotten into what I call "bookkeeping" mode. "You did this first, and I only did that because you did so and so." That drops away, and a couple who is having trouble can, for the first time in a very long time, recapture their original empathy and love for each other. They're able to see each other not as an enemy but as a friend and lover, which may have become lost. I've seen that happen very often.

One of the most important potential uses for MDMA is in the treatment of post-traumatic stress disorder. This is where it really should be used. It can be an aid in the context of all sorts of traumas, whether sexual or physical abuse in childhood or postwar trauma. MDMA is the perfect agent for opening up these areas and really being able to look at them, assimilate them, and get rid of a lot of the symptoms of having repressed the memory for so long.

JH: Ann, you performed MDMA-assisted psychotherapy, didn't you?

AS: I performed MDMA-assisted psychotherapy as a lay therapist for about three years, and I probably worked with about fifteen individuals and maybe half a dozen couples. About five of these people had completely repressed memories of early sexual abuse. Interestingly, four of them had gone into careers where they were helping children who had been sexually abused. They had no memory of their own abuse, but they had been driven unconsciously to become therapists. MDMA is superb for uncovering repressed memories.

JH: Do either of you think there is any use for MDMA outside psychotherapy?

AS: Oh, I do. I think that it's a lovely, gentle way for people to connect with each other. People who have no problems in their relationship but would just like to spend an evening together, just being loving toward each other. It should be emphasized that ninety-nine percent of the people I've met would agree that MDMA is not a sexual drug. It is almost impossible for most people to have a sexual response, but it opens up the ability to feel love.

SS: There is an incredible magic for the first few times you use MDMA, and that magic sometimes is lost. People try to recover it; sometimes there's a temptation to go to a larger dose to try to recapture that magic. It's the kind of drug that cannot be used frequently.

AS: I've been warning people that if they're going to use this material, first, they should be careful, because it is illegal. Second, I would advise them not to use it more than four times a year. If you use it more often than that, you're going to lose the magic. It seems to be a pretty permanent loss for most, but not all, people. Some people can go a year without taking it and then come back and revive that feeling. But for most people, once they have overused it, it is very difficult to get back to that original state.

The more you use it, the less effective it is. That's why it is best used in therapy. Many people need only one or two sessions. It isn't something you would take every time you go to the therapist. And it isn't something casual. Our particular group of people who occasionally took psychedelics or MDMA together would always do a blessing beforehand. It's considered a sacred journey.

JH: What do you think about the current rave culture?

SS: My feeling about the rave culture is that it is a representation of an inevitable form of behavior of people who are coming into adolescence and young adulthood. It's a way of becoming an independent person—not having to answer to authority, to parents, and establishing oneself as an individual. In that age group of fifteen to twenty-five years, you are immortal, and you don't care for the older generation. As the old saying goes, "Don't trust anyone over thirty." And I don't think it is unique to the rave community; it is specific to that stage of development. Everyone through the entire history of human beings has experienced that same rebellion against authority. It happened to express itself in this generation as rave culture, but in another, it might be jazz music at Golden Gate Park [in San Francisco].

AS: I think Sasha's absolutely right, but I have another point to add about the use of MDMA at raves. Most raves, but not all, are held in or near large cities. In most large cities in the United States and in other countries, young people learn to be very cautious and careful when they're out in public. We all know not to meet the eyes of a stranger when we're out in the streets. This becomes magnified in a place like New York. We are cautious to the point of near paranoia. We learn to be extremely careful and alert and aware, whether it's of the potential pickpocket or of someone whose sanity may be just on the edge. The only time these young people can totally relax these feelings of suspicion and caution and distrust is when they go to a rave, where you don't have to be worried about strangers. Everybody is on the same wavelength. People can touch and hold hands and be affectionate with people they've never met before. Whether this is wise is not the important point; they feel that they can be trusting.

SS: There is another aspect of MDMA use that has never received much attention. Whether it still occurs, I don't know. Years ago it did happen, when there were sports contests between England and other European countries, soccer primarily. In the early days, these young sports enthusiasts would end up drinking alcohol and getting into fights, and there would be property damage and injuries. And then, after many years, there was a tendency to move toward intoxication not with alcohol but with MDMA. This changed the entire flavor of the post-game celebration. This phenomenon was written up by Nicholas Saunders [1993].

JH: I don't know if you're familiar with Terence McKenna's theory of how mushrooms were possibly an evolutionary tool in early man [1975], but I'm wondering whether MDMA isn't some sort of evolutionary tool in modern man.

SS: It certainly has made people adopt a different attitude toward other people and interpersonal interactions. I think the blending and integration of interactions between people is an extremely healthy evolutionary adaptation.

Instead of being defensive and protecting yourself, be cautious, but not necessarily by putting up a barrier that could be interpreted as being angry or challenging. I think it's an excellent direction in which to go. In some ways, it may be emulating the use of marijuana over the past couple of generations. That was something shared by people, and it was *shared* rather than used competitively. MDMA may be playing that role now.

JH: The other thing I think it's mirroring is the Internet, the interconnectivity of people around the world.

SS: I hadn't thought of that, but it's a very nice parallel. The barriers are dropped—not physical or territorial barriers but communication barriers. The Internet is achieving a unification through communication that has never been seen before. MDMA can do this too.

AS: Of course, critics are going to point out that MDMA and the Internet can be misused by people who are damaged or dangerous, but so can anything in the world.

SS: That's the nature of humans. There's a small percentage of these people everywhere.

AS: In other words, nothing is a cure for all the problems of humankind. There's no single thing that can fill that role. But the idea of connectivity is something that we have almost entirely lost in this modern world—at least in the West. There is a complete lack of the extended family living together, and people are very isolated, especially in big cities. I think that the Internet has helped and is part of the answer. MDMA is also an answer for the younger generation, though young people are not the only ones using MDMA.

JH: Is there anything that you regret that has happened in the past twenty years with MDMA?

SS: My general response to that is that I very seriously regret the overall approach to drug use and drug abuse as a criminal issue, as opposed to a medical or a spiritual issue. The bifurcation of this entire area into that which is use and abuse, that which is legal and illegal, is a great disservice to the integrity of this country and our constitution.

AS: There's another point, which also applies to other countries where the authorities are desperate to hold on to power and to control the population, because they have total distrust of their citizens. In the old Soviet Union certain music wasn't allowed because of the message it conveyed. China and other countries with authoritarian dictatorships have tried to repress religious freedom and prevent individual expression of various opinions or even emotions. The authorities try to maintain control over people's thinking, their perceptions, and their expression of emotions, which may not be healthy for the dictatorship. I think it's the same impulse here that makes the government criminalize certain kind of drugs. They're trying to control the thinking and perceptions and feelings of the people over whom they wield power.

JH: Drugs are subversive. They make those in power very nervous.

SS: Also, those in power see changing consciousness as something they do not wish to do, because they will lose control. Therefore, they tend to bar that from happening, partly out of their own fear and inability to alter where they stand and how they think.

AS: In other words, it's a projection of their fear of their own unconscious.

SS: It's more than that, though. By having this degree of control, by being able to seize and confiscate things and arrest people and put people you don't like into prison, you're gaining power, money, and control. And that is the overwhelming drive of anybody who is in authority—to get as much control and power and money as you can. The war on drugs is providing an unparalleled example of a mechanism for doing just that.

JH: What is your opinion about the way the media has been handling MDMA over the past several years?

AS: I'm a media freak. I watch a lot of news programs. There has been a change, though, just within the beginning of this century. The establishment media, the non-cable shows, wore themselves out with documentaries on "the killer drug" Ecstasy—they never called it MDMA— and the rave scene. Then John Cloud's *Time* magazine cover story (2000) came out with a different article, paying more attention to both sides of the issue. All of a sudden we were getting calls from the networks wanting to pursue the idea of MDMA in therapy. They weren't doing it out of the goodness of their hearts or greater wisdom, but perhaps because it would help boost their ratings. CBS especially took a stab with a segment on *48 Hours*, even though they included some horrific stupidities in that program. At least they kept the Sue Stevens section intact, showing an MDMA-assisted psychotherapy session, and that was really well done. And this trend is absolutely new; it would have been unthinkable five years ago. I haven't seen any positive mention of the war on drugs in the main media in 2001.

SS: On the other hand, the President of Uruguay gave two press conferences, in his country and in Mexico, at which he recommended that his country and other South American countries repeal their drug laws. Even though members of the press from the United States were present at that speech, no one in this country ran the story.

AS: The important thing to me is that he said it and he intends to do it, but the important thing to Sasha is that no one reported it! But the report at least is making the rounds on the Internet. And that takes a lot of courage, because most of these countries have become dependent on American money.

JH: We gave a billion dollars to Colombia—they better look as if they're tough on drugs.

AS: Right. And in our country, I don't know who is worse, the Republicans or the Democrats.

SS: Senator Dianne Feinstein, who is a Democrat from California, introduced a horrible methamphetamine bill, which multiplies everything into more severe penalties.

AS: Feinstein also attempted to put into two different bills a penalty for publishing information on drugs.

JH: That information ban drove me crazy and made me very nervous until it was struck down. People were e-mailing me and saying, "Are you still going to go ahead with the book?"

AS: Thank heaven somebody with sense took that portion out of the bill.

SS: And yet every even-numbered year, people have to be elected to Congress and every even-numbered year another bill comes up with the same things in it. One of these days it's going to pass.

AS: Having gone to the Shadow Convention in Los Angeles, I am very hopeful, because the Black Caucus has become more aware all of a sudden that the majority of people in jail on nonviolent drug offenses are young black men. There were many people speaking out against the war on drugs at that convention, including Congressmen Charles Rangel from New York and John Conyers from Michigan. I don't know that they're going to continue to go along with higher penalties if an entire generation of black men are being disenfranchised.

SS: You asked me how I feel about the past twenty years. Am I happy about where MDMA stands now? No, I am quite sad. Here is a compound, an incredibly safe compound when used appropriately, that has the potential of giving pleasure to the user and of being of medical value to those who have certain psychological problems. It is thus both an affirmative and a curative agent. And yet, for political and self-serving reasons, the authorities have demonized it and made it a felony to possess and use. In effect, they forbid information about its virtues to be made available. I am proud to have had some hand in uncovering its value, but I am sad to see it become illegal and thus effectively unavailable to those who could benefit from it. A good analogy is the total ignorance shown by an entire generation of German youth to Mendelssohn's music in Nazi Germany in the mid-thirties to early forties because he happened to be a Jew and his music was politically forbidden by the police state. It was unavailable to those who might have enjoyed it.

JH: What are your hopes for the future regarding MDMA?

SS: My hope is that it be relocated from a legal and criminal arena to the medical and personal arena—that it be removed from legal control and be placed in personal control.

AS: I think that MDMA should be made available for psychotherapy, just as there's a push for marijuana to be made available as a prescription medicine. That's what we hope will happen.

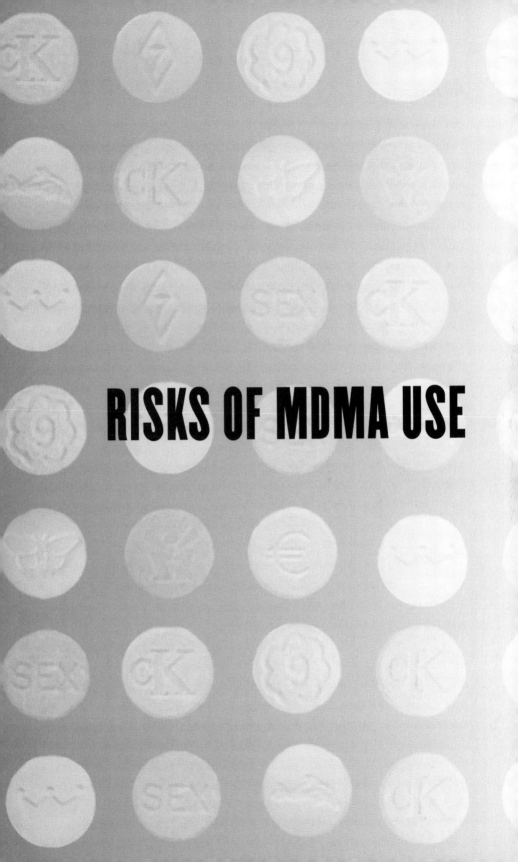

RISKS OF MDMA USE

Introduction

Not long ago, I had breakfast with a friend of mine, the mother of a sixteen-year-old girl who had vomited on the family room couch after coming home drunk from a party. She asked how this book was coming along and voiced concern about some of the information I was planning to include. "Why teach people how to use Ecstasy more safely?" she asked. "Millions of people around the world are using this drug," I explained. "They are going to use it whether we like it or not, and there are ways to keep them safe and keep them alive. Didn't you explain to Aisha about the dangers of alcohol? Didn't you tell her about not drinking too much or not driving when she had been drinking?" That is harm reduction. Wearing seat belts while driving in cars, helmets while riding on motorcycles, and even wrist guards while inline skating are all examples of harm reduction. Teaching safe sex is harm reduction; preaching abstinence is not. Offering simple advice to people who are using Ecstasy is harm reduction; reminding them to "just say no" is not.

There are several areas of concern when it comes to minimizing the risks associated with MDMA. First, there is no guarantee that when someone buys a tablet of so-called Ecstasy at a club or elsewhere it is, in fact, MDMA. Pill testing at raves and other venues can lessen the risk of ingesting adulterants that either are more dangerous than MDMA or mix badly with MDMA. In the chapter "Minimizing Risk in the Dance Community," Emanuel Sferios describes a group called DanceSafe, which sets up tables at raves and tests pills for their contents. This is clearly a controversial subject, and parents frequently are frightened by the idea that their children are being given a go-ahead from this group. By disseminating information about how to minimize the injury associated with Ecstasy use, especially in the rave setting, this group probably has saved countless lives.

The second crucial message to be passed along concerns dosage. More is not better when it comes to MDMA. Like any potent medicine, or any illicit drug, there is a dose that is safer and one that is more dangerous. All of the side effects of MDMA occur, to a greater extent, at higher doses, and most anecdotal evidence suggests that the desired effects do not increase in the same manner. There is some evidence to support what can be called "cumulative tolerance" to MDMA. This means that the longer people take MDMA, the less they feel the euphoria they are looking for and the more they notice unwanted side effects, such as jitteriness and jaw tightening. This phenomenon also has been referred to as "loss of magic." Unfortunately, some people still try to chase the elusive high they experienced early on with MDMA, and they take more of the drug. The risks of depression, neurological damage, and possible memory changes all have been linked to ingesting hundreds of doses of MDMA. When used in small doses, infrequently (often only once or twice in a lifetime) in a therapeutic setting, reports of adverse effects have been minimal. As Bruce Eisner said in the 1980s, "When you get the message, hang up the phone." The lessons learned from MDMA need to be integrated into every day of our lives, without the drug.

Taking multiple tablets of Ecstasy at one time and dancing for hours without rest or fluids has been associated with reports of hyperthermia, an elevated body temperature that can lead to seizures, muscle breakdown, kidney failure, and even death. The latest animal research shows that when high doses of MDMA are taken in an overheated environment, hyperthermia is more likely to occur than when the animals are kept cool. The third lesson to be learned is to stay cool, take breaks from dancing, and replace any fluids lost by drinking about a liter of water or isotonic sports drink an hour. It is possible to drink too much water, however, and there has been at least one reported death due to overhydration.

The debate surrounding the neurotoxicity associated with MDMA is complex. Most data have been gathered from studies in which animals were given large doses, usually twice a day for four days. While therapeutic doses of MDMA never have been shown to cause neurotoxicity, there are probably some people whose recreational use is excessive to the point that it mirrors those doses given to laboratory animals.

In the practice of medicine, when doctors offer a particular treatment to a patient, they typically perform a risk/benefit analysis. The potential pitfalls of the medication in question are balanced against the expected advantages. I have chosen to place the risk section of this book ahead of the benefits section, because I want it clearly understood that there are indeed inherent risks in MDMA use, as with any other potent medication. Just as there are risks with too high a dose of lithium or too many sessions of radiation therapy, MDMA has its own set of therapeutic guidelines.

Look in any medical textbook of pharmacology and you will see that each medicine has certain indications for its use and certain contraindications, situations in which its use is proscribed. So it is for MDMA. Not only are there potential medical complications from MDMA use but there are psychological issues to consider as well. Because MDMA allows for the exploration of repressed traumatic memories, it is possible that the release of this psychological material can trigger anxiety and panic reactions.

Also of concern is the potential for sexual promiscuity. Because some people, especially in clubs, find Ecstasy to be an aphrodisiac and because some people become less inhibited, or more enamored of others, there is a real risk of transmission of sexually transmitted diseases. People who usually use condoms or refrain from casual sex may make poorer choices or take more chances while using Ecstasy. Last, because it is a Schedule I drug, a very real risk of Ecstasy use is criminal prosecution and perhaps imprisonment.

The least risky way to use MDMA would be under medical supervision in a therapeutic context. In therapy, the setting is controlled, the amount of MDMA administered is appropriate, and the quality and purity of the drug are not in question. Because the patient is resting comfortably during the session, there is no risk of overheating, and because fluids would be needed to a much lesser degree, there is no risk of overhydrating. It should be noted that during MDMA's long tenure as a catalyst used during therapy, there were no adverse events reported among the underground therapists. It is likely that the time taken to prepare the patients for what they would be experiencing went a long way toward minimizing the potential for untoward psychological reactions. Clearly the safest way to use MDMA is as a single oral dose in the context of ongoing therapy with a supervising physician or psychiatrist.

Estimated U.S. Deaths in 1998 attributed to:	
tobacco	400,000
alcohol	110,000
prescription drugs	100,000
aspirin and over-the-counter-painkillers	7,600
MDMA	9

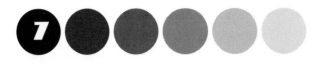

MEDICAL RISKS ASSOCIATED WITH MDMA USE

John A. Henry, M.D., and Joseph G. Rella, M.D.

A critical evaluation of the morbidity and mortality associated with MDMA use is limited by the type and amount of information that has been reported to date. Morbidity refers to the harm that comes to a patient and mortality refers to deaths. Most laboratory research examining the effects of MDMA has been done primarily on animals; only a few studies have focused on humans. Much of the literature on the harm in humans consists of reports of individual cases that do not represent much more than collective anecdotal experience. The major limitation to these reports is that, often, no toxicology studies are done using the patient's blood or urine to identify all the drugs that were ingested before admittance to the emergency room or before visiting the physician. The most that can be said about these cases is that they are Ecstasy exposures, as poison centers define exposures, since patients report having ingested Ecstasy, but the presence of MDMA within their bodies was never verified by a blood test. It is important to remember that illicitly manufactured so-called Ecstasy contains a range of ingredients of widely differing concentrations; even tablets with the same brand name may have varying concentrations of ingredients (Sherlock et al. 1999).

The pharmacological makeup of tablets sold as Ecstasy varies widely. While some pills contain MDMA, others may contain MDA (methylenedioxyamphetamine); or the stimulants amphetamine sulfate (speed), caffeine, or ephedrine; or the dissociative anesthetics, ketamine or dextromethorphan; or mixtures of these drugs and other substances in differing amounts. The effects and toxicity of what is sold as Ecstasy therefore may be quite distinct in different places and at different times. Because of the uncertainty about the contents of the tablets, these contaminants may be responsible for many of the toxic reactions reported. But although tablets sold as Ecstasy have been found to contain various adulterants, there is little solid evidence that major toxic effects have resulted from constituents other than the MDMA group of chemicals, mostly owing to limitations in identifying the drugs involved.

Adverse drug reactions to MDMA were first reported in the mid-1980s. Consistently reported findings include rapid heart rate, high blood pressure, teeth grinding, tense muscles, nausea, sweating, difficulty urinating, and headache (Buchanan 1985; Greer and Tolbert 1986; Hayner and McKinney 1986; Bryden et al. 1995). These effects, which may result in part from increased adrenaline (alpha-adrenergic activity), can last from hours to days after MDMA use and occur even after a single dose. Other reported effects of MDMA use have included psychosis, panic, and depression. [See "Mental Health Problems Associated with MDMA Use" for further information on psychiatric complications.] Not surprisingly, people whose only complications from using MDMA are teeth grinding or sweating almost never have to go to the hospital. One report indicates, however, that a large proportion of people who do go to emergency departments are first-time users who are experiencing what might be considered typical adverse effects, or "side effects" (Williams et al. 1998).

Hyperthermia

Hyperthermia is an increase in body temperature to the extent of endangering life; it can be a cause of significant morbidity and mortality. The condition usually occurs at temperatures over 40 degrees Celsius or 104 degrees Fahrenheit. A commonly reported scenario involves an Ecstasy user who spends time at a dance club, where the ambient temperatures may be high, usually dancing for many hours without adequate fluid replacement. This behavior leads to collapse or convulsions (seizures) (Simpson and Rumack 1981; Henry 1992b; Singarajah and Lavies 1992; Logan et al. 1993; Maxwell et al. 1993; Tehan et al. 1993; Satchell and Connaughton 1994). Clinical examination shows dilated pupils, sweating (though in severe cases sweating may have ceased), marked sinus tachycardia (a heart rate increase to 140–160 beats per minute is not uncommon), hypotension (low blood pressure), and core temperature of 39–42°C (102.2–107.6°F). Cases such as this represent an acute medical emergency.

As the body temperature rises, the normal response to stop activity and to cool down is blunted, possibly owing to the effects of MDMA. These patients may arrive at the hospital with core body temperatures as high as 109°F. At these temperatures, organ dysfunction ensues and may include liver failure, kidney failure, and cerebral edema (swelling of the brain), any one of which can cause death. One dangerous complication of hyperthermia is rhabdomyolysis, which is muscle breakdown that damages the kidneys and can lead to high potassium levels that cause fatal heart rhythms (Brown and Osterloh 1987; Chadwick et al. 1991; Campkin and Davies 1992; Fahal et al. 1992; Henry 1992a; Screaton et al. 1992; Nimmo et al. 1993; Montgomery and Myerson 1997). Another commonly reported complication of hyperthermia is disseminated intravascular coagulopathy (DIC), a blood-clotting disorder that can cause the patient to bleed to death. Once DIC has become established, management is difficult; this complication is the most common reason for death in patients with hyperthermia who have taken Ecstasy.

In the early 1990s, several case reports of fatal hyperthermia following Ecstasy ingestion appeared in the British literature. The patients collapsed, sometimes with seizures; when they were examined in the hospital, they tended to have a very fast heart rate and low blood pressure and body temperatures as high as 43°C (109.4°F). Attention was drawn to the importance of high body temperature as a predictor of fatal outcome in hyperthermia. The mean recorded temperature in fatalities was 41.6°C (106.9°F), compared with 40.5°C (104.9°F) in the survivors (Miller et al. 1997). Although there is a single case report of a survivor who had a recorded body temperature of 42.9°C (109.2°F), generally the body cannot sustain the massive cardiovascular and metabolic stress of a high body temperature.

Hyperthermia seems to be a particularly dangerous complication of Ecstasy, but it may be associated more closely with the behavior that follows its use. It seems apparent that cases of severe hyperthermia and deaths from heatstroke were due mainly to prolonged dancing without rest and without drinking enough liquid to allow for normal temperature control through sweating. Henry (1992) writes that the most seriously ill patients in his experience were people at crowded parties where Ecstasy was used as a dance drug. He concludes that the severe toxicity of MDMA may be "due mainly to the circumstances in which it is misused." This conclusion is well reflected in the case reports that have been published since 1992, since many of them include a brief or at least a partial description that links ill patients with hyperthermia to dancing at clubs (Brown and Osterloh 1987; Smilkstein et al. 1987). Hyperthermia has been reported in laboratory animals given MDMA (Schmidt et al. 1990a). [Recent animal studies have noted that the ambient temperature is a crucial factor in whether laboratory animals show toxic effects from MDMA. Also, the degree of hyperthermia has been shown to correlate with the degree of serotonin depletion in rats (Malberg and Seiden 1998).—Ed.]

It is commonly noted that people who have undergone MDMA-assisted psychotherapy do not suffer from hyperthermic reactions. One study of human volunteers who were not exercising vigorously did not report any subjects with complications of high body temperature, though temperature was not specifically measured (Downing 1986). [Personal communication with several researchers produced the following information: Grob (UCLA) found a 1°F increase in core temperature; Camí/Farré (Spain) found a slight increase in temperature that was not statistically significant; Jones (UCSF) found no change in core temperature but a decrease in skin temperature; Vollenweider (Switzerland) found no change in temperature; Tancer's (Wayne State University) data are pending.—Ed.]

Management of Ecstasy-Induced Hyperthermia

The main objectives in management of the patient with acute hyperthermia are to cool the body; to facilitate thermoregulation, usually with intravenous fluid replacement; and to prevent the development of DIC. Full supportive care should be provided, and an anticonvulsant, such as intravenous diazepam (Valium), may be needed if the patient is having seizures.

The most urgent priority is to restore the blood volume, since extracellular fluid volume tends to be depleted grossly by prolonged sweating. Once a high core temperature has been confirmed, one liter of normal saline (0.9 percent) should be given immediately, without waiting to measure central venous pressure. If this treatment brings down the pulse rate and raises the blood pressure, another liter can be given, after which the central venous pressure should be measured and more fluids given, as required. The fluid replacement usually achieves thermoregulation through sweating and vasodilation without the need for active cooling in milder cases of hyperthermia. Sedation and active cooling, such as an ice bath, should be strongly considered for more serious cases, those with temperatures above 106°F. Since severe hyperthermia reduces the calcium requirement for excitation-contraction coupling (the muscles' mechanism of action), further heat production may develop from muscle contractions, even in the absence of exertion, once hyperthermia has developed. This can be prevented by administration of dantrolene, which acts as a calcium antagonist at the level of the sarcolemmal membrane in the muscle.

Ecstasy-Induced Hyponatremia

Another problem seen in Ecstasy users is acute hyponatremia, a low plasma sodium level due to dilution of the blood with water. Sodium levels are often 125 mmol/L or lower (137–147 mmol/L is a normal plasma sodium range). This complication occurs among patients who have taken Ecstasy and who also have drunk large amounts of water without losing as much fluid by sweating. This raises a theoretical concern for those users of Ecstasy who are commonly advised by friends to drink plenty of fluids, possibly to guard against hyperthermia and dehydration. The problem is that MDMA causes secretion of antidiuretic hormone. ADH, also known as vasopressin, is a hormone that inhibits urination by promoting increased water reabsorption by the kidneys. An experimental study in healthy volunteers has shown that administration of 40 mg of MDMA (a very low dose) produced a marked rise in levels of ADH in plasma, which was accompanied by a small fall in the sodium concentration (Henry et al. 1998). One case of MDMA-induced hyponatremia has been documented in which the ADH level was measured, and it was confirmed that this level was inappropriately raised. In this case the ADH concentration was 4.5 pmol/L. (Holden and Jackson 1996), whereas the normal range is 1–2.5 pmol/L.

The combination of excess water intake and increased absorption of water from elevated ADH may contribute to a dangerous decline in serum sodium.

This can lead to mute states, headache, and vomiting. The low sodium also may cause nausea, cramps, weakness, fatigue, confusion, and seizures that may be very difficult to control. Low levels of sodium in the body lead to cerebral edema, a condition where the brain cells swell with water. It is a major cause of death in hyponatremia. In cases of Ecstasy-related hyponatremia, patients did not have elevated temperatures. There are several reports of hyponatremia in people attending rave parties; two people experienced seizures. In many of these cases, the patient was reported to have drunk copious amounts of water, which likely contributed substantially to their illness (Maxwell et al. 1993; Satchell and Connaughton 1994; Ajaelo et al. 1998). These reports, however, are far outnumbered by those of patients who experience hyperthermia.

Patients with hyponatremia show signs of severe illness within twelve hours of ingestion of Ecstasy, suggesting that there is an acute drop in serum sodium as the result of unrestricted fluid ingestion. The resultant low sodium level may be relatively close to normal, because the change has occurred suddenly and the cells have had less time to adapt to the low plasma osmolality (a measure of dilution). Severe symptoms may develop with plasma sodium levels of 130 mmol/L or less, and the urine is inappropriately concentrated, with raised osmolality due to excessive production of ADH.

Ecstasy-induced hyponatremia can be compared to the syndrome of inappropriate secretion of antidiuretic hormone (SIADH). SIADH is a syndrome marked by diluted blood and concentrated urine; it is typically seen when someone who has taken MDMA drinks excess water, which contains no solutes (as opposed to isotonic sports drinks such as Gatorade), to replace fluid lost from sweating, which does contain these salts. If ADH is inappropriately secreted, less urine is excreted, and the overall water-to-salt balance in the body is disrupted. Since MDMA has been shown to enhance the production of ADH, it is probable that the syndrome of inappropriate ADH secretion is mediated by the serotonergic system. [A syndrome of inappropriate ADH secretion also is seen in people who take antidepressants known as serotonin reuptake inhibitors, and it may be mediated through serotonin 2A and 2C receptors (Liu et al. 1996; Spigset and Mjorndal 1997).—Ed.]

Table I. Reasons for the acute hyperthermic and hyponatremic effects of MDMA

Reasons for hyperthermia

Prolonged exertion, warm environment

Amphetamine-like effect

   Promotion of repetitive activity like dancing

   Disregard for body signals (thirst, exhaustion)

Mood-enhancing effect

   Euphoria

   Feeling of energy

Serotonergic effect

   Increased muscle tone, heat production

Reasons for hyponatremia

Harm reduction message to drink fluids

Amphetamine-like effect

   Dry mouth and throat

   Repetitive behaviors, including compulsively drinking water

Mood-enhancing effect

   Reduced inhibitions and impaired judgment possibly leading to excessive water intake

Serotonergic effect

   Reduced renal response to water load (SIADH)

Management of Ecstasy-Induced Hyponatremia

In most cases stopping all fluid intake and providing supportive care is all that is required. Patients with Ecstasy-induced hyponatremia will often have mental status changes but will typically be cool to the touch; hyponatremia and hyperthermia never co-exist. A serum sodium level will assist in making the diagnosis. Fluid restriction is the first level of treatment for minor cases of hyponatremia. Hypertonic saline should be given intravenously in more severe cases, or for serious complications, such as treating seizures due to hyponatremia. Dr. Henry recommends treating severe Ecstasy-induced SIADH with mannitol and diuretics, but Dr. Rella cautions that this treatment may actually exacerbate the fluid and electrolyte problems the patient may be experiencing.

The Serotonin Syndrome

The use of MDMA triggers an excess release of serotonin (McKenna and Peroutka 1990; Rudnick and Wall 1992), which can cause the serotonin syndrome, one of the more serious complications associated with Ecstasy use. This syndrome is a rare, drug-induced event characterized by confusion, difficulty walking, increased sweating, diarrhea, heightened deep tendon reflexes and myoclonus (muscle jerks), poor control of heart rate and blood pressure, shivering and increased muscle tone and rigidity, which can lead to hyperthermia and death (Sternbach 1991; Ames and Wirshing 1993). This syndrome carries a mortality rate of about 10 to 15 percent. Drugs known to affect serotonin metabolism include amphetamines, cocaine, and many different kinds of antidepressants. The occurrence of serotonin syndrome as the result of Ecstasy use may explain some hyperthermic fatalities among patients who engaged in minimal physical exercise. However, since muscle rigidity, a common feature of serotonin syndrome, is not noted in all case reports, it can be difficult to distinguish patients with serotonin syndrome from those with hyperthermia stemming from exercising or dancing.

There have been reports describing potential cases of serotonin syndrome after Ecstasy use (Brown and Osterloh 1987; Smilkstein et al. 1987; Henry et al. 1992; Screaton et al. 1992; Nimmo et al. 1993; Tehan et al. 1993; Mueller and Korey 1998). Of the eleven patients in these studies who reportedly had serotonin syndrome, five died. It is important to understand that these reports are biased, in that they cite only the worst cases and outcomes. When serotonin syndrome is the result of drugs other than MDMA, its effects usually resolve within 24 hours, and the condition requires only general medical support to prevent progressive ill effects or death. Sedation and active cooling are the mainstays of treatment for serotin syndrome as with hyperthermia from overactivity. Patients with MDMA-associated serotonin syndrome often have a rapid, severe course, and death may result from complications of hyperthermia. Heat production can be stopped by paralysis and ventilation of the patient. Since there are no medical personnel at clubs to ensure that people do not become ill, patients may not get medical attention until it is too late. Patients may have hyperthermia for a long time, resulting in severe complications. Their clinical appearance also may be disguised by the use of other club drugs, such as GHB (gamma hydroxy butyrate) or ketamine (dissociative anesthetics), or by another drug that the user consumed believing it was MDMA, such as methamphetamine or dextromethorphan.

Cardiac Complications

Cardiac complications include hypertension (increases of 40 mm Hg in systolic blood pressure), tachycardia (increases of 30 beats/minute) (Mas et al. 1999), cardiac arrhythmias (irregular heart rhythms), and contraction band necrosis (cell death of a specific part of the heart muscle), as seen in catecholamine-induced myocardial injury (such as cocaine-related heart attacks) (Milroy et al. 1996). A case of QT-interval prolongation (an electrocardiogram abnormality) has been reported (Drake and Broadhurst 1996). Ecstasy has been known to induce fatal cardiac arrhythmias (Dowling et al. 1987).

Liver Abnormalities

Another serious adverse reaction to Ecstasy use is hepatitis, inflammation of the liver. There have been several reported cases (Henry et al. 1992; Dykhuizen et al. 1995), but they do not conclusively define MDMA as the inciting agent, and the specific mechanism of action by which MDMA might cause the damage has not been described. [In twenty-eight-day toxicology studies in the rat and dog, Frith and Chang (1987) did not report any liver damage from MDMA administration.—Ed.] Liver damage after Ecstasy use has been reported, but it appears to be unrelated to hyperthermia and may be due to an idiosyncratic drug reaction (Karch 1996; Milroy et al. 1996).

In 1992 a case series of seven patients with liver damage associated with Ecstasy use was reported (Henry et al. 1992). Several isolated cases also have been reported, including two cases of acute hepatitis (Delentre et al. 1994; Dykhuizen et al. 1995) and one case of accelerated hepatic fibrosis (hardening of the liver) (Khakoo et al. 1995). A series of twelve cases of hepatic damage has been reported from the Institute of Liver Studies at King's

College Hospital (Ellis et al. 1996); it was suggested in this report that the incidence of Ecstasy-induced hepatitis was increasing. A spectrum of severity seems to exist, with histologic changes varying from mild to moderate lobular hepatitis to features of massive hepatic parenchymal collapse with areas of nodular regeneration. An immunologic mechanism of action appears to be the most likely cause of the sporadic cases of hepatitis that have been seen in Ecstasy users. This means, however, that hepatitis due to Ecstasy use is unlikely to be dose dependent and also that it is likely to be highly unpredictable. It is also possible that with the current degree of Ecstasy use, leading to repeated re-exposure, the incidence of cases of liver damage may rise with time. Young people who have unexplained jaundice or hepatomegaly should be asked about their possible use of Ecstasy.

The Liver Enzyme CYP2D6

There are no reports that people who take MDMA repeatedly build tolerance to adverse events and will no longer experience any complications. In general, it cannot be predicted who will experience side effects. Why do some people seem to be more susceptible to the effects of even a single dose of the drug while others seem relatively resistant? One possible explanation may be genetic polymorphism, which is how scientists describe the way everyone's genetic makeup differs. Since some people have different genes, they have different enzymes and therefore different abilities to metabolize, or break down, drugs. Scientists have found that MDMA is broken down by a specific enzyme in the liver that is known to be genetically deficient in a small percentage of the population. [CYP2D6 is the enzyme that breaks down MDMA. It is inactive in 5 to 10 percent of Caucasian and 1 to 2 percent of Asian people.—Ed.] In a person who is deficient in the enzyme, the effects of MDMA may last longer in the body and cause damage to the organs, and that person would not be able to detect the deficiency beforehand. It should be made clear that this is only a theory of how a rare event may occur in a very small part of the MDMA-taking population.

A recent study has shown that this liver enzyme theory may not be accurate and that small increases in the dose of MDMA ingested can translate to a disproportionate increase in MDMA plasma concentrations (de la Torre et al. 2000a). The half-life of MDMA is about eight hours (Ecstasy TOXBASE). The lethal dose (LD_{50}, the dose at which half the laboratory animals die) has been studied in various animal models and by various routes of administration. Studies in rats have shown the drug's LD_{50} is 49 mg/kg when administered parenterally (through routes other than the gastrointestinal tract) and 325 mg/kg when taken orally. Nonhuman primate studies have shown an LD_{50} of 22 mg/kg parenterally. While no LD_{50} studies in humans will ever be carried out, serum levels assayed in patients with toxic effects of MDMA ingestion have approached or, in some cases, exceeded the primate LD_{50} dose (Rochester and Kirchner 1999).

Neurological Complications

The potential for neurotoxicity resulting from the use of MDMA has been investigated in some detail over the past ten to fifteen years. These investigations suggest that MDMA poisons special nerves in the brain that use the chemical serotonin. Studies of rats found that they had lower levels of brain serotonin for up to a year or more after they were given the drug. The levels in monkeys remained altered for an even longer period of time. Scientists also found that some damaged nerves grew back and reorganized in unpredictable ways in both species and that these effects persisted longer in monkeys than in rats (Ricaurte et al. 1992). Some of these experiments were conducted simulating the way some people use MDMA and not in an artificial, purely experimental manner, such as using extremely high doses (Fischer et al. 1995; Ricaurte et al. 1988a,c).

Among the few studies involving humans, one documented diminished levels of serotonin in the cerebrospinal fluid (CSF—the fluid that bathes the brain) of people who used Ecstasy compared with people who did not use Ecstasy (McCann et al. 1994). This is similar to the findings in the animal studies mentioned earlier. But it is difficult to determine how these changes in serotonin levels affect the way people live and think and feel, because there is no straightforward test that can examine its effects. The same study that found decreased serotonin levels in the CSF of Ecstasy users further evaluated its subjects for pain response and for impulsive and hostile personality traits. Previous studies have associated lower serotonin levels in humans with alterations in pain sensation and with impulsive and hostile personality characteristics. Researchers hypothesized that since users of Ecstasy have lower serotonin levels, they also might have these alterations in pain sensation and impulsive and hostile personality traits. They found that there was no difference in pain sensitivity; moreover, Ecstasy users with lower levels of serotonin were actually less hostile and impulsive than might otherwise have been predicted. This study therefore was able to show a difference in serotonin levels in humans, but it did not confirm any other effects of this difference. [For a thorough evaluation of the neurotoxicity debate, see "Does MDMA Cause Brain Damage?"]

Other serious reported neurological complications of Ecstasy use include intracerebral hemorrhage (ICH, or bleeding into the brain). One report cited four cases of ICH related to the use of Ecstasy (Harries and DeSilva 1992). Of these four patients, one was found to have a congenital anomaly that may have caused the bleeding, and another did not actually take MDMA. Two other patients were said to have used MDMA, but use was never confirmed by a blood test. Another report cites five deaths related to MDMA use (Dowling et al. 1987). In one case a user climbed an electrical utility tower and was electrocuted. In another case, a twenty-five-year-old man was driving home from his physician's office when he died of a heart attack; no information is offered concerning whether the man was experiencing the effects of MDMA while at the doctor's office. The third man apparently died of an asthma attack, and the fourth died of a sudden fatal heart rhythm. The fifth person cited in the report died from complications of a congenital heart problem. Levels of MDMA were found in all of these patients. None of these reports, however, contain any data regarding signs or symptoms of MDMA use in the patients before their deaths, such as rapid heart rate or high blood pressure. While it is possible that the effects of MDMA may exacerbate an underlying condition, such as heart disease, or assist an individual in doing something foolish, such as climbing an electrical tower, the data in these reports only suggest a possible association between death and MDMA and cannot confirm a direct causal relationship.

Table 2. Effects of MDMA

Minor adverse effects (relatively common and generally short-lived reactions, which occur shortly after taking a dose)

Mydriasis (dilated pupils)

Photophobia (discomfort when looking at bright lights)

Headache

Anorexia (diminished appetite), nausea, dry mouth, abdominal cramps, diarrhea

Sweating, tachypnea (rapid breathing), tachycardia (rapid heart rate), palpitations, tremor

Bruxism (grinding of teeth)

Trismus (uncomfortable rigidity of the jaw muscles)

Gait disturbance, ataxia (difficulty walking)

Serious acute adverse effects (uncommon reactions)

Hallucinations, severe anxiety, agitation, panic attacks, paranoia

Hypertension (increased blood pressure)

Cardiac arrhythmias (irregular heart rhythms)

Severe central chest pain (probably due to intercostal muscle spasm)

Severe abdominal cramps

Urinary retention (due to alpha-adrenergic stimulation of bladder neck) (Bryden et al. 1995)

Adverse effects only in certain circumstances

Overexertion, dehydration, collapse

Hyperpyrexia (increased body temperature)

Convulsions (seizures)

Rhabdomyolysis (muscle breakdown)

Disseminated intravascular coagulation (blood clots throughout the body)

Cerebrovascular accident (stroke), intracerebral hemorrhage

Acute renal failure

Polydipsia (excessive drinking), low sodium levels, and stupor

Road traffic accidents

Facial dermatosis (pimples) (Wollina et al. 1998)

Delayed reactions to exposure

Jaundice, hepatotoxicity

Tooth wear (Redfearn et al. 1998)

Possible congenital anomalies (McElhatton et al. 1999)

Poor concentration and attention, memory impairment, depression

Sleep disturbance

Weight loss, exhaustion

General Management of MDMA Toxicity

Treatment of the symptomatic patient is mainly supportive. Gastric lavage (pumping the stomach) is not necessary, but it is advisable to give oral activated charcoal if the drug was taken within the previous hour. Monitoring of the blood pressure, electrocardiogram, and body temperature for a minimum of twelve hours is recommended. Diazepam may be given to control anxiety and agitation. Chlorpromazine (Thorazine) and haloperidol (Haldol), antipsychotic medications, should be avoided, since they are likely to reduce the threshold for seizures and exacerbate hypotension (low blood pressure). Symptomatic narrow complex tachycardia in adults should be treated with beta-blockers (for example, 5–10 mg metoprolol given intravenously, only if there is certainty that cocaine was not ingested), and hypertension should be treated with calcium channel blockers (for example, 5–10 mg nifedipine taken orally) or alpha-adrenergic antagonists (for example, 2–5 mg phentolamine intravenously, only if there is certainty that cocaine was not ingested). If the rectal temperature exceeds 39°C (102.2°F), rehydration is essential. In severe cases, dantrolene can be considered, though its effects are not immediate. Any period of time wasted not actively cooling the patient risks worsened end organ damage and death. If these measures are not effective, the patient should be paralyzed and ventilated. Laboratory evaluations should include serum sodium level, liver function tests, creatinine phosphokinase, plasma potassium, blood fibrin degradation products to test for DIC, and urine for myoglobinuria. Acidosis should be corrected with intravenous sodium bicarbonate.

Assessing the Risk of MDMA Use

The exact number of MDMA users remains unknown, though most researchers and clinicians think that the overall use of MDMA is on the rise. The incidence of adverse effects of MDMA therefore will remain unknown, and any useful clinical information will continue to rely on the accurate recording of data from patients who come to medical attention. The reports of morbidity and mortality can be difficult to interpret, rendering the determination of safety of MDMA use difficult as well.

Those who assess whether MDMA is safe, such as the government, the media, or researchers, are necessarily biased by various factors. In 1985, the government classified MDMA as a Schedule I drug, meaning that it has no therapeutic value. This decision was based on limited data concerning MDA, a drug structurally similar to MDMA, and presumably was implemented for the public good. The media declared MDMA to be dangerous based partly on their interpretation of the extant scientific research and partly on their desire to make headlines. The sensationalizing of the deaths of two young women, one in England and another in Australia, which might have been related to hyponatremia associated with drinking too much water after Ecstasy use, clearly illustrates a desire to sell newspapers rather than cogently inform. These cases are unfortunately unavailable for critical review, since the medical literature does not include the proper names of patients, to maintain confidentiality.

Scientific research is done for the public good, though it, too, can be influenced by various factors. Most human reports are gathered retrospectively, that is, data are collected after the fact. For this reason, collected data are often incomplete. For example, not all serotonin syndrome cases record the patient's muscle tone, and not all hyperthermia case reports included information about whether the patient had been dancing. Such missing pieces limit any conclusion that may be drawn from the report. An especially powerful bias in the medical literature is that only severe or unusual cases are ever reported in the first place.

There is not now, nor will there ever be, a collection of case reports of those who used MDMA and never became ill. Researchers consider only very sick patients and exceptional cases interesting enough to write about, which likely accounts for the fact that nearly half of all patients with serotonin syndrome whose cases were reviewed here died. What can the reader learn who wishes to know more about the safety of MDMA based on the reports of morbidity and mortality? The data may not be as good as we would like it to be, but a few facts still can be gleaned. Intuitively, we know that the incidence of adverse outcomes is likely low, since emergency departments are not being overrun each weekend by people dying from Ecstasy use. The risks of Ecstasy-related problems may be reduced by encouraging users, if they insist on taking the drug, to apply the following precautions:

- Do not take more than one pill.

- Avoid dancing for prolonged periods of time. Take regular rests and relax in a cool place for a while. Many clubs have "chill out" areas for this purpose.

- Drink electrolyte-rich fluids to replace lost fluid but avoid overhydration. Do not drink extra fluids if you are not exercising.

- Wear light loose clothes.

- Seek medical help early if you begin to experience unusual or worrying symptoms.

Given the many reports of the unpredictable and potentially lethal complications sometimes associated with Ecstasy use, it is easy to see that further controlled studies of MDMA are required to define its effects on humans before any conclusion can be drawn concerning its potential usefulness and safety as a therapeutic tool in a controlled setting. Dr. Henry and colleagues (1992) mentioned a single case of a patient who was reported to have ingested forty tablets of MDMA, did not engage in vigorous physical activity or drink copious amounts of fluids, and never experienced hyperthermia or hyponatremia. This case supports the idea that the manner in which MDMA is used poses the greatest danger to the patient.

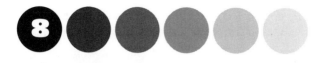

MENTAL HEALTH PROBLEMS ASSOCIATED WITH MDMA USE

Karl L. R. Jansen, M.D., Ph.D.

Like other mind-altering drugs, MDMA was perceived as one with few adverse effects when it was first introduced. However, as its use spread from psychotherapy into the general community, it became linked with a variety of mental health problems. When MDMA was used as an aid to psychotherapy in the late 1970s, therapists characterized the effects as feelings of empathic understanding for others and a release of emotions. Since then, however, there have been reports of confusion, anxiety, amnesia, panic attacks, depression, mania (excessive excitation), suicide, insomnia, nightmares, depersonalization (feeling unreal), derealization (feeling that the surroundings are unreal), hallucinations, flashbacks, post-traumatic stress disorder (PTSD), paranoia and other persistent false beliefs, other types of psychosis, automatic or repetitive behavior, dissociative disorders, irritability and aggression with mood swings, tolerance, dependence, and increased risk of problems with other drugs (McCann et al. 1996; Jansen 1997; Spatt et al. 1997).

The reader may have noted that this is a remarkably long, diverse, and nonspecific list. When widespread consumption of a drug results in nonspecific problems embracing a large slice of general psychiatric complaints, as has happened with MDMA, we may be recording, to some extent, the mental disorders that usually exist in the general population. Some of these problems have been attributed wrongly to consumption of the drug, and some, of course, have been quite correctly ascribed to drug use. The more mental health problems are attributed to use of a drug, and the more the sample size grows to reflect the general population, the more wary we should be of false assumptions about cause and effect. The association may be entirely coincidental. Some of these reports have more to do with the psychological characteristics of the person reporting them than with any particular effect of the drug upon the mind or the brain.

Animal studies have shown that taking large quantities of MDMA can result in persistently low serotonin levels. Attempts to explain the adverse effects linked with MDMA use in terms of neurochemical changes, however, ignore the role of psychological changes due to the emotional effects of the drug. MDMA could upset the balance of the mind by releasing disturbing material from the unconscious. The release of such material can be useful in psychotherapy, but there may be some risk of accompanying neurotic symptoms, such as anxiety, insomnia, and nightmares. Psychological explanations may be highly relevant, since many of the adverse effects were reported after just one or two modest doses. In addition, some of these reports cite an entirely false attribution of symptoms to the drug. Widespread use eventually leads to a lack of connection, in some cases, between the dose size and frequency and the reporting of neurotic symptoms. For example, a typical case would be a person who takes half a pill of Ecstasy once and then reports two years of panic attacks, attributed to taking the pill (which, if it had been tested in a laboratory, may not even have contained a psychoactive dose of MDMA). With a primarily physical cause, one usually would expect to see at least some link between the development of symptoms and the dose size and frequency; that is, neurochemical factors may be responsible for midweek problems, such as low mood and irritability, following heavy weekend use.

The 1990s saw general recreational use of Ecstasy, resulting in reports of an apparent link between its ingestion and a diverse range of mental health problems (McGuire et al. 1994; Kemmerling et al. 1996). It was reported that large doses of MDMA repeatedly injected into animals lowered serotonin levels and damaged the nerve terminals from which serotonin is released. The relevance of these studies to the situation of humans taking one or two doses occasionally always has been doubtful, but persons taking large quantities for several days may be at risk. Because low serotonin levels have been linked to depression (Maes and Meltzer 1995) and anxiety (Lesch et al. 1992; van Praag 1994), it has been suggested that heavy users may be at increased risk of these disorders. Against this theory are the observations that a low serotonin level is linked with aggressive behavior (Cleare and Bond 1995; Mann 1995; Coccaro et al. 1997), and yet heavy Ecstasy users are believed to be less aggressive than average, rather than more aggressive (McCann et al. 1994).

Explanations for adverse reactions to Ecstasy thus have focused on possible brain chemical changes, often ignoring the fact that MDMA may release emotions that alter the psychodynamic balance of the mind. The psychodynamic model maintains that anxiety-provoking material unacceptable to the waking consciousness is repressed in the unconscious and that defenses are erected against it. Some types of psychotherapy may involve bringing such material to the surface so that it can be worked through and discharged. MDMA has been used in therapy to remove such defenses. What happens if defenses against disturbing material in the psyche are removed in a non-therapeutic context? The results will depend partly on the set and setting. While no eventual harm may result and the defenses may rebuild themselves as the drug wears off, it is also possible that some of the liberated material will not easily be repressed. There may be little chance of working through the material or containing it. For instance, if a person were to realize that she had been the victim of incest in childhood, it would be wholly traumatic to the psyche. Possible consequences might include the range of symptoms associated with the neuroses: anxiety, mood disorders, insomnia, nightmares, drug use in an effort to anesthetize the pain, and dissociative or conversion disorders (such as hysteria, where mental anxiety may be converted into a physical or psychological symptom).

The frequent lack of lasting changes in animal behavior (other than a behavioral tolerance to the drug) following long-term, high-dose injection of MDMA also indicates that an exclusive focus on neurochemistry to explain adverse effects probably is misguided. Many of the communications received from persons who have suffered mental health consequences linked with the use of Ecstasy describe ingestion of only a few doses. Where psychosis (delusions, hallucinations, disorganized speech) is concerned, it is more likely that neurochemical factors are important. The release of dopamine in a manner similar to amphetamine could lead to a link between long-term, high-dose Ecstasy use and the development of a brief paranoid psychotic illness, as sometimes can be seen with amphetamine itself. An excess of dopamine is thought to be involved in producing paranoid symptoms, as predicted by the dopamine hypothesis of schizophrenia.

Problems with Reports of MDMA Use and Consequences

The limited information we have is largely in the form of personal accounts, interviews, single case reports, and short case series in which there is no control group. (A control group is a group that is exactly the same as the MDMA group, except that the controls have not taken the drug. Matching the two groups on use of other drugs is particularly important.) There are several key issues to bear in mind when considering reports of this type.

Was the Drug Taken Actually MDMA?

Authors who allege that a person took MDMA should attempt to present toxicological proof to support this claim (tests of the tablets taken or at least a urine drug test). Pills may contain other drugs, such as MDE, MDA, MBDB (N-methyl-1-[3,4-methylenedioxyphenyl]-2-butanamine), 2CB (4-Bromo-2,5-Dimethoxyphenethylamine), ketamine, amphetamine, LSD, pseudoephedrine, or other pharmaceutical agents (Saunders 1995, 1997). Some pills contain no psychoactive substances at all. MDE has a shorter duration of action (two hours) and is more of a stimulant, with fewer emotional effects. MBDB is similar to MDMA, but the effects are described as less intense, with a greater cognitive component as distinct from an empathogenic/emotional one. MDA is more psychedelic (LSD-like) and is considered to be more toxic. 2CB is more psychedelic than MDMA but less so than MDA (Shulgin and Shulgin 1991). Amphetamine is a very common additive in Ecstasy tablets, and the links between amphetamine use and a brief period of paranoid psychosis are well established (Connell 1958; Bell 1965). MDE is very common in the United Kingdom. It may be closer to amphetamine in its effects than to MDMA and may possibly have a profile more similar to amphetamine in terms of adverse effects. Ketamine, another common additive, has been given to experimental subjects to produce model schizophrenia; it can be profoundly hallucinogenic (Jansen 1993, 2001). The current tendency in the United

Kingdom to attribute problems to MDMA rather than to other drugs is due to a psychology of negative-effects reporting, which is in the mind of the media-influenced doctor as well as the patient.

The Role of Polydrug Use

The majority of persons who take Ecstasy also use other drugs, a point that rarely is emphasized in reports attributing a disorder to MDMA use. In such reports use of other drugs often is dismissed in a few lines. The concurrent use of large amounts of cannabis, LSD, alcohol, cocaine, ketamine, or amphetamine, for example, often is pushed into the background. Many habitual weekend Ecstasy users are also daily or near daily users of cannabis. This is an important factor to bear in mind when conducting research in this area. The use of cannabis has been linked to relapse in schizophrenia (Mathers and Ghodse 1992). For example, there is a case report of persistent depersonalization syndrome after ingestion of only one Ecstasy pill (Wodarz and Boning 1993). It subsequently was pointed out that this patient had a history of daily alcohol and cannabis use, and serious doubt was cast upon the role of MDMA in the case (Gouzoulis 1994).

The Role of Set and Setting

"Set" refers to the personality, early imprinting and learning, past experiences (including previous drug experiences), temperament, mood, motivations, attitudes, and expectations of the drug user. "Setting" refers to the conditions of use, including the physical, social, and emotional environment and the behavior, understanding, and empathy of the other persons present. An optimistic set and pleasant setting are more likely to have a positive outcome, while a fearful set and unpleasant setting are more likely to have a negative outcome. In general, MDMA effects are less susceptible to the influence of set and setting than psychedelic drugs, such as LSD. Nevertheless, expectations do play an important part in all drug effects. There are many who want to dance simply because they have been conditioned to associate dancing with Ecstasy use, irrespective of the actual content of the pill they have swallowed. Expectations sometimes can lead to a negative outcome. For example, from a statistical perspective, serious physical effects from MDMA are rare. Nevertheless, a perception on the part of consumers that they are experiencing such effects has increased considerably in the wake of fear spread by the media. As a result, there has been an increase in the number of persons seeking treatment with the false belief that they are in physical extremis. The real diagnosis is likely to be panic.

The Probability of a Chance Association

Many of the published reports draw cause and effect conclusions that are not justified by the data; that is, they conclude that Ecstasy consumption caused—rather than was associated with—the symptoms. It is important to recognize that among the large group of drug users within the general population, a proportion will become mentally ill regardless of any supposed psychotomimetic properties of drugs (Poole and Brabbins 1996). Depression and anxiety are common conditions in the general population. It is a statistical certainty that many persons who take MDMA will show signs of depression regardless of drug use. The one-year incidence of major depression in the general population is 80–200 per 100,000 for men and 240–600 per 100,000 for women (Gelder et al. 1995). Anxiety, panic attacks, and all of the other symptoms associated with MDMA use also have an incidence, sometimes substantial, in the general population.

Poor Pre-morbid Adjustment

A poor adjustment to life circumstances is associated with an increased likelihood of drug use and a worse prognosis when major mental illness develops. Drug use may be a symptom of impending or actual mental illness as a result of "self-medication" of distress, or it may be due to impaired judgment. Preexisting mental illness and a family history of mental illness are common in persons who show signs of psychiatric illness in apparent association with drug use.

Preexisting Neurochemical, Genetic, and Personality Differences

Each year brings new reports linking inherited genes to behavioral patterns, including alcoholism and the need for high levels of stimulation (thrill seeking), both of which are thought to involve dopamine receptors. It is possible that persons who take drugs may have preexisting, genetically determined underfunctioning of serotonergic or dopaminergic systems, and this less than optimal functioning increases the likelihood of depression and anxiety and creates an inner drive to take drugs that provide relief. Thus, retrospective studies of the serotonin and dopamine systems in long-term users of high-dose Ecstasy, compared with non-using controls, may be seriously confounded by preexisting differences between the two groups (Jansen and Forrest 1999). This is a point that researchers taking cerebrospinal fluid measures of serotonin or its metabolites and performing *d*-fenfluramine challenge tests rarely take into account.

The Role of the Media

The media have played a highly significant role in the psychology of adverse drug effect reporting. There is the historical case of LSD, which has implications in terms of the situation with MDMA. In the 1960s and 1970s, an astonishing range of mental and physical disorders was attributed to LSD use. Psychiatrists were as influenced by the media's emphasis on LSD as the general public. Sometimes persons with schizophrenia, bipolar disorder (manic-depression), dissociative conversion disorders (such as hysteria), PTSD from a traumatic LSD experience, neuroses, and problems stemming from the use of other drugs were diagnosed as having conditions induced by LSD. Although LSD use is now at very high levels in the United Kingdom (10 to 12 percent among fifteen- to twenty-nine-year-olds) (McMiller and Plant 1996; President of the Council 1998), LSD is no longer generally accepted as a major cause of an extended list of complaints.

The 1990s saw a remarkable rerun in the United Kingdom of 1960s-style media hysteria based on Ecstasy. A single death, that of Leah Betts, who had drunk too much water after swallowing a pill, was front-page news for months. It rarely was pointed out that the actual risk of death from all causes in association with taking MDMA was in the region of 1 in 650,000 to 1 in 3 million risk exposures (Saunders 1995, 1997). In the same week that Leah Betts died, an average of a thousand people died from the health consequences of alcohol, and more than two thousand people died from the health consequences of cigarette smoking in the United Kingdom. In that week, alcohol played a part in at least 30 percent of reported motor vehicle deaths, suicides, and murders. There was a complete loss of perspective on the "killer drug Ecstasy." This type of media and political attention, regardless of the drug, almost always results in an increase in the number of persons seen at hospitals and by doctors in the belief that they are suffering serious effects from taking the drug in question.

What Are the Risks in Numerical Terms?

The actual risk that a serious psychiatric condition will develop following the use of MDMA is unknown, but it is likely to be relatively low once the person has recovered from the acute effects of the drug. The relative risk of any particular outcome should be determined by dividing the total number of outcomes that occur by the total number of doses consumed (risk exposures). Many case reports make no attempt to provide a statistical perspective, but it is necessary to tolerate this deficiency, because such estimates are very difficult to provide. We do not know how many cases of MDMA-associated psychiatric disturbance are treated by the medical community but never reported, and even more inaccessible are those that are never treated at all.

Another method of gaining perspective on the general importance of MDMA-induced mental disorder is to tour emergency rooms and the wards of psychiatric hospitals. This pragmatic investigation will produce at least one clear conclusion: the drug that is principally associated with suicidal depression, homicide, cognitive deficits, schizophrenic relapse, and psychosis in this society is alcohol, by an enormous margin. It is often several weeks before a single case associated with consumption of toxicologically proven MDMA is seen in these institutions, and even longer before a case is seen that does not involve other drugs and a personal or family history of preexisting psychiatric disorder. Nevertheless, one study of self-reported immediate and long-term effects (months or years after ingestion) in five hundred people cited high levels of reported adverse psychological effects (Cohen 1995). The immediate effects reported included paranoia in 20 percent, anxiety in 16 percent, and depression in 12 percent, while the long-term/ recurring effects included depersonalization in 54 percent, insomnia in 38 percent, depression in 38 percent, and flashbacks in 27 percent.

Adverse Psychological Effects of MDMA

As noted, current research evidence is sparse and retrospective (which means that research is carried out by looking into the past, after the side effect has appeared, rather than giving a person the drug to see what will happen). Research also generally is uncontrolled (there is no properly matched group of people for comparison who have not taken the drug) and typically lacks toxicological confirmation of the drugs taken. Moreover, we usually are not told what happened next—the course of the disorder and the long-term outcome for the person. Follow-up is very important in terms of excluding underlying schizophrenia or manic-depression, for example, each of which occurs in roughly 1 percent of the population worldwide. The studies rarely relate the person's mental state to the toxicological results (for example, the continuing presence of drug metabolites in the urine), and they depend heavily on single case studies. Nevertheless, they frequently conclude cause-and-effect relationships from what may be chance associations, athough it is also possible that there is a cause-and-effect relationship.

Psychosis

MDMA may produce a state of intoxication that mimics paranoid psychosis (Williams et al. 1993; Kemmerling et al. 1996), but this does not usually last for more than a few days and appears to be relatively rare. Although MDMA does not act like a hallucinogen in most people, it can cause hallucinations on occasion, especially at higher doses. I have seen a person in a state of toxic delirium after taking no more than 200 mg of pure MDMA and no other drugs. She was completely disoriented, had marked difficulty walking (she collapsed several times, injuring herself), and spent several hours trying to pick up nonexistent objects from the floor and talking to people who were not present. She had no history of psychosis, although her mother had suffered from depersonalization disorder (discussed later). She was an experienced MDMA user and had not had episodes of this nature previously. It is worth noting that this person had experienced depersonalization with a single dose of fluoxetine (Prozac).

Ecstasy use may sometimes alter the clinical picture of a preexisting psychosis. Some people with schizophrenia or manic-depression take Ecstasy;

the peak age of onset of schizophrenia is twenty to thirty, an age at which experimentation with drugs is relatively common. It is unknown whether MDMA can induce a relapse of preexisting schizophrenia or manic-depression, beyond the increased risk of relapse attached to any substantial emotional stressor. MDMA experiences are typically emotional events, and for this reason alone one would expect to see an association with increased risk of relapse in both these illnesses.

MDMA enhances dopamine availability, as do amphetamine and cocaine (Nichols and Oberlender 1989); as such, these drugs might be expected to raise the risk of psychotic illness if used over the long term. Some investigators report that they have repeatedly found clear links between the onset of psychotic symptoms and the use of Ecstasy (McGuire and Fahy 1991). This study is based on two cases, other substances were involved, and there was no toxicological confirmation of pill content. However, there are several other reports citing the same effects (Nuñez-Dominguiez, 1994; Schifano 1991; Winstock 1991; Williams et al. 1993; Schifano and Magni 1994). Taken together, the evidence is indicative of some risk of psychosis, though it is likely small, given the incidence with which it is reported compared with the prevalence of Ecstasy use.

Decisions about classifying MDMA effects should be made by those who can differentiate intoxication (that is, the effects that are experienced by most persons who have taken that drug) from psychosis and other adverse effects. If the majority of persons experience a particular effect when given MDMA, this effect is intoxication and not an adverse reaction. It is also important to look closely at psychotic beliefs (delusions) versus a person's beliefs; delusions must be incompatible with what is held to be true and possible in a person's particular culture or religious sect.

Can MDMA cause a true "drug-induced psychosis"? Poole and Brabbins (1996) have argued that this term should be restricted to psychotic symptoms arising in the context of drug intoxication but persisting beyond elimination of the drug and its metabolites from the body. Such a psychosis should recur only on reexposure to the drug and must have a different course and outcome from the major functional psychoses (such as schizophrenia and manic-depression). The authors go on to state that the common assumption that a specific, amphetamine-induced psychosis meeting these criteria has been established is in doubt. The most often cited study is that of Connell (1958); however a close reading of his work indicates that he did not describe such a syndrome. Connell showed that psychosis occurred only with intoxication, confirmed by measures of amphetamines in the blood. According to Connell, psychosis wholly due to amphetamines tends to resolve as the urine clears. Where the psychosis does not resolve, long-term follow-up studies usually find schizophrenia or manic-depression rather than a condition caused by amphetamine. However, Sato (1992) has reported that long-term use of methamphetamine produces a lasting vulnerability to paranoid delusional psychosis with schizophrenia-like hallucinations. It extends beyond the excretion of the drug in the urine, and reuse of methamphetamine and alcohol, along with stressors, leads to recurrence of psychosis with clinical features matching the previous methamphetamine-linked episodes.

I have reported the case of a person who injected 250 mg of MDMA powder intravenously up to four times daily for six months without experiencing any psychotic phenomena. This person became acutely psychotic on injecting dextroamphetamine (Jansen 1998). This finding suggests that we should be cautious in transferring generalizations based on amphetamine data to MDMA, tempting as this may be. It is also important to note that drug use may sometimes be a signal of psychological distress, rather than a cause of that distress. People may try to medicate themselves with drugs during the early stages of psychosis or a relapse, so the drug use is not causal but symptomatic. They also may be more likely to use drugs when they are ill, as a result of impaired judgment; this is seen commonly in certain phases of mania and in psychosis.

Anxiety Disorders and Panic Attacks

We are currently limited to a handful of case reports (Greer and Tolbert 1986; Whitaker-Azmitia and Aronson 1989; Pallanti and Mazzi 1992; Hermle et al. 1993; McGuire et al. 1994, Kemmerling et al. 1996; McCann et al. 1996; Jansen 1997) of adverse Ecstasy reactions categorized as anxiety disorders. The communications I have received from persons who have experienced adverse effects suggest that anxiety disorders are more common than depression as a long-term outcome. This is confirmed by the published reports in which forms of anxiety disorder currently appear to be more common than depression, once the acute effects of the drug have passed. It is possible that the serotonergic terminals involved in anxiety control are distinct from those principally involved in mood control and that MDMA may preferentially affect the former. It is more likely that the real explanation lies in the psychological effects of MDMA in terms of impairing psychic defenses against anxiety-generating material in the unconscious, as discussed previously.

Depersonalization and Derealization

Depersonalization refers to feeling that one is detached from the surroundings, not "real," unable to feel emotion, and separated from the world by a glass wall. Derealization is a state in which the environment appears unreal and meaningless; surrounding people may be described as cardboard-like. These phenomena have been reported in association with Ecstasy use (Wodarz and Boning 1993), but there are many other possible explanations, such as fatigue, depression, anxiety, schizophrenia, epilepsy, and, most likely of all, other drugs, such as ketamine, which is particularly associated with this effect (Jansen 2000, 2001). Depersonalization and derealization disorder also may occur spontaneously in the general population.

Depression and Mania

A brief period of low mood associated with coming down from the effects of the drug is common (Curran and Travill 1997). A longer lasting form of depression also has been reported (Benazzi and Mazzoli 1991; McCann et al. 1998). Drug use may be a form of self-medication of preexisting depression or latent depression, rather than a cause of depression. Depression may be predicted on theoretical grounds, owing to links between mood and serotonin. Animals with extensively damaged cortical serotonergic nerve terminals, however, generally show little difference in their behavior relative to control animals several weeks later. It is possible that this is because MDMA appears to alter one type of serotonin terminal preferentially (the "thin" fibers), and not those of a second system in the brain (the "fat" fibers) (Molliver et al. 1989). It may be this second system that controls mood, appetite, sleep, and sex drive. Chemical changes last for a week in this second system, but the structural changes typically are not seen (Molliver et al. 1989). This pattern matches the weekly cycle of findings in humans, where low mood may occur for a few days after Ecstasy use.

Cognitive Deficits (Impaired Memory, Attention, and Concentration)

Conducting good research into persisting (as distinct from acute) drug-induced problems with memory, attention, and concentration is very difficult. The number of alternative explanations for any problem is always high. For example, it is essential to control for the use of other drugs, particularly regular cannabis smoking and excessive alcohol consumption, and for the effects of any mood disorder that affects cognition. It is crucial that all claims of persistent problems be accompanied by evidence that the urine tests of the subjects are clear of all drugs and their metabolites, including cannabis metabolites, which can take at least four weeks to disappear from urine in habitual smokers. It is not possible to test for alcohol use in this way, but liver function tests should show normal results. Reported subtle memory deficits that are not accompanied by published urine test data may be due to cannabis. Krystal et al. (1992) noted subtle memory deficits in association with Ecstasy use, and there is a related report by Parrott et al. (1998). [See appendices for more details on memory studies.]

Persistent problems are those that are still present once all drug breakdown products (metabolites) have been completely eliminated from the body. The self-report of subjects regarding personal drug use is often inaccurate and is unacceptable for research of this nature. Despite the best of intentions, people often lapse and use various drugs while taking part in studies and then deny any use to the experimenters, because they do not wish to disappoint them or be excluded from the study. It is not enough for authors to say that subjects were asked to abstain from drugs for several weeks. Nor is it enough to say that urine tests were carried out. The actual results of the drug tests must be published, along with the rest of the report.

When I was studying long-term users of high-dose Ecstasy, many of the urine tests were positive for cannabis. I recall carrying out a six-hour neuroendocrine test at the laboratory one Saturday morning. I left the room for a few minutes; on my return, I found that both subjects had risen from their beds—where they were supposed to be lying still—and were leaning out the window smoking cannabis. It seemed better science, in the end, not to publish these test results, owing to the extent of the uncontrolled variables and contamination of the data from various sources.

It is also important to eliminate the possible effects of depression, anxiety, and other mental health problems on testing cognition. It is well recognized that depression and anxiety impair memory, attention, and concentration. Where investigators have not excluded these factors, they may contribute significantly to the results of a study.

If subjects have been told to abstain from all drugs before cognitive testing takes place, a withdrawal syndrome may result (going "cold turkey"), which could confound tests conducted during this withdrawal period. For example, even stopping regular coffee intake can result in headaches, fatigue, and impaired function. There is some controversy concerning the effect of abstaining from long-term daily cannabis use. Irritation and anxiety are sometimes noted.

It is essential to have a control group that is a genuine match for the subject group. It is particularly important to match carefully for the use of other drugs. In many drug studies, there is a subtle bias for the control group to have used fewer drugs and to function at a higher level than the subjects.

The Pandora's Box Syndrome

Persons who have taken large quantities of such drugs as LSD, MDMA, and ketamine for a prolonged period may show signs of a mental state that involves a high level of internal mental imagery but no perceptual disorder (Jansen 2000, 2001). It is as if perforations have been made in the defenses that usually separate conscious from unconscious processes, with material percolating through the conscious mind where it would not normally be found. I have named this syndrome after the legend of Pandora's box: once opened, it proved impossible to push back in everything that flew out. The condition is not serious. It does not prevent the afflicted person from going to work or going about the normal business of life. Attention and concentration are impaired, however, and this may lead to an apparently poor memory due to failure to attend to new information. The person may be said to have lost their edge or lack focus.

Flashbacks and Post-traumatic Stress Disorder

Ecstasy users have described flashbacks (Creighton et al. 1991; McGuire and Fahy 1992). The term "flashbacks" is used widely but rarely defined. Researchers who use this term should define exactly what they mean. The term commonly refers to episodes of a few seconds' duration in which the person reexperiences some of the subjective effects of taking the drug in question, after an intervening period of normality. This is clearly very different from the media-generated impression that a flashback is a complete, unprovoked reliving of the full drug experience. The term flashback covers a potentially wide range of possibilities and should be subdivided into categories. A persistent perceptual disorder has not yet been described in the literature in connection with MDMA, as opposed to LSD.

We can learn more about drug-related flashbacks by considering another condition in which flashbacks occur: PTSD. The Tenth International Classification of Diseases (ICD-10) (World Health Organization 1992) defines PTSD as a delayed and/or protracted response to a stressful event of an exceptionally threatening or catastrophic nature, which is likely to cause distress in almost anyone. A small number of MDMA experiences may be very stressful and perceived as catastrophic. Predisposing factors, such as personality problems or a history of neurosis, may make the development of PTSD more likely or aggravate its course, but they are neither necessary nor sufficient to explain it.

ICD-10 describes the typical symptoms of PTSD as including episodes of repeated reliving of the trauma in the form of intrusive memories (flashbacks) or dreams. Flashbacks are more likely after very traumatic drug experiences. In a case series of Ecstasy-associated flashbacks, one of the three cases cited by Creighton et al. (1991) described a woman who had been abducted and raped while under the influence of Ecstasy. The other two cases involved heavy daily cannabis users with LSD-like features, which Creighton suggests may have been due to such substances in the pills. This underscores the importance of considering polysubstance use and conducting drug analysis.

It is unlikely, but not impossible, that flashbacks are due to persisting changes in the brain. There is a view that some forms of PTSD lead to underlying brain changes, albeit of a resolving nature (Stein et al. 1997). It may be the extreme stress that produces this change rather than a neurochemical effect specific to the drug, since a wide array of drugs with quite different mechanisms of action in the brain (for example, LSD and ketamine) also have been linked to flashbacks. There is no evidence to support the notion that lingering drug quantities in the brain cause flashbacks.

Other drug-related flashbacks may be a form of psychological conversion disorder (formerly known as hysteria), where anxiety with a neurotic basis is "converted" into psychological symptoms, just as it may be converted into physical symptoms, such as a "paralyzed" arm. It is worth noting that persons who have never taken any illicit drugs but who are prone to severe anxiety and panic attacks may describe visual and other phenomena that bear some resemblance to the flashbacks described by some drug users.

Sleep Disturbance

Insomnia that persists for several days after taking Ecstasy is relatively common, but in a few cases it has lasted for months, with excessive dreaming and sometimes nightmares (McCann and Ricaurte, 1991a). A minor but persistent reduction in the second stage of sleep has been verified in a sleep laboratory, although the subjects in this investigation were not considered to be suffering from sleep disorders or to be in distress (Allen et al. 1993).

Ecstasy—A Stepping-Stone to Other Drugs?

The use of Ecstasy may be associated with the use of other drugs for a variety of purposes, particularly to overcome the stimulant effects of Ecstasy and allow for sleep (to "come down" from the drug) or to prolong and strengthen the stimulant effects and avoid sleep. For the first purpose, benzodiazepines (minor tranquilizers, such as diazepam which is also known as Valium), alcohol, and cannabis often are used. There also has been a rapid rise in smoking heroin for this purpose in the United Kingdom, possibly owing to a massive increase in supply. For the second purpose, amphetamines and cocaine are used. There is a link between taking Ecstasy and a desire to smoke cigarettes excessively, which may be related to the effect of these drugs upon dopamine pleasure systems in the brain.

Tolerance and Dependence

The use of almost any substance can become compulsive and excessive in some people, and there are certainly a few people who have taken Ecstasy on a daily basis, regardless of tolerance, for prolonged periods (McGuire and

Fahy 1991; Jansen 1998). I have described the case of a person who injected 250 mg of MDMA powder intravenously, up to four times a day for six months. Eventually, 250 mg taken orally had almost no effect at all (Jansen 1998). It is far more common, however, for habitual and troubling Ecstasy use to involve consumption of 20–40 pills of the drug in binges lasting from Thursday night until Monday morning, with four recovery days between. If people have had a reasonable amount of sleep, not consumed large quantities of other drugs, and not gone "clubbing," many feel elevated in mood the day after taking Ecstasy. By the third day, however, low mood, which may be quite severe, and irritability sometimes are seen. This continues into the fourth day, with relative recovery of mood on the fifth day. The cycle often repeats itself, with Ecstasy use on the fifth, sixth, and seventh days and another round of recovery. Thus, some persons may be said to be affected continually by the drug, even if they take it only on weekends.

The so-called love effect fades with repeated use, and the subsequent effects may become more amphetamine-like (Peroutka 1990). This may explain in part some of the escalation in dose levels seen in recent years: some users are vainly attempting to recover the mental state that they experienced initially, now impossible owing to neurochemical and psychological changes in the brain and mind resulting from repeated use. There are other possible reasons for escalating dose levels, among them, the substantial drop in price of the drug and the fact that underfunctioning of serotonergic nerve terminals can result in increased use of amphetamine-like substances for pharmacological reasons, as has been found in animal studies (Lyness et al. 1981).

It is not necessary to take a drug every day to cause a dependency syndrome, nor is physical withdrawal essential. The possibility that MDMA is associated with tolerance, psychological dependence, and withdrawal syndromes will surprise those Apollonian users who take the drug only occasionally in controlled circumstances (as distinct from the Dionysian, three-day party, "stacking" group). In this context it is valuable to recall the history of amphetamine itself. In the late 1930s, the American Medical Association approved the use of amphetamine for a wide range of disorders, and the pharmaceutical company Smith, Kline and French reassured physicians that no serious reactions had been found. Between 1932 and 1946, the pharmaceutical industry found thirty-nine licensed uses for amphetamine, including the treatment of schizophrenia and tobacco smoking [for review, see Lukas 1985]. It was not until the late 1960s, after numerous case reports, that it was officially accepted that amphetamines were addictive and that amphetamine-associated paranoid psychosis was relatively common among heavy users.

The extreme fatigue, excessive sleeping, anxiety, insomnia, and depression that follow cessation of long-term amphetamine use are regarded as a bona fide withdrawal syndrome. It has not yet become apparent which aspects of this clinical picture may be shared by long-term users of high-dose Ecstasy. MDMA has an effect on dopaminergic systems that is similar to that of stimulants associated with dependency, and it activates dopamine-based pleasure systems in a manner resembling amphetamine and cocaine (Nichols and Oberlender 1989).

It was once believed that MDMA would be free of any dependency risk because of the rapid loss of the empathogenic effect with repeated use (Peroutka 1990). While loss of this effect may lead to declining use in an older group of people who take MDMA for its empathogenic properties, younger users in the dance culture may come to appreciate the more amphetamine-like qualities and have different expectations. This group rarely takes pure compounds and may have been conditioned from the outset to expect amphetamine-like effects from a pill, since many pills are, in fact, amphetamine or MDE, rather than MDMA [for review, see Saunders 1995]. Because polydrug use is very common, many of those who party throughout the weekend deliberately take amphetamine and other drugs in addition to Ecstasy. This creates a milieu in which the particular effects that distinguish MDMA from other pleasurable stimulants are diminished.

A questionnaire administered to one hundred Ecstasy users in Sydney, Australia, found that 2 percent of the sample considered themselves to be dependent (Solowij et al. 1992). The value of such a self-report is questionable, however. Forty-seven percent of respondents in the study expressed the belief that it was possible to become dependent on MDMA. The animal evidence suggests a dependency potential, and presumed changes in serotonergic nerve terminals do not result in reduced frequency of MDMA self-injecting behavior in monkeys (Lamb and Griffiths 1987). In fact, impaired serotonergic function has been linked to increased self-administration of amphetamine, because of a complex interaction between serotonergic systems and dopaminergic pleasure systems in the brain's pleasure centers (Lyness et al. 1981).

Treatment

Most Ecstasy-associated problems resolve over time without special treatment. Where outside help is sought, the approach should address biological, psychological, social, and spiritual issues. People should be encouraged to take responsibility for themselves, in tandem with professional assessment and advice. For problems that do not involve psychosis, drug-free treatments are a good long-term investment in terms of remaining well, avoiding side effects, and placing the locus of control inside the person rather than outside. It should be possible for most literate persons at least to buy a self-help book on overcoming anxiety, panic attacks, depression, and sleeping problems; there are many such books.

It is best to avoid automatically accepting the conclusions of the drug-using person or the family, who may be only too ready to make an attribution to drug use—vastly preferable to a diagnosis of schizophrenia or bipolar disorder, which suggests something more fundamental and potentially uncontrollable. It is also worth bearing in mind that people who show psychotic symptoms in the context of Ecstasy use may be more prone to schizophrenia and mania in any case. That is, they may have an inherent predisposition unmasked by the effects of the drug, or the drug may have precipitated a relapse of a preexisting condition. Most people can absorb substantial quantities of all types of drugs without stepping very far over the line between intoxication and psychosis. The reverse error is also possible: in an acutely intoxicated state, a misdiagnosis of schizophrenia or mania may result in inappropriate treatment with antipsychotic drugs and the risk of committal to a psychiatric hospital.

To Talk Down or to Medicate?

In an acute situation, while the person is still affected by the drug, there are three main options: doing nothing (which is the usual approach—people may recover while waiting to see a doctor), talking down, and medicating. It must be established that the person is physically safe and has not taken unknown quantities of sedating drugs, such as alcohol, GHB, opiates, or tranquilizers. If the person has taken these then psychological care must be secondary to physical concerns, which may involve monitoring and nursing in an appropriate care unit to ensure physical safety. Panic is the most likely diagnosis of most persons seen by health and emergency services. This condition can be treated by placing the affected person in a quiet room, with reassurance and, possibly, administration of lorazepam (Ativan, a fast-acting relative of diazepam) if the person has not already taken sedatives.

Because of the link between traumatic drug experiences and subsequent flashbacks and PTSD, the use of talking down (nonjudgmental verbal reassurance in a low-stimulation environment) requires serious reevaluation. If a person who has taken a psychedelic or dissociative drug is having a very unpleasant experience and has sought professional help, early consideration should be given to administration of lorazepam as an intramuscular injection to relieve anxiety, possibly with oral diazepam to follow. This will substantially lower the risk of subsequent PTSD and other anxiety-related conditions in a way that talking down does not.

Antipsychotic drugs, such as chlorpromazine (Thorazine) and haloperidol (Haldol), should not be used, regardless of agitation or psychosis. It is not widely appreciated that the antipsychotic effects of such drugs as haloperidol usually take several weeks to manifest. Antipsychotic drugs should also be avoided because their anticholinergic and numerous other side effects may be additive to those of MDMA and whatever else the person may have consumed. The increasing likelihood that several substances have been taken is another argument against the use of haloperidol. Haloperidol is also a cause of the rare neuroleptic malignant syndrome, which may be linked to the overheating syndromes associated with several Ecstasy-related deaths (Ames and Wirshing 1993).

Psychotherapy

For some conditions, counseling, psychotherapy, and cognitive/behavioral therapy is indicated. This can be considered for persistent effects once the acute situation has passed. Denial can be dealt with using facts from the person's life rather than research findings. The therapist might say, for example, "Let's examine the effect that taking ten Ecstasy pills every weekend is having on your studies . . . on your finances . . . on the way you feel by Wednesday afternoon . . . on your life in general now that you have been arrested and charged with intent to supply because you bought a big bag of pills to save money . . . on your increasing tendency to smoke heroin to come down." This approach is bound to be more effective than discussions about serotonergic nerve terminals. Where the symptoms have a strongly neurotic character, psychodynamic psychotherapy or formal psychoanalysis is worth considering. The approach involves a gradual exploration of the unconscious, and a working through of difficult psychic material. The focus is not usually on the drug-taking behavior itself.

Medication

It is possible that the person who abuses Ecstasy may be self-medicating an underlying disorder that should be treated separately, such as depression, anxiety disorder, personality disorder, or incipient psychosis. If such a condition is identified or suspected, treatment should be aimed at it. Antidepressants, such as fluoxetine (Prozac) and paroxetine (Paxil), can be useful treatments for depression, anxiety, panic attacks, and sleep disorders (Windhaber et al. 1998). As noted earlier, however, after the acute crisis has passed, it is usually best to try nondrug approaches first, including emphasizing good sleep hygiene, avoiding caffeine, and eating and exercising properly. Benzodiazepines can be used for a short period to treat panic attacks and severe anxiety if nondrug methods fail to bring results, but these drugs are potentially addictive and are best not used for more than a few weeks at a time.

If it becomes clear over the course of time that psychotic symptoms fail to resolve after several drug-free days, an antipsychotic drug is required; the drug of choice is olanzepine (Zyprexa), which is sedating and can be taken once only, at night. When making an assessment, however, it is important to bear in mind that a drug-induced psychosis should not be diagnosed simply because a patient with psychosis has been using drugs. Incorrect attribution of psychotic symptoms to the use of Ecstasy may have the effect of withholding proper care and education about their illness from persons with schizophrenia or manic-depression. These patients are not prescribed long-term medications to prevent relapses and do not avail themselves adequately of services; moreover, their families are not appropriately educated. The result is a very high relapse rate. It is thus important to take a careful history, speak with relatives, and avoid jumping to hasty conclusions. There may be an underlying psychiatric disorder that is associated with drug use by chance. A urine drug screen is essential when psychotic symptoms are seen in association with drug use. It is also important to note that the overwhelming majority of Ecstasy users are polydrug consumers, and care must be taken not to attribute symptoms to the wrong drug.

Meditation, Relaxation, Martial Arts, and Physical Exercise

Relaxation exercises may be useful for persons with anxiety problems. Tapes are widely available. Meditation involves learning to attend to a single stimulus without allowing the attention to wander. This is useful for a range of disorders, particularly Pandora's Box Syndrome. Martial arts are also useful for strengthening the "signal-over-noise" ratio and improving attention and concentration. They are demanding and require a change of lifestyle from weekend-long raving. They can also meet high stimulus needs, provide an endorphin rush, and encourage self-control. Most forms of physical exercise and gym work can be valuable for persons who wish to stop the regular use of psychostimulants.

Antioxidants and Food Supplements: Tryptophan and Tyrosine

Some Ecstasy users also take high doses of antioxidants, such as vitamin C and vitamin E. There is evidence that free radicals may play a part in neurotoxicity [see "Does MDMA Cause Brain Damage?"]. The supplements tyrosine and tryptophan may elevate levels of serotonin, but the use of tryptophan is severely restricted in some countries. Bananas, chocolate, milk, and turkey are rich sources of tryptophan, and it is a valid suggestion that persons taking MDMA may profit from eating these foods. It is also possible to obtain a product called "5-HTP serotonic." 5-HT is another term for serotonin, and 5-HTP is actually one step closer than tryptophan to serotonin in the biochemical pathway that forms serotonin.

Conclusions

The true levels of serious adverse psychological effects linked to taking Ecstasy are unknown. Many of the disorders that have been reported may be related to both psychological and neurochemical events. The cause-and-effect conclusions drawn by single case studies must be viewed with caution, but this does not mean that these studies should be disregarded. There is still a widespread tendency to diagnose persons as suffering from MDMA or psychedelic-induced psychosis when they are suffering from such conditions as schizophrenia, manic-depression, borderline personality disorder, or problems related to the use of different drugs, such as alcohol or methamphetamine. This tendency is strengthened by the natural inclination on the part of sufferers to seek an explanation external to themselves, over which they can have some control.

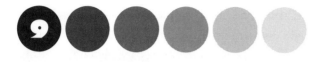

DOES MDMA CAUSE BRAIN DAMAGE?

Matthew Baggott
and John Mendelson, M.D.

Introduction

The acute toxic effects of MDMA are well documented by hundreds of case reports of adverse events reported among illicit users of the drug. Considering how many people use Ecstasy, serious acute adverse events seem rare. MDMA, in general, appears to be similar to such psychostimulants as methamphetamine (speed) with respect to the risks of acute toxicity. With trained personnel, properly screened volunteers, and established protocols for monitoring and treating adverse events, these acute risks seem to be modest and do not present a strong argument against carefully conducted clinical research with MDMA.

On the other hand, the risks associated with possible long-term brain damage are more difficult to assess. Numerous studies in animals have shown that MDMA can produce long-lasting declines in brain functions involving the neurotransmitter serotonin. The meaning of these changes is unclear. Lasting behavioral changes in MDMA-exposed animals seldom have been detected and are fairly subtle when they are found. Though limited in scope, studies of Ecstasy users suggest a strong probability that similar serotonergic changes occur in many humans. Studies comparing Ecstasy users and nonusers support an association between modestly lowered scores on tests of mental abilities (cognitive performance tests), and Ecstasy use, but clinically significant performance impairments have not been detected. In other words, there is no increased incidence of clinical complaints or findings.

The modest findings of MDMA neurotoxicity in certain behavioral studies have led some people to dismiss concerns about MDMA neurotoxicity as politically motivated and alarmist. It is commonly pointed out that even though fenfluramine and methamphetamine generate similar changes, their status as prescription medications was not affected by this finding. It is reasonable to note, however, that the truly long-term effects of MDMA exposure are unknown. In fifteen years of research on MDMA neurotoxicity, no published studies have investigated whether MDMA exposure can cause significant toxicity that becomes apparent only with aging. This fact must be taken into account when considering the risks and benefits of possible clinical studies. Perhaps the single most worrisome issue surrounding MDMA neurotoxicity is that there may be significant impairment associated with serotonergic changes that is undetected at present. Although millions of people have taken millions of doses of Ecstasy, controlled studies of users have not been sufficiently large to detect any but the most common long-term adverse effects. Possible adverse effects, such as a higher than normal incidence of affective disorders, like depression, may have gone unnoticed.

Because so little is known about the possible long-term clinical implications of MDMA neurotoxicity, we believe that it is important to minimize the risks in research volunteers. It is hoped that the information presented here will contribute to assessments of, and perhaps reductions in, the risks associated with MDMA use. In this chapter we discuss the nature and meaning of MDMA-induced serotonergic changes, their possible mechanisms of action, factors influencing the severity of these changes (such as dose, route of administration, species and animal strain, and environment), and the time course of the changes and recovery from them. Later in the chapter we focus on the implications of long-term MDMA-induced serotonergic changes in terms of the behavioral and functional effects of these changes in animals. We also discuss studies comparing Ecstasy users to nonusers in terms of personality, cognitive, and functional assessments, and we review available data from clinical studies in which MDMA was administered and potential strategies for limiting risk to human volunteers.

Limitations of space prevent a full discussion of every important article about and aspect of this complex topic. For a broader sense of the range of views on MDMA neurotoxicity, the reader is advised to consult other review articles (McKenna and Peroutka 1990; Steele et al. 1994; Green et al. 1995; Seiden and Sabol 1996; Sprague et al. 1998; Hegadoren et al. 1999; Boot et al. 2000; Burgess et al. 2000; Morgan 2000; O'Callaghan and Miller 2001). There is also an entire issue of the journal *Neuropsychobiology* (vol. 42, 2000) dedicated to MDMA neurotoxicity.

Long-Term Serotonergic Changes with MDMA

Before discussing MDMA-induced changes and their meaning, it is necessary to define a few terms. In this chapter, drug doses and dosing patterns used in research that produce long-term serotonergic changes are referred to as "neurotoxic regimens." Neurotoxic regimens often consist of four to eight injections of MDMA given over the course of one to four days; however, a single injection of MDMA also can give rise to these changes. In this chapter, any changes noted at seven or more days after drug administration is considered "long-term." Many studies examining the brains of animals after longer time periods (often at two, four, or eight weeks) have established that the MDMA-induced changes at seven days are primarily long-term in nature.

The term "neurotoxicity" is more difficult to define. Although no universal definition exists, most definitions are broad enough to encompass both short-term alcohol-induced headaches and the permanent nerve cell damage caused by the drug MPTP. A more useful approach to the question of whether MDMA is neurotoxic is to describe the nature and mechanisms of action of the long-term changes it can cause. Using this approach, it becomes evident that some neurotoxic MDMA regimens cause both changes in the serotonin-containing nerve cells and acute damage to the brain by free radicals (reactive chemicals that can damage cells) and thereby precipitate loss of nerve cell axons. This suggests that MDMA neurotoxicity is a type of drug-induced damage, even though the consequences of this damage are unknown.

MDMA produces long-lasting changes to the serotonergic system at some doses. These long-term changes include decreases in brain concentrations of the neurotransmitter serotonin (5-HT) and its metabolite, or breakdown product, 5-hydroxyindoleacetic acid (5-HIAA). Levels of tryptophan hydroxylase (TPH), the enzyme that begins the synthesis of 5-HT within the serotonergic nerve cell, are lowered by MDMA. There are also fewer serotonin reuptake transporters (SERT), proteins on the membrane of serotonergic neurons that recycle released 5-HT by pulling it back into the cell. Most studies suggest that MDMA primarily causes long-term changes in serotonergic axons that have their cell bodies in an area of the brain stem called the dorsal raphe nucleus.

Long-lasting decreases in these serotonergic markers suggest either that serotonergic axons are permanently lost, or that some type of "down-regulation" has occurred, meaning that the nerve cell is making and maintaining fewer of the markers. The question of whether MDMA is truly neurotoxic stems from this issue. Down-regulation suggests an active adaptation to drug effects, whereas axonal loss indicates that true damage may have occurred. Determining which really happens can be difficult. SERT density may change in response to drugs, but this has been difficult to establish (Ramamoorthy et al. 1998; Le Poul et al. 2000). Similarly, diet and other factors can influence 5-HT levels. Because MDMA has been shown to inactivate the enzyme TPH rapidly, diminished 5-HT levels would be expected until TPH activity returns to normal. Thus, decreased 5-HT synthesis and subsequent SERT down-regulation at first appear to be a plausible explanation for MDMA-induced serotonergic changes. By examining the structure of serotonergic axons in MDMA-exposed animals, however, it is clear that MDMA also can cause axonal loss.

Serotonergic Changes Accompanied by Structural Changes to Axons
An important approach to understanding MDMA-induced serotonergic changes involves staining brain slices from MDMA-exposed animals. By attaching a marker to the 5-HT molecule through a process called immunocytochemistry, 5-HT is stained, allowing serotonergic axons and terminals to be seen under a microscope. This technique shows irregular swelling and fragmentation of fine serotonergic axons shortly after a neurotoxic regimen of MDMA or MDA (Kalia et al. 2000; O'Hearn et al. 1988; Scallet et al. 1988). Later measurements, taken two or four weeks after neurotoxic MDMA

regimens, also show a persistent decrease in stained axons (O'Hearn et al. 1988; Scallet et al. 1988; Slikker et al. 1988; Wilson et al. 1989). The initial swelling suggests some type of axonal damage, while the later decrease in stained axons indicates axon loss. Some researchers have argued, however, that immunocytochemistry cannot determine whether measured differences in 5-HT are accompanied by changes in the axons themselves. Because of this limitation, it is necessary to confirm the apparent loss of axons using techniques that do not rely on serotonergic markers.

Transport of materials within axons is crucial for maintaining cell structure and function. Lasting reductions in axonal transport suggest a drastic impairment of axonal functioning and, more likely, loss of axons. One can assess axonal transport by measuring the movement of compounds between brain regions that serotonergic axons should connect. For example, if injected into the cortex (the outer layer of the brain) the fluorescent dye Fluoro-Gold should be transported along serotonergic axons into cell bodies in the brain stem. Axonal transport studies have been carried out after neurotoxic regimens of MDMA (Ricaurte et al. 2000) and parachloroamphetamine (Fritschy et al. 1988; Haring et al.1992). The results suggest that a loss of axons takes place after at least some neurotoxic regimens of MDMA and related drugs.

Another method of assessing loss of nerve terminals involves measuring the vesicular monoamine transporter type II (VMAT2). This is a protein on the storage compartments, or "vesicles," inside the nerve's axon terminals. Because the amount of VMAT2 does not appear to be adjusted in response to drug exposure (Vander Borght et al. 1995), it is sometimes used as an indirect measure of nerve terminals in research on such neurodegenerative disorders as Parkinson's disease. In other words, diminished levels of VMAT2 would suggest that nerve terminals and axons have been lost. Neurotoxic regimens of MDMA (Ricaurte et al. 2000) or methamphetamine (Frey et al. 1997) have been shown to decrease VMAT2. Therefore, at least some neurotoxic regimens of MDMA are associated with structural changes to cells.

These data consistently indicate that MDMA can cause serotonergic axons to degenerate and that this explains at least some of the MDMA-induced decline in serotonergic markers. Further evidence of axonal degeneration comes from studies in which recovery from MDMA neurotoxicity is associated with apparent sprouting and regrowth of axons (discussed in more detail later herein). Why, then, has MDMA neurotoxicity been the subject of controversy? One reason is that attempts to measure MDMA-induced cell damage itself yield ambiguous results.

Serotonergic and Axonal Changes: Evidence of Damage?

In general, neural cell damage can be detected by two techniques: silver staining and measuring the expression of glial fibrillary acidic protein (GFAP). Not all neurotoxic regimens using MDMA show increased silver staining or GFAP expression. These techniques seem to detect MDMA-induced alterations only at doses higher than those needed to affect serotonergic function (Commins et al. 1987; O'Callaghan and Miller 1993). Furthermore, the MDMA-induced cell damage detected by silver staining appears to occur in non-serotonergic cells (Commins et al. 1987; Jensen et al. 1993) as well as in what are likely serotonergic axons (Scallet et al. 1988). These inconsistencies are difficult to interpret. Some researchers believe that they are evidence that MDMA-induced serotonergic changes result from down-regulation of the serotonergic system rather than damage (e.g., O'Callaghan and Miller 2001). Others have argued that the techniques for measuring cell damage are simply insensitive to selective serotonergic damage (Axt et al. 1994; Bendotti et al. 1994; Wilson and Molliver 1994).

Because studies of axonal transport and VMAT2 changes have provided strong evidence of MDMA-induced axonal damage, it appears that serotonergic down-regulation cannot explain in full the long-term effects of MDMA. Structural changes to serotonergic axons also must be explained. Although we are not aware that this hypothesis has been advanced, one could argue that loss of axons represents a non-neurotoxic form of neuroplasticity or benign change in the nerve cell in response to drugs. Non-neurotoxic (though not necessarily beneficial) morphologic changes can occur in the brain as the result of alterations in serotonin levels (reviewed in Azmitia 1999). It appears to be more likely, however, that these changes are, in fact, the result of damage, specifically damage involving oxidative stress.

The Role of Oxidative Stress in MDMA Neurotoxicity

Free radicals are highly reactive chemicals that contain one or more unpaired electrons. Free radicals can damage neural molecules through reactions called reduction and oxidation and thereby alter the ability of these molecules to carry out their normal cellular function. Neurotoxic regimens of MDMA increase oxidative stress in the brain. In this chapter, the term "oxidative stress" is used to refer to both the increase in reactive chemicals, including free radicals, and the burden they place on cellular functioning.

MDMA-induced oxidative stress has been shown in two ways. First, researchers have examined the brains of MDMA-treated animals for thiobarbituric acid–reacting substances (Sprague and Nichols 1995b; Colado et al. 1997a; Jayanthi et al. 1999). Increases in these substances suggest that neural lipids, or fat molecules in the brain cells, have been oxidized. Second, researchers have perfused the brains of live animals with either salicylate or d-phenylalanine. These substances react with hydroxyl radicals to form 2,3-dihydroxybenzoic acid and d-tyrosine, respectively. By measuring formation of these compounds, researchers have shown that neurotoxic MDMA regimens increase the amount of extracellular hydroxyl radicals of the striatum (Shankaran et al. 1999a,b) and hippocampus (Colado et al. 1997b, 1999b), two areas of the brain where serotonergic neurotoxicity occurs.

There is strong evidence that oxidative stress plays a part in MDMA neurotoxicity. Antioxidants are substances that inactivate free radicals; the antioxidants ascorbate and cysteine each reduce MDMA neurotoxicity in rats without altering levels of MDMA or MDMA-stimulated dopamine release, which suggests that the nontoxic effects of MDMA are not being altered by the addition of antioxidants (Schmidt and Kehne 1990; Gudelsky 1996). The free radical scavenger N-tert-butyl-alpha-phenylnitrone decreases both MDMA-induced hydroxyl formation and MDMA neurotoxicity in rats; the latter effect, however, may be due in part to an attenuation of MDMA-induced high body temperature, or hyperthermia (Che et al. 1995; Colado et al. 1998; Colado and Green. 1995; Yeh 1999). Pretreatment with the antioxidant alpha-lipoic acid blocks both MDMA-induced serotonergic neurotoxicity and GFAP expression in the rat hippocampus without altering MDMA-induced hyperthermia (Aguirre et al. 1999). Mice that have been genetically altered to have large amounts of the human antioxidant enzyme copper/zinc superoxide dismutase are protected from MDMA-induced dopamine depletions, probably because of the enhanced trapping of superoxide radicals (Cadet et al. 1994; Cadet et al. 1995; Jayanthi et al. 1999). At the same time, these genetically modified mice are protected from the acute inactivation of antioxidant enzymes and free radical changes seen in normal mice after a neurotoxic MDMA regimen (Jayanthi et al. 1999).

Early evidence that MDMA causes significant oxidative stress came from Stone and colleagues (1989a), who reactivated TPH, which had been inactivated in rats at three hours after administration of high-dose MDMA, by using sulfhydryl-reducing conditions. This experiment showed that acute inactivation of TPH by MDMA was due to intracellular oxidative stress. Intracellular oxidative stress appears to be an effect of MDMA that requires sustained brain concentrations of MDMA (or a centrally formed metabolite). While a single injection of MDMA into the brain had no effect on TPH activity, slow infusion of 1 mg/kg MDMA into the brain over one hour produced enough oxidative stress to reduce TPH activity immediately (Schmidt and Taylor 1988). The immediate decline in TPH activity is an early effect of MDMA and can be seen fifteen minutes after administration (Stone et al. 1989b). TPH inactivation also can be produced by non-neurotoxic MDMA doses (Schmidt and Taylor 1988; Stone et al. 1989a,b). It therefore appears that MDMA rapidly induces oxidative stress but only produces neurotoxicity when the brain's free radical scavenging systems become overwhelmed.

In summary, MDMA neurotoxicity involves an initial period of oxidative damage, when an increase in free radicals damages neural lipids and inactivates enzymes. This damage seems to be part of the sequence of events causing serotonergic neurotoxicity, since treatments that curb MDMA-induced oxidative stress also lessen the long-term serotonergic changes (Aguirre et al. 1999). While MDMA can cause loss of axons, a certain degree of serotonergic downregulation cannot be ruled out. Research on methamphetamine-induced dopaminergic neurotoxicity has led some researchers to conclude that long-term dopaminergic changes can take place without significant axonal loss (Wilson et al. 1996; Harvey et al. 2000). Whether this is also the case with MDMA is unknown. For now, it seems reasonable to conclude that long-term serotonergic alterations after MDMA exposure indicate that a degree of damage has occurred, while remembering that one is also measuring the response of the serotonergic system to short-term drug effects and loss of axons.

Proposed Sources of Oxidative Stress

Several possible sources of neurotoxic oxidative stress have been proposed. First, the sustained effects of MDMA may deplete neuronal energy sources and/or impair energy metabolism within the neuron (Huether et al. 1997). Second, both MDMA and dopamine can be metabolized to highly reactive quinone-like molecules. Quinones are molecules that are often very reactive, can form free radicals, and are thus potentially damaging to neural molecules. There is not yet conclusive evidence to implicate any of these possible causes, and it is possible that some combination of mechanisms of action is at work. The possible roles of energy exhaustion or impairment, MDMA metabolites, and dopamine metabolites are discussed later herein. It also has been proposed that 5-HT metabolites or increased levels of intracellular calcium, nitric oxide, or glutamate (all potential sources of cell damage in other instances) contribute to MDMA neurotoxicity, but current evidence provides little support for these theories.

Cellular energy exhaustion or impairment may cause MDMA neurotoxicity. Normal activity of the neuron causes a certain degree of oxidative stress. A sustained increase in neuronal activity therefore would be expected to magnify oxidative stress. More important, increased neuronal activity is accompanied by increased energy consumption that could eventually lead to depletion of neuronal energy sources. This sequence of events can impair the energy-requiring mechanisms that maintain and repair neurons. Furthermore, the most important source of energy in each cell, the mitochondria, can be impaired by oxidative stress (Crompton et al. 1999). Mitochondria produce adenosine triphosphate (ATP), the source of energy for most cellular processes. Insufficient ATP will lead to cell damage or death.

Whether energy exhaustion or impairment actually plays a role in MDMA neurotoxicity is not yet clear. MDMA does enhance the activity of the enzyme glycogen phosphorylase (Poblete and Azmitia 1995), which suggests that MDMA could reduce glial stores of glycogen, an important source of energy in the brain. MDMA-induced alterations in mitochondrial functioning have been reported (Burrows et al. 2000), but it is not yet clear if these alterations are sufficient to impair mitochondria and damage cells. One study found that ATP levels were unaltered up to three hours after MDMA administration (Hervias et al. 2000), but since ATP levels at later times were not examined, it remains possible that they diminish over time.

MDMA breakdown products, or metabolites, also may play a role in MDMA neurotoxicity, but it is difficult to investigate this possible role. Hypothetically, a given metabolite may be toxic only in the presence of MDMA, when there are high concentrations of the metabolite in the brain for several hours, or in the context of certain acute effects of MDMA. In such situations, administering the toxic metabolite on its own would not necessarily lead to toxicity. Thus, it is hard to interpret the results of many studies in which an MDMA metabolite was administered and no evidence of neurotoxicity was found (McCann and Ricaurte 1991b; Steele et al. 1991; Elayan et al. 1992; Johnson et al. 1992; Zhao et al. 1992). The MDMA metabolite, alpha-methyl dopamine, may contribute to neurotoxicity as it is metabolized into compounds that can deplete 5-HT (Miller et al. 1997).

It also has been suggested that some of the dopamine released by MDMA may be transported by SERT into serotonergic axons (Faraj et al. 1994) and subsequently oxidized (Nash 1990; Schmidt and Kehne 1990; Sprague and Nichols 1995b). The oxidation of dopamine can form hydrogen peroxide, which, in turn, may produce hydroxyl radicals. A quinone-like dopamine metabolite also may be formed, with potential to generate more free radicals (Graham et al. 1978; Cadet and Brannock 1998). Among many other possible toxic effects on cells, dopamine oxidation products have been shown to impair mitochondrial functioning (Berman and Hastings 1999). At present there is little direct evidence to support the role of dopamine metabolites in MDMA neurotoxicity. Some dopaminergic drugs alter MDMA neurotoxicity, but it is not clear that this effect is due to increasing or decreasing dopamine release. Many dopaminergic drugs are now thought to affect MDMA neurotoxicity through nonspecific mechanisms of action, such as altering body temperature (Malberg et al. 1996; Colado et al. 1999a) or scavenging free radicals (Sprague and Nichols 1995a,b; Sprague et al. 1999). Dopamine release, however, does seem to play a poorly understood role in MDMA neurotoxicity (Stone et al. 1988; Schmidt and Kehne 1990; Nash and Brodkin 1991; Shankaran et al. 1999b).

Dependence of the Extent of Neurotoxicity on Dose, Route of Administration, and Species

The extent of neurotoxicity is dose-dependent. Long-term changes occur in rats at doses approximately five to ten times higher than those known to be psychoactive (Commins et al. 1987; O'Shea et al. 1998). Most MDMA neurotoxicity studies have used regimens involving multiple doses, usually giving eight doses over a four-day period. These studies show that "binge" use of MDMA carries a greater risk of neurotoxicity than single doses. When administered repeatedly, a non-neurotoxic dose of MDMA can become neurotoxic (Battaglia et al. 1988; O'Shea et al. 1998). Multiple-dose neurotoxic regimens appear to produce more profound and possibly more lasting serotonergic changes than single-dose MDMA (Battaglia et al. 1988). The results of multiple-dose studies are difficult to compare across species, since the same interval between doses can have very different effects in two species with different clearance rates of MDMA.

The effect of the route of MDMA administration on long-term serotonergic changes has been investigated. In the rat, subcutaneous injection and oral administration of MDMA produce comparable 5-HT depletions in the hippocampus (Finnegan et al. 1988). Studies of nonhuman primates have yielded less consistent results. In the squirrel monkey, Ricaurte et al. (1988a) found that repeated oral administration of MDMA resulted in only one half to two thirds as much 5-HT depletion as the equivalent subcutaneous dose. In contrast, Kleven et al. (1989) reported that repeated oral administration of MDMA in the rhesus monkey produced twice the decrease in hippocampal SERT activity as was produced by repeated subcutaneous injections. These apparent differences between nonhuman primate species magnify the difficulty of assessing the risk of oral MDMA administration in humans.

Different animal strains and species differ in sensitivity to MDMA neurotoxicity. For example, Logan et al. (1988) were unable to detect neurotoxicity when 25 mg/kg of MDMA was administered to randomly bred albino rats. In contrast, in dark agouti rats 5-HT depletions appear at a threshold between 4 and 10 mg/kg of injected MDMA (O'Shea et al. 1998). These apparent strain differences also may be influenced by differences in ambient temperature and animal housing (Gordon and Fogelson 1994; Dafters 1995).

Compared with rats, nonhuman primates seem to be more sensitive to MDMA neurotoxicity, suffering more damage at lower doses (Insel et al. 1989; Ricaurte and McCann 1992; Ricaurte et al. 1992; Ali et al. 1993; Fischer et al. 1995; see also De Souza et al. 1990 for slightly different results). Many MDMA neurotoxicity studies have used squirrel monkeys as subjects. The threshold dose for producing long-term 5-HT depletions in this species is between 2.5 and 5 mg/kg of oral MDMA. Two weeks after a single 5.0 mg/kg oral MDMA dose, 5-HT levels declined to 83 percent of control levels in the hypothalamus and 79 percent of controls in the thalamus but were not changed in other examined brain regions (Ricaurte et al. 1988a). In contrast, no long-term serotonergic changes were seen in squirrel monkeys after 2.5 mg/kg of MDMA was given orally every two weeks for four months (Ricaurte unpublished observations, cited in Vollenweider et al. 1999a). [The therapeutic dose of 125 mg of MDMA in a 150-pound person equals 1.66 mg/kg.—Ed.]

Another commonly studied nonhuman primate species is the rhesus monkey. It is difficult to determine the threshold dose for 5-HT depletions in this species, since all published studies using rhesus monkeys have employed multiple-dose neurotoxic regimens. In one study, 1.25 mg/kg of oral MDMA did not produce any long-term serotonergic changes when given twice daily for four consecutive days. Similarly repeated doses of 2.5 mg/kg of MDMA lowered hippocampal 5-HT levels (to about 80 percent of controls) but did not affect levels in six other brain regions after one month (Ali et al. 1993). In another experiment, Insel et al. (1989) found that 2.5 mg/kg of MDMA given intramuscularly to rhesus monkeys twice daily for four days produced extensive (possibly short-term) 5-HT depletions but did not alter SERT density at sixteen to eighteen hours after the last drug exposure. Since SERT density was unaffected, the researchers concluded that axonal loss had not occurred, despite the 5-HT depletions.

In a study that raises interesting questions about possible tolerance to MDMA neurotoxicity, Frederick and associates (1995) investigated the long-term effects of escalating doses of MDMA in rhesus monkeys. Intramuscular MDMA (0.1–20 mg/kg) was given twice daily for fourteen consecutive days at each dose level, followed by three dose-response regimens using single MDMA doses up to 5.6 mg/kg. One month after the final dose-response determination and twenty-one months after the initial escalating dose regimen, animals were sacrificed. Few significant serotonergic effects were found. MDMA exposure did not cause significant 5-HT depletions in any brain region and reduced SERT to about 60 percent of control levels only in the hippocampus (not in two other brain regions). Thus, data on rhesus monkeys are complex, and perhaps all that can be said with certainty is that the threshold dose for long-term 5-HT depletions appears to be above 1.25 mg/kg of oral MDMA in this species.

Reasons and Possible Justifications for High-Dose Administration of MDMA in Animals

Research on MDMA neurotoxicity sometimes has been criticized for the high-dose regimens that are commonly used. Some critics have questioned whether repeated injections of 20 mg/kg of MDMA in rodents can provide useful information about the toxicity of single oral MDMA doses of 1.7–2.0 mg/kg in humans. It is true that many of the neurotoxic regimens are not designed to be clinically relevant but were intended to maximize the serotonergic neurotoxicity of MDMA to better understand its mechanisms of action and consequences.

Comparing dose on the basis on body weight, however, can be misleading. In general, smaller species excrete drugs more quickly and form metabolites in greater amounts than larger species. This is due to many factors, including the proportionally larger livers and kidneys and faster blood circulation times in smaller mammals (Mordenti and Chappell 1989; Lin 1998). As a result of such factors, the time it takes to lower the plasma levels of MDMA by half is about 1.5 hours in a rat (Cho et al. 1990) and about eight hours in a human (Mas et al. 1999). This suggests that small species may require higher doses to achieve drug exposures comparable to those seen in larger species. These considerations justify, at least in part, the apparently high doses commonly used in rodent toxicity studies. Unfortunately, higher doses tend to alter the character of the drug exposure. While they lengthen the time smaller animals are exposed to the drug, they also tend to produce higher peak blood concentrations of drug and greater acute effects than occur in larger species at lower doses.

Many techniques have been developed for estimating equivalent drug doses in different species (Mordenti and Chappell 1989; Ings 1990; Lin 1998; Mahmood 1999). One of the most commonly used techniques, allometric interspecies scaling, involves administering a drug to different species and measuring resulting blood concentrations of drug. These measurements are used to determine the relationships of species weight, drug exposure, and dose. Drug exposure in humans then can be estimated from these relationships. Equivalent drug exposures are assumed to produce equivalent drug effects, including neurotoxicity. Ricaurte and associates (2000) estimated that as little as 1.28 mg/kg of MDMA may cause long-term 5-HT depletions in humans if interspecies dose conversions for MDMA follow a pattern that is common for drugs that are not extensively metabolized. Estimates of this sort are useful for emphasizing that the MDMA dose required to bring about neurotoxicity in humans may be within the range of commonly administered doses, despite the seemingly higher doses used in rodent studies.

Such estimates require making assumptions about the mechanisms of neurotoxicity. For example, it is necessary to assume that different species experience comparable drug effects when blood concentrations of drug are the same. This may not be true. In addition, species may differ in the brain concentration of drug produced by a given blood concentration. It is not known if this is the case with MDMA, though it does seem to be true for fenfluramine (Campbell 1995). Furthermore, if MDMA neurotoxicity is caused by a toxic metabolite, as some researchers have suggested, then the more extensive metabolism of MDMA expected in smaller animals will lead to increased neurotoxicity. Formation of specific drug metabolites in different species is difficult to predict, and few data are available on MDMA. Research on species differences in fenfluramine metabolism have led some researchers to conclude that no nonhuman species provides a good model of possible human fenfluramine neurotoxicity (Marchant et al. 1992; Caccia et al. 1995). Because current data suggest that both MDMA and metabolite exposure may mediate neurotoxicity, more data are needed from more species before interspecies dose conversions can be made with any confidence.

Data from clinical MDMA studies show that there is a complex relationship between MDMA dose and blood levels of the drug and its metabolites (Mas et al. 1999; de la Torre et al. 2000). It appears that MDMA inactivates one of the enzymes in the liver that is important to its metabolism (cytochrome

P450 isozyme 2D6 or CYP2D6) (Brady et al. 1986; Wu et al. 1997). As a result, small increases in dose can lead to large increases in drug exposure. When the dose was increased from 125 mg to 150 mg, drug exposure almost doubled in human volunteers (de la Torre et al. 2000a). Formation of some metabolites remained approximately constant, however. These complex, dose-dependent pharmacokinetics in humans amplify the difficulty of estimating dose conversions between species. Nonetheless, these human studies with MDMA suggest that doses above 125 mg may be associated with unexpectedly elevated levels of drug exposure and therefore risks of toxicity.

Influence of Environment, Especially Ambient Temperature, on Neurotoxicity in Rats and Mice

Several studies have explored the relationships among environmental temperature, animal core temperature, and neurotoxicity. In rats, MDMA can impair temperature regulation in a dose-dependent manner (Gordon et al. 1991; Dafters 1994, 1995; Broening et al. 1995; Colado et al. 1995), perhaps through alterations in the functioning of the hypothalamus and thermoregulatory behaviors. Resulting changes in animal temperature can alter neurotoxicity; hyperthermia increases and hypothermia decreases serotonergic depletions. Thus, the degree of hyperthermia has been found to correlate with long-term 5-HT depletions in adult rats (Colado et al. 1993, 1995; Broening et al. 1995; Malberg and Seiden 1998) and with long-term dopamine depletions in mice (Miller and O'Callaghan 1994). In addition to the ambient temperature, the degree of hyperthermia is influenced by the thermal conductivity of animal housing and hydration status (Gordon and Fogelson 1994; Dafters 1995).

The mechanisms of action by which temperature affects MDMA neurotoxicity are unclear. Plasma levels of MDMA in rats (Colado et al. 1995) and brain levels of MDMA in mice (Campbell 1996) do not appear to be influenced by changes in animal core temperature. MDMA-induced neurotransmitter release may be temperature-sensitive (Sabol and Seiden 1998), though studies examining the temperature dependence of methamphetamine-induced dopamine release have reported conflicting findings (Bowyer et al. 1993; LaVoie and Hastings 1999). It also may be that elevated temperature nonspecifically increases the rate of chemical reactions and contributes to oxidative stress; this effect is seen in the neurotoxicity that accompanies decreased blood supply (Globus et al. 1995). Prolonged hyperthermia has been shown to decrease the number or curb the function of mitochondria in some brain regions, suggesting diminished energy stores (Burrows and Meshul 1999). Hyperthermia on its own, however, does not selectively damage the serotonergic system.

In spite of the apparent relationship between hyperthermia and MDMA neurotoxicity, it would be a simplification to think that avoiding hyperthermia ensures that humans who have taken MDMA will not experience long-term serotonergic changes. Inducing hypothermia does not always completely block MDMA neurotoxicity (Broening et al. 1995). The link between temperature and neurotoxicity has been investigated primarily in rodents and remains to be confirmed in primates.

Time Course of Changes and Extent of Recovery

High doses of MDMA have complex effects on serotonergic functioning, causing acute declines followed by partial recovery and then long-term declines. For example, after a single 10 mg/kg dose of MDMA in a rat, release of 5-HT leads to depletion of tissue levels of 5-HT and its metabolite 5-HIAA within three hours of dosing (Schmidt 1987; Stone et al. 1987b). Approximately six hours later, levels begin to return to normal, but this recovery is not sustained. About twenty-four hours after dosing, 5-HT levels begin a second, sustained decline and remain significantly lower than baseline two weeks later. This sustained reduction is thought to be associated with axonal damage.

The intracellular enzyme TPH follows a similar time course—activity decreases within fifteen minutes of drug administration. But there is less short-term recovery of TPH activity compared with 5-HT activity. The recovery of TPH activity appears to involve regeneration of enzyme that was inactivated by oxidation rather than synthesis of new enzyme. SERT functioning also is altered. When rats were given a subcutaneous dose of 15 mg/kg of MDMA and sacrificed an hour later, the uptake of serotonin decreased by 80 percent (Fleckenstein et al. 1999). It should be noted that significant immediate 5-HT depletions are not necessarily produced by all active doses of MDMA. Schmidt and colleagues (1986) reported that 2.5 mg/kg of MDMA did not cause an immediate decrease in 5-HT or 5-HIAA in Sprague Dawley rats three hours after injection. Kish and associates (2000) did find striatal 5-HT depletions in a long-term Ecstasy user who died shortly after Ecstasy ingestion. This suggests that at least some of the doses administered by humans are sufficient to cause 5-HT depletions.

This discussion focuses on serotonergic changes because these are used to measure toxicity. Many other short-term neurochemical changes occur after MDMA exposure. For example, dopamine is released (Stone et al. 1986), and dopamine transporter reuptake activity declines within one hour of administration of high-dose MDMA (Metzger et al. 1998; Fleckenstein, et al. 1999). MDMA also can increase dopamine synthesis immediately (Nash et al. 1990). Mice are selectively vulnerable to MDMA-induced dopaminergic neurotoxicity (Stone et al. 1987a; Logan et al. 1988; Miller and O'Callaghan 1994). In some studies, long-term alterations in dopaminergic functioning have been seen in other species (such as rats in Commins et al. 1987).

The time course of damaging events in rats can be assessed by administering antidepressant selective serotonin reuptake inhibitors (SSRIs), such as fluoxetine (Prozac) and citalopram (Celexa), after MDMA. Pretreatment with fluoxetine or citalopram has been shown to block the neurotoxicity of MDMA (Schmidt 1987; Schmidt and Taylor 1990; Battaglia et al. 1988; Shankaran et al. 1999a), probably by obstructing interactions of MDMA with SERT. Fluoxetine remains almost fully protective if given three to four hours after MDMA. By four hours after administration, most of the MDMA-induced release of 5-HT and dopamine has already taken place (Hiramatsu and Cho 1990; Gough et al. 1991), and increases in extracellular free radicals (Colado et al. 1997b; Shankaran et al. 1999a) and lipid peroxidation (the alteration of fat molecules by free radicals) (Colado et al. 1997a) can be measured. Nevertheless, the administration of fluoxetine at this point decreases subsequent extracellular oxidative stress (Shankaran et al. 1999a) and long-term 5-HT depletions (Schmidt 1987; Shankaran et al. 1999a). Fluoxetine is still partially protective if given six hours after MDMA, but it has no protective effect twelve hours after administration (Schmidt 1987). This shows that neurotoxic MDMA regimens initiate a series of events that become increasingly damaging between three and twelve hours after drug administration in rats.

Slow recovery of serotonergic functioning can be seen following a neurotoxic dose of MDMA. The extent of recovery is different in different species. In rats, there is extensive recovery of indicators of serotonergic functioning one year after drug exposure (Battaglia et al. 1988; Scanzello et al. 1993; Lew et al. 1996; Sabol et al. 1996), though there are significant variations in recovery between individual animals (Fischer et al. 1995). In primates, there is some recovery of serotonergic function, but it is less extensive than in rats. Altered serotonergic axon density was still detectable seven years after MDMA exposure in one study of squirrel monkeys (Hatzidimitriou et al. 1999). Therefore, despite some recovery, MDMA-induced serotonergic changes are likely permanent in this primate species. This apparent species difference may be related in part to the more severe initial serotonergic damage usually seen in primates compared with rats. It also likely indicates a species difference in regrowth of serotonergic axons.

Behavioral and Functional Correlates of MDMA Exposure in Animals

Many studies have looked for evidence that MDMA neurotoxicity causes lasting behavioral or functional changes in laboratory animals. These studies are summarized in Table 1 [see appendices] and are perhaps impressive for the limited nature of their behavioral findings. It is clear that neurotoxic MDMA exposure can alter neurochemical functioning and the response of animals to subsequent drug exposures, but to date only two published studies suggest that MDMA-exposed animals have behavioral alterations or functional impairments at seven or more days after their last MDMA exposure. Dafters and Lynch (1998) found that MDMA-exposed animals experience lasting thermoregulatory impairment. Fourteen weeks after exposure to a neurotoxic MDMA or placebo regimen, rats were placed in a warm environment. MDMA-exposed rats had significantly larger increases in core temperature than control rats. It has been known for many years that individuals who experience heatstroke have heightened susceptibility to subsequent episodes for some time (Shapiro et al. 1979), and it seems possible that the same phenomenon is being detected in these rats.

Another study has suggested that neurotoxic MDMA exposure may cause cognitive impairment in rats. Marston and coworkers (1999) found drug-free alterations in performance of a delayed memory task. In contrast, Ricaurte and associates (1993) and Robinson and colleagues (1993) were unable to ascertain any long-term effects of MDMA neurotoxicity on spatial navigation memory tasks in rats. Robinson, however, did detect short-term residual effects of MDMA on this task when animals were tested two days after their last MDMA exposure.

The cautious interpretation of behavioral studies of MDMA neurotoxicity in animals is that we should not expect gross behavioral effects of MDMA neurotoxicity in humans, even with extensive serotonergic changes. It also must be remembered that we do not completely understand the role of 5-HT in the brain (reviewed in Lucki 1998) and that this makes it more difficult to detect 5-HT-related changes. Findings from studies of Ecstasy users may allow more focused and hypothesis-driven studies of animals.

Studies Comparing Ecstasy Users and Nonusers

More than thirty-five studies have retrospectively compared illicit Ecstasy users to nonusers. Before discussing the findings of these studies (reviewed in Morgan 2000), it is worth noting their limitations. Retrospective studies are difficult to interpret, since it is always possible that there were preexisting differences between the users and nonusers. It is almost trivial to suggest that frequent users of illicit drugs are different from those who do not use drugs. Thus, one might evaluate studies by considering to what extent they differentiate between typical characteristics of frequent illicit drug users and those specifically associated with Ecstasy users. [It is also important to realize that Ecstasy users may not be ingesting MDMA at all, since there is no guarantee that Ecstasy purchased on the street contains MDMA. Moreover, use of other drugs, including ketamine and dextromethorphan, may affect cognitive testing results.—Ed.] Other common methodologic limitations of these studies include poorly described recruitment and matching of volunteer groups, reliance on self-reports of drug use, failure to separate residual effects of recent drug use from long-term effects, use of the same volunteers in several studies, and difficulty in relating serotonergic differences to toxicity. Despite these limitations, a few conclusions can be drawn from studies comparing Ecstasy users and nonusers. Findings can be grouped into personality, neurofunctional, and cognitive performance differences. These areas are discussed below.

Reports consistently link repeated Ecstasy use to depressed mood (Solowij et al. 1992; Cohen 1995; Curran and Travill 1997; Davison and Parrott 1997; Gerra et al. 1998, 2000; Parrott and Lasky 1998; Morgan 1999; Gamma et al. 2000a; Parrott 2000). Because depressed mood is a known residual effect of other psychostimulant drugs (Coffey et al. 2000), it is likely that Ecstasy use plays a causal role in this phenomenon. In a survey of 158 polydrug users, Williamson et al. (1997) found that similar numbers of users reported depression, anxiety, and related adverse effects after cocaine compared with MDMA.

In addition, there are several case reports of psychiatric disorders, such as psychosis, depression, and panic attacks, in Ecstasy users (reviewed in McGuire 2000). Given that other psychostimulants are associated with psychiatric disorders in illicit users, it would not be surprising if this were also true of MDMA. For example, it is well established that stimulant-induced psychosis can occur in cocaine or methamphetamine users (Angrist 1994). Reports of MDMA-related psychosis also have been published (Creighton et al. 1991; McCann and Ricaurte 1991a; McGuire and Fahy 1991, McGuire 2000). These psychiatric disorders need not be related to the selective neurotoxicity discussed in this chapter. For example, methamphetamine can produce chronic behavioral disturbances resembling psychosis in primates using regimens that are not neurotoxic to dopaminergic or serotonergic systems (Castner and Goldman-Rakic 1999).

Personality Differences Between Ecstasy Users and Nonusers

While Ecstasy users sometimes have been found to have personalities that are different from those of nonusers, it is not clear that this is an effect of MDMA exposure. Many of the reported personality differences between Ecstasy users and volunteers who do not ordinarily use illicit drugs likely reflect preexisting differences. Higher levels of novelty seeking (Gerra et al. 1998), venturesomeness, and impulsivity (Morgan 1998) have been reported in Ecstasy users, but this can be expected in users of illicit drugs compared with nonusers. Several authors have pointed out the possibility of preexisting differences. For example, Gerra et al. (2000) suggested that the enhanced novelty seeking (measured with the self-report Tridimensional Personality Questionnaire) characteristic of Ecstasy users undergoing substance abuse treatment reflected a preexisting trait. Similarly, the higher direct aggression scores on the Buss-Durkee Hostility Index (BDHI) of Ecstasy users in substance abuse treatment (Gerra et al. 2000) and the lower BDHI indirect hostility scores in untreated Ecstasy users (McCann et al. 1994) may be explained in part by social circumstances and the values of the rave subculture, respectively. To minimize the influence of traits generally associated with illicit drug use, one could compare Ecstasy users with different total Ecstasy exposures, or one could compare multiple-drug users with and without Ecstasy experience. Findings from the comparisons cited here are ambiguous, and such comparisons can provide at best only limited support for possible MDMA-induced alterations in personality. Studies in which the same individuals are examined at different time points are necessary to examine this issue properly.

There is mixed evidence that MDMA use is associated with increases in self-reported impulsive behavior. Morgan (1998) reported that a post hoc comparison of more experienced (more than thirty tablets ingested) and less experienced (twenty to thirty tablets ingested) Ecstasy users showed heightened levels of impulsivity (measured with Eysenck's self-report IVE [impulsiveness, venturesomeness, empathy] questionnaire) in the more experienced group. Parrott (2000) reported a nonsignificant trend toward greater IVE impulsivity in polydrug-using Ecstasy users with an average of 371 (varying from thirty to one thousand) exposures compared with a group of users with an average of 6.8 (one to twenty) exposures. Tuchtenhagen and colleagues (2000) found that Ecstasy users with an average of 93.4 ± 119.9 (twenty to five hundred) exposures had significantly higher scores for impulsivity (measured with the self-report Barratt Impulsiveness Scale) compared with controls matched for other drug use. The researchers also noted a trend toward increased experience seeking (measured with the self-report Sensation-Seeking Scale), which reached statistical significance only when Ecstasy users were compared with nonusers. These findings differ from those of McCann et al. (1994), who compared Ecstasy users with an average of 94.4 ± 90.6 (twenty-five to three hundred) reported Ecstasy exposures to nonusers (without controlling for other drug use). McCann reported decreased impulsivity (measured as increases in the Control subscale of the Multidimensional Personality Questionnaire) but did not find significant differences in self-reported impulsivity with a second questionnaire (the self-report Eysenck Personality Questionnaire).

There are fewer data examining impulsive behavior, which is thought to be different from self-reported impulsivity (Evenden 1999). Using the same volunteers as in the Tuchtenhagen (2000) report, Gouzoulis-Mayfrank et al. (2000) did not find evidence of impulsivity in Ecstasy users undergoing a cognitive test battery. In contrast, Morgan (1998) reported that Ecstasy users made more errors in a Matching Familiar Figures task, a difference he interpreted as evidence of increased impulsiveness. Morgan suggested that his behavioral findings indicated an impaired capacity to cope with high-level cognitive demands.

Neurofunctional Differences Between Ecstasy Users and Nonusers

Studies also have established an association between Ecstasy exposure and altered neurofunctioning. Reported neurofunctional differences summarized in Table 2 [see appendices] include putative serotonergic measures as well as more general measures, such as EEG findings. While retrospective studies, technically speaking, cannot establish causality, many of these user/nonuser differences correlate with extent of Ecstasy exposure. Correlations have been reported between Ecstasy exposure and such measures as cerebrospinal fluid 5-HIAA levels (Bolla et al. 1998), SERT density (McCann et al. 1998), brain myo-inositol increases (Chang et al. 1999), and EEG alterations (Dafters et al. 1999). A primary difficulty in interpreting the results of these studies is that we do not know the real meaning of many of these neurofunctional differences.

At a minimum, we certainly can conclude that the brains of these Ecstasy users are different from those of nonuser volunteers. Does this mean that serotonergic neurotoxicity has taken place? This seems the most likely possibility. Several studies have shown differences in measures of serotonergic functioning between users and nonusers. Two groups have reported diminished cortical SERT binding in Ecstasy users (McCann et al. 1998; Semple et al. 1999), though there is some question about the specificity of the measurement technique (Kuikka and Ahonen 1999; Heinz and Jones 2000). Three of four studies have found cerebrospinal fluid levels of 5-HIAA to be lower in users than in nonusers (decreased in McCann et al., 1994, 1999b; Ricaurte et al. 1990; unchanged in Peroutka et al. 1987). These differences are consistent with the results of animal studies, in which neurotoxic MDMA exposure similarly altered these indicators (Ricaurte et al. 1988b; Insel et al. 1989; Scheffel et al. 1998).

Such parallel findings in humans and nonhumans provide evidence that selective serotonergic neurotoxicity has occurred, but it must be noted that all published studies in humans have been retrospective. Without knowing what Ecstasy users were like before using drugs, we can only guess whether unusual serotonergic functioning is the result of damage. Unfortunately, these serotonergic measures are sufficiently new that we do not know the full range of so-called normal values for them. This makes it difficult to decide whether the values seen in Ecstasy users are truly abnormal and indicative of damage. Alternatively, they may be simply unusual for nondrug users but usual for the kind of person who is likely to ingest Ecstasy repeatedly. [People with depression have been shown to have a lower density of SERT in certain brain regions (Mann et al. 2000) and decreased levels of 5-HT and 5-HIAA (Meltzer 1990) before being treated with antidepressants.—Ed.] In addition, typical indicators of serotonergic function may be affected by influences other than neurotoxicity. Some theories suggest that individuals who abuse psychostimulants are more likely to have unusual serotonergic functioning (Zuckerman 1996; Laviola et al. 1999). These interpretive difficulties can be illustrated using studies that investigate the amount of hormone released after serotonergic drug administration in different populations.

Measuring the amount of hormone released in response to a serotonergic drug is one way to test for changes in the serotonergic system. This tactic has uncovered statistically significant user/nonuser differences in four of six studies (differences detected in Gerra et al. 1998, 2000; McCann et al. 1999a; Verkes et al. 2000; no significant differences in Price et al. 1989; McCann et al. 1994). Other studies have established that both personality and use of other drugs, such as cocaine, may modulate this serotonergic measure. People who are more prone to sensation seeking have been shown to have blunted hormone responses to the partial $5-HT1_A$ agonist ipsapirone (Netter et al. 1996). Similarly, the hormone prolactin's response to the 5-HT releaser fenfluramine in a group of cocaine-dependent individuals was significantly higher between the first and third weeks after discontinuing cocaine use (Buydens-Branchey et al. 1999), suggesting recovery from cocaine-induced alterations. One could argue that factors other than MDMA neurotoxicity might explain some apparent serotonergic differences between users and nonusers. This issue can be solved only through prospective studies that assess the same individuals at different time points.

One strong argument that many human users experience MDMA neurotoxicity is simply that estimated ingested doses exceed those known to produce 5-HT depletions in squirrel monkeys (Ricaurte et al. 1988a). Given that approximately similar doses are associated with similar changes in serotonergic indexes in nonhuman species and in humans, it seems likely that the same phenomenon is occurring in all species. Furthermore, in administering MDMA to humans, it may be more important to be conservative in risk assessment than to wait for conclusive scientific proof of neurotoxicity. This is especially important in light of the fact that some individuals may be more susceptible to neurotoxicity than others. Studies comparing Ecstasy users to nonusers suggest that neurotoxicity may occur when MDMA is self-administered by humans. MDMA neurotoxicity and its largely unknown possible long-term consequences must therefore be considered when evaluating the risks of clinical MDMA research.

Cognitive Differences Between Ecstasy Users and Nonusers

Repeated Ecstasy exposure is associated with decreased performance on cognitive tests. Tests of declarative verbal memory frequently have been used to detect this decline (Parrott and Lasky 1998, Parrott et al. 1998; Gouzoulis-Mayfrank et al. 2000; Morgan 1999; Reneman et al. 2000a). However, user/nonuser differences have been detected using a broad range of cognitive tasks (McCann et al. 1999b; Gouzoulis-Mayfrank et al. 2000; Rodgers 2000). Some researchers have suggested that specific alterations in executive functioning and working memory may explain the observed differences (Dafters et al. 1999; Gouzoulis-Mayfrank et al. 2000; Wareing et al. 2000), but there is no conclusive evidence.

Perhaps the most thorough study published so far was conducted by Gouzoulis-Mayfrank et al. (2000). In this study, users of both Ecstasy and cannabis were compared with cannabis users and drug-free volunteers.

Extent of Ecstasy use was correlated with impaired performance in a range of tasks. Performance among Ecstasy-using volunteers remained, on average, at the low end of clinically normal functioning. This is not particularly reassuring, given that these users appeared to have fairly common use patterns (1.4 ± 0.9 tablets taken 2.4 ± 1.6 times per month). If modestly diminished cognitive performance is an effect of MDMA, it is likely one experienced by many people. Does Ecstasy use cause this poor cognitive performance? The available data are inconclusive, but they suggest that this is so. Many, but not all (e.g., Morgan 1998), studies have found that long-term Ecstasy users perform worse on many cognitive tests than nonusers and that users with more Ecstasy exposure perform worse than those with less exposure (Bolla et al. 1998; Dafters et al. 1999; McCann et al. 1999b; Gouzoulis-Mayfrank et al. 2000).

It is likely that there are differences between Ecstasy users and nonusers that predate illicit drug use. Schifano (2000) described unpublished survey data taken from high school students in Italy; these data indicated that students attending less academic secondary schools were 2.89 times more likely to have used Ecstasy than those attending schools with a more highly academic focus. In another survey of 737 Italian Ecstasy users, there was evidence of inverse relationships between the tendency to take higher Ecstasy doses and both lower schooling level and lower family income (Schifano 2000).

The association between Ecstasy exposure and lower cognitive performance also may be caused in part by factors correlated with Ecstasy exposure, such as repeated sleep and nutrient deprivation associated with attending late-night dance events. Nonetheless, the few scientific studies that looked at these possible factors (Dinges and Kribbs 1991; Kretsch et al. 1997; Cho et al. 2000) would not lead us to expect an effect comparable to what we see in studies of Ecstasy users. These other possible factors are likely significant only if the Ecstasy-using volunteers in these international studies engage in a particularly hard-partying lifestyle. In the first published study that properly controlled for lifestyle, Verkes and co-workers (2000) found that moderate Ecstasy users (with 73 ± 68 reported exposures to Ecstasy) had lower performance scores than nonusers who had attended a similar number of "raves" in the previous twelve months.

It seems unlikely that preexisting differences and effects of lifestyle can fully explain the reported cognitive performance differences. Average performance in immediate declarative verbal memory tasks declined by about 0.8 standard deviation units in several studies (Parrott and Lasky 1998; Parrott et al. 1998; Morgan 1999; Gouzoulis-Mayfrank et al. 2000). This means that the average Ecstasy-using volunteer in these studies scored in the bottom 21 percent of expected scores, based on the comparison volunteers. While it is possible, it seems improbable that the fourth of the population with the worst memories go on to use Ecstasy several times a month (and participate in these studies).

Use of drugs other than MDMA has not always been taken into account properly in studies of Ecstasy users. In particular, Ecstasy-using volunteers often have been found to use more cannabis than Ecstasy-naive volunteers. This is significant, because long-term cannabis use can cause long-lasting residual impairments in cognitive performance (Pope and Yurgelun-Todd 1996). Three studies have compared users of both Ecstasy and cannabis to users of cannabis alone (Croft et al. 2001; Gouzoulis-Mayfrank et al. 2000; Rodgers 2000). Two of these studies have suggested that MDMA use is associated with cognitive performance lower than that expected with cannabis (Gouzoulis-Mayfrank et al. 2000; Rodgers 2000). In contrast, Croft and associates (2001) were unable to detect performance differences between cannabis users and users of both cannabis and Ecstasy on a battery of cognitive tests. Further statistical analysis suggested that performance declines were related more closely to cannabis than to Ecstasy use. In another study that attempted to control for the influence of other drugs, Morgan (1999) detected lower memory performance in Ecstasy-experienced polydrug users compared with Ecstasy-naive polydrug users. However, matching of drug use between comparison groups was imperfect in this study. It is clear that future studies should control for use of cannabis and that the apparent magnitude of the MDMA-associated cognitive performance decline likely is exaggerated by cannabis use. [None of these studies specifically addressed the issue of ketamine, which is frequently used at raves, is known to affect memory, and is being investigated as a chemical model for dementia.—Ed.]

The lower cognitive performance of Ecstasy users may be due to serotonergic neurotoxicity or to some other neurochemical alteration. It has been shown that acute serotonergic depletion (by dietary manipulation) can impair declarative verbal memory in healthy volunteers (Riedel et al. 1999). Three studies of Ecstasy users have reported correlations between alterations in serotonergic measures and decreased cognitive performance (Bolla et al. 1998; Reneman et al. 2000a; Verkes et al. 2000). This finding suggests a relationship between lower cognitive performance and MDMA-induced serotonin depletions or neurotoxicity. On the other hand, if MDMA-induced loss of serotonin or damage to serotonergic axons were sufficient to impair memory to the degree suggested by human studies, one would expect this effect to be detected readily in prospective animal studies.

It seems possible that the reported lower cognitive performance is related to the volunteers' long-term, repeated patterns of Ecstasy use. MDMA exposures are limited (usually four consecutive days or fewer) in most animal experiments, and this could explain the apparent discrepancy between these studies and Ecstasy user studies. Furthermore, it is well established that long-term psychostimulant use impairs cognitive performance (McKetin and Solowij 1999; Ornstein et al. 2000). For example, repeated cocaine use is associated with impaired cognitive functioning (O'Malley et al. 1992; Beatty et al. 1995; Bolla et al. 1999), though cocaine use per se does not necessarily produce deficits (Bolla et al. 1999). Cocaine is not a selective neurotoxin, but, like MDMA, it can cause both serotonergic (Little et al. 1998; Jacobsen et al. 2000) and cerebrovascular (Bartzokis et al. 1999; Herning et al. 1999) alterations. Since repeated exposure to other psychostimulants can impair cognitive functioning, it is credible that repeated MDMA use might be associated with cognitive deficits. This suggestion leaves open the question of whether this effect is due to repeated neurotoxic damage or residual drug effects.

Specific evidence linking lower-level cognitive performance of long-term Ecstasy users to serotonergic neurotoxicity could come from studies of the time course of these differences. Residual drug effects might be expected to improve more quickly than changes due to serotonergic neurotoxicity. Unfortunately, too few studies have looked for evidence of recovery to draw any conclusions. Morgan (1999) reported that a subset of three Ecstasy users who had not taken Ecstasy in more than six months had significantly better immediate and delayed recall (of ideas from stories taken from the Rivermead

Behavioral Memory Test) than users with more recent history of drug use. In contrast, Wareing and colleagues (2000) were unable to find evidence of a significant abstinence-related improvement in working memory and executive functioning tasks when ten current Ecstasy users were compared with ten volunteers who reportedly had not used Ecstasy in six months. It is therefore not clear if there is recovery from this lower cognitive performance.

In conclusion, repeated Ecstasy exposure is associated with diminished cognitive performance. The apparent magnitude of the effect may be exaggerated by limitations in published studies, particularly the confounding effects of cannabis [as well as ketamine and dextromethorphan—Ed.] on performance. There are insufficient data to decide whether there is recovery of performance with abstinence. It is an open question whether this is due to a residual drug effect or a frank neurotoxic change.

Possible Significance of Cognitive Differences and MDMA Neurotoxicity

How severe are these cognitive changes? They do not indicate impairment in day-to-day activities. The differences are seen in cognitive tests in which young, healthy people perform well. Thus, these differences are generally small in magnitude despite their statistical significance. In fact, neither the investigators nor the Ecstasy-using volunteers themselves appeared to be aware of any cognitive impairment (McCann and Ricaurte 1991b; Rodgers 2000). These studies raise questions about whether the Ecstasy-using volunteers have experienced serotonergic neurotoxicity that eventually might be associated with more severe symptoms. Such symptoms could become prominent as Ecstasy users age. Additionally, larger impairments in specialized areas of functioning may exist but simply have not been discovered yet.

Studies of individual variation in symptoms associated with neurodegenerative disorders have led to two relevant concepts. First, there is a threshold of damage that must be exceeded in some brain systems before symptoms develop. This has been investigated primarily with reference to dopaminergic cell loss and Parkinson's disease (Calne et al. 1985; Brownell et al. 1999; Di Monte et al. 2000). There are fewer data on the serotonergic system. In a rat study using the serotonergic neurotoxin 5,7-DHT, Hall et al. (1999) concluded that a loss of more than 60 percent of serotonergic neurons was necessary to decrease extracellular 5-HT levels in the striatum. Alterations in behavior were seen with slightly smaller depletions (51 percent or more), possibly as the result of regional variations in neurotoxicity. One might speculate that even smaller depletions do not affect many serotonergic-related behaviors, though the maximal serotonergic response to drugs or other stimuli is likely to be reduced. (Reduced electrically stimulated 5-HT release in MDMA-exposed rats was documented by Gartside et al. 1996).

Second, the concept of cognitive reserve has been developed to explain why higher education or intelligence or greater brain size is associated with less severe impairment in conditions such as Alzheimer disease, AIDS, and normal aging (Graves et al. 1996; Stern et al. 1996; Alexander et al. 1997; Coffey et al. 1999). This cognitive reserve may be seen as a surplus of processing capacity that protects a person against loss of functioning when that capacity decreases. Cognitive reserve could be the result of more extensive functional brain tissue, density of neural connections, or cognitive strategies for problem solving. People with less cognitive reserve could be expected to undergo larger cognitive declines from MDMA exposure than users with greater cognitive reserve. Support for this possibility comes from Bolla and associates (1998), who reported a significant interaction between drug dose and vocabulary (measured with the Wechsler Adult Intelligence Scale-Revised). Ecstasy users with lower vocabulary scores showed greater deficits in delayed visual memory performance, while users with higher vocabulary scores had largely preserved performance. Although the absolute magnitude of performance decline was small, this study suggests that cognitive reserve could play a role in expression of MDMA neurotoxicity.

It is difficult to predict whether symptoms of MDMA neurotoxicity are likely to increase as users age. Some researchers have speculated that aging Ecstasy users might have a higher risk of depression and other affective disorders. From a neurochemical perspective, age-related declines in SERT density appear modest (estimated at 4.3 percent per decade by van Dyck and colleagues 2000), while 5-HT receptors undergo more complex age-related changes (reviewed in Meltzer et al. 1998). One would hope that these changes would not cause Ecstasy users to exceed a hypothetical threshold for showing symptoms of neurotoxicity, but we simply do not understand 5-HT or affective disorders sufficiently to make predictions with any confidence. Late-onset affective disorders probably are influenced by many nonserotonergic factors, such as social isolation and cerebrovascular disease.

These are serious and legitimate concerns, and there is insufficient research to address them adequately. On the other hand, there is no direct evidence to support these concerns. Neurotoxic phenethylamines have been self-administered by humans for more than sixty years. In this time, no evidence has been published suggesting that methamphetamine or amphetamine increases the risk of Parkinson's disease, despite the fact that they damage dopaminergic axons. In contrast, the link between Parkinson's disease and MPTP, a dopaminergic neurotoxin, was discovered immediately (Davis et al. 1979; Langston et al. 1983). This suggests that there may be fundamental differences between neurotoxic phenethylamines, which selectively damage a subset of the brain's axons but not cell bodies, and other neurotoxins. Similarly, concerns about the selective serotonergic neurotoxicity induced by MDMA and other drugs are not fueled by a toxic syndrome identified in users. Instead, they are motivated by the intuition that the dramatic decreases in indexes of serotonergic functioning must have some adverse behavioral consequences.

Findings in Prospective Clinical MDMA Studies

Few peer-reviewed reports are available that examine volunteers in clinical MDMA studies for evidence of neurotoxic changes. This section therefore significantly relies on unpublished data kindly supplied by researchers who are in the process of preparing reports on their findings. The reader is advised to consider this discussion as preliminary and subject to revision in more definitive peer-reviewed publications.

Preliminary retrospective analysis of data from studies conducted by Dr. Franz Vollenweider and colleagues reportedly has found no evidence that one or two oral exposures of up to 1.7 mg/kg MDMA is associated with lasting cognitive or neurofunctional alterations. Measures in this retrospective analysis include EEG, regional cerebral blood flow, mood, cognitive functioning, and indexes of information processing, such as event-related

EEG potentials and pre-pulse inhibition (Franz Vollenweider, personal communication). Most important, Vollenweider and colleagues conducted a prospective study in which six MDMA-naive volunteers were administered a single oral dose of 1.5 or 1.7 mg/kg MDMA. Positron emission tomography (PET) measures of SERT density (using the same technique employed by McCann et al. 1998) were made before and four weeks after MDMA administration. No significant changes were noted. It would appear that long-term serotonergic changes either do not occur or are too small to measure using this technique after one exposure to up to 1.7 mg/kg MDMA in healthy volunteers. These data will need to be replicated using a larger sample size before this conclusion can be made with confidence.

Data collected by Dr. Charles Grob and colleagues are more difficult to interpret. These researchers administered two doses (separated by two weeks or more) of up to 2.5 mg/kg MDMA to Ecstasy-experienced volunteers and carried out cognitive testing in fourteen people before and approximately two weeks after study participation. No alterations in cognitive performance were detected (Charles Grob, personal communication). MDMA-induced decreases in regional cerebral blood flow were seen, however, in a subset of eight volunteers assessed ten to twenty-one days after their last MDMA exposure (Chang et al. 2000). Cerebral blood flow was measured using single-positron emission computed tomography (SPECT) scans co-registered with magnetic resonance imaging (MRI), and significant decreases were found bilaterally in the visual cortex, caudate, superior parietal, and dorsolateral frontal regions. Therefore, doses as low as 1.25 mg/kg MDMA may reduce cerebral blood flow at two or three weeks after drug exposure.

It is not clear how long these declines last. Two volunteers who underwent repeated SPECT scans showed evidence of possibly increased cerebral blood flow at later time points (forty-three and eighty days after taking MDMA, respectively). This finding suggests that the impaired cerebral blood flow is either a subacute drug effect of limited duration or part of a lasting biphasic effect (with decreases followed by increases). Chang states that diminished regional cerebral blood flow was generally less severe in volunteers with greater time since the last MDMA exposure, providing evidence of recovery. In addition, the authors did not find differences in cerebral blood flow when twenty-one Ecstasy-experienced volunteers were compared with twenty-one nonusers (Chang et al. 2000). Similarly, Gamma (2001) saw no significant differences between sixteen Ecstasy users (most of whom had used Ecstasy at least one hundred times) and seventeen nonusers when regional cerebral blood flow was measured during a vigilance task using $[H_2O^{15}]$-PET. Finally, it should be pointed out that Gamma and colleagues reportedly did not detect changes in regional cerebral blood flow using $[H_2O^{15}]$-PET in a retrospective analysis of a study in which volunteers received 1.7 mg/kg MDMA (Alex Gamma, personal communication).

One possible mechanism of action of subacute alterations in regional cerebral blood flow is suggested by two preliminary reports of a study by Dr. Liesbeth Reneman and colleagues (2000a,b). These researchers used SPECT scans to measure cortical $5\text{-}HT2_A$ receptors and found evidence of fewer $5\text{-}HT2_A$ receptors in ten Ecstasy users 7 ± 5 weeks after their last Ecstasy exposure. In contrast, a group of five Ecstasy users showed a trend toward increased cortical $5\text{-}HT2_A$ binding, which did not reach statistical significance, at least two months after their last reported exposure (18 ± 15 weeks). Reneman suggests that MDMA-induced 5-HT release may have led to down-regulation of $5\text{-}HT2_A$ receptors. Indeed, Scheffel and associates (1992) reported transient down-regulation of these receptors in rats after a neurotoxic regimen of MDMA. Changes in $5\text{-}HT2_A$ receptors are thought to play a role in the regulation of cerebral blood vessel constriction (Nobler et al. 1999). In support of this idea, Reneman et al. (2000b) reported correlations between apparent $5\text{-}HT2_A$ density and regional cerebral blood volume in the occipital cortex and globus pallidus (areas involved in vision and movement) of a subset of five Ecstasy users in whom cerebral blood volume was measured using MRI. Thus, the diminished cerebral blood flow/volume seen in Grob's volunteers and Reneman's Ecstasy users may be the result of transient $5\text{-}HT2_A$ down-regulation due to MDMA-induced 5-HT release.

This hypothesis does not, however, explain the trends toward increased cerebral blood flow or volume seen by both research groups at later time points. Given that this trend occurred in very few volunteers, it must be interpreted with caution until it is confirmed in a more detailed study. Nonetheless, the duration of this possible increase is cause for concern. Even though one could hypothesize non-neurotoxic mechanisms of action, long-term increases in cerebral blood flow have been associated with serotonergic neurotoxicity. Specifically, a rodent study by McBean et al. (1990) found that a neurotoxic regimen of MDA heightened regional cerebral blood flow in rats at six to nine weeks after drug exposure. It seems possible, therefore, that one or more of the doses received by these two volunteers (the two that had increased SPECT in Grob's study) is sufficient to produce neurotoxicity. The two volunteers each received 2.0 mg/kg MDMA in one session and either 1.75 or 2.25 mg/kg in another session. Increases in cerebral blood flow after MDMA may not be permanent, since the MDMA-experienced volunteers in Grob's study did not have enhanced cerebral blood flow compared with nonusers (Chang et al. 2000). Nonetheless, researchers may wish to consider carefully the risks and benefits of exposing volunteers to a drug that may have detectable effects eighty days later.

Overall, preliminary findings from clinical studies suggest that cognitive functioning is not likely to be significantly altered by one or two exposures to MDMA in a clinical context, but there may be changes in cerebral blood flow lasting several weeks or longer. Although the mechanism of action of these changes has not been investigated directly, MDMA neurotoxicity cannot be ruled out as a possible explanation for any changes lasting several months. Of course, it must be noted again that the numbers of volunteers in the studies described in this section are small and any conclusions must be tentative. Further research is necessary.

Potential Strategies for Reducing Risk of Neurotoxicity in Clinical Settings

Because the range of psychoactive but non-neurotoxic MDMA doses appears to be narrow in most species and the possible long-term consequences of neurotoxicity are unknown, researchers and therapists may be well advised to consider strategies for limiting the risk of neurotoxicity. For example, although high ambient temperature and humidity are unlikely in clinical settings, it is probably worth noting that these factors may raise body temperature, which is associated with enhanced MDMA neurotoxicity in rats. In addition, MDMA dose and frequency of administration should be kept to the minimum required. Even if all active doses of MDMA do not produce measurable neurotoxicity, they likely cause a degree of oxidative stress in the brain. Furthermore, the nonlinear pharmacokinetics of MDMA suggests that small increases in dose may lead to large increases in plasma MDMA levels

(Mas et al. 1999; de la Torre et al. 2000a) and, possibly, the risk of neurotoxicity. Administration of a small booster dose to lengthen MDMA intoxication may also magnify risk, given the apparently saturable metabolism of MDMA. The possible benefits of such booster doses should be carefully weighed against this risk.

Anecdotal reports suggest that many Ecstasy users already employ pharmacological interventions that have been found to be neuroprotective in rodent MDMA studies. These interventions include antioxidants, SSRIs, and 5-HTP (5 hydroxytryptophan). Because rodent studies showing neuroprotection almost exclusively have used several injections of high-dose neuroprotective agents, it is not clear that humans can achieve comparable neuroprotection with oral dosing. This is particularly true for vitamin C, which has saturable absorption and increased clearance at high doses in humans (Blanchard et al. 1997; Graumlich et al. 1997). Similarly, in rodent studies using 5-HTP, another drug typically also is administered to curb peripheral metabolism of 5-HTP, allowing more to reach the brain. Oral administration of 5-HTP in humans therefore may not achieve adequate brain levels.

Keeping in mind the almost complete lack of controlled studies examining these interventions in humans, some seem sufficiently promising to warrant further consideration when designing protocols. Administering an SSRI when subjective MDMA effects have become minimal could be considered. Liechti and associates (2000a) have shown that pretreatment with 40 mg of the SSRI citalopram lessens the effects of 1.5 mg/kg MDMA. This study shows that these drugs can be co-administered safely in a clinical setting, despite the fact that a previous case report describes a possible adverse interaction between these compounds (Lauerma et al. 1998). Thus, giving an SSRI at three to four hours after MDMA administration could be considered, if MDMA pharmacokinetics are not being measured and SSRIs are not otherwise contraindicated in the relevant patient or volunteer population.

Antioxidant supplements also may prove useful. Aguirre and colleagues (1999) reported that twice-daily administration of high-dose alpha-lipoic acid for two days completely blocked the neurotoxicity of a subsequent single dose of MDMA in rats. Because the acute inactivation of TPH can occur after non-neurotoxic MDMA doses and is due to oxidative stress, it is plausible that antioxidants also may enhance recovery from even low MDMA doses. One consideration with antioxidants is that high doses of some acids, such as ascorbic acid (vitamin C), may alter urinary pH and thus affect excretion of MDMA. Aside from such possible pharmacokinetic interactions, doses of antioxidants that are known to be well tolerated appear unlikely to increase the risk of adverse events and may decrease the risks of long-term toxicity.

Although these potentially neuroprotective strategies are worth considering, the appropriate doses and timing of their administration are largely unknown. It would be technically and ethically difficult to establish whether a given intervention has been successful in lessening MDMA neurotoxicity. These interventions therefore should be considered experimental and should not be used to reassure potential research volunteers that the risks of MDMA neurotoxicity are reduced.

The Need for More Research

People who have read this far likely need little convincing that more research is needed. More animal studies could investigate possible symptoms of MDMA neurotoxicity and the potential influence of the aging process on these symptoms. Measuring blood and brain levels of MDMA and its metabolites after neurotoxic and non-neurotoxic exposures in different species would allow us to predict potential neurotoxic MDMA doses in humans with more accuracy. There is a particular need for primate studies to establish threshold doses for neurotoxicity and measure MDMA pharmacokinetics. Now that MDMA pharmacokinetics have been characterized in humans and rats, it would be possible to design drug dose regimens that expose rats or nonhuman primates to the same MDMA plasma concentrations that are seen in humans after commonly used MDMA doses. Once nonhuman primate pharmacokinetics are established, similar studies could be carried out in those species. Such studies would make great advances in our understanding of the risks of MDMA neurotoxicity to humans.

Long-term follow-up studies in humans should investigate whether MDMA exposure is associated with clinically significant symptoms, such as a higher risk of affective disorders. The hundreds of patients who underwent MDMA-assisted psychotherapy in the 1970s and early 1980s are one important population who could be assessed. Prospective studies of Ecstasy users are needed to establish definitively the extent to which MDMA impairs cognitive performance and whether abstinence from MDMA is associated with recovery. Both human and animal studies should investigate the time course of MDMA-induced changes in regional cerebral blood flow and its relationship to serotonergic functioning.

Summary

High- or repeated-dose MDMA regimens can produce long-term changes in serotonergic and axonal functioning in animals. More and more evidence supports the view that these changes, at least in part, are the result of damage. The magnitude of these serotonergic changes varies with dose, species, and route of administration. Rodent studies have shown that changes in the core temperature of animals can increase or decrease MDMA neurotoxicity. While a degree of recovery does occur, a study in squirrel monkeys suggests that there may be permanent changes in axonal distribution in some areas of the brain. Oxidative stress appears to play an important role in MDMA neurotoxicity, though the exact mechanisms of action are poorly understood. The sustained pharmacological effects of MDMA may exhaust neuronal energy sources and antioxidant defenses, leading to damage. Metabolites of MDMA are another possible source of oxidative stress. Very few behavioral correlates of MDMA exposure have been found in drug-free laboratory animals, despite dramatic serotonergic changes, alterations in neurofunctioning, and changes in response to drugs. A growing number of studies describe differences between Ecstasy users and nonusers. These studies have serious limitations, but they suggest that some Ecstasy users experience serotonergic changes and cognitive alterations. In contrast to studies of illicit Ecstasy users, the few controlled clinical trials with MDMA in healthy volunteers reportedly have not found evidence of cognitive changes, despite the cerebral blood flow alterations that were documented in one study. The possible risks of neurotoxicity must be considered when assessing the potential administration of MDMA to humans.

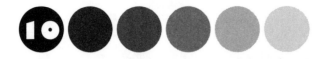

THE LEGAL STATUS OF MDMA AROUND THE WORLD

Julie Holland, M.D

In the United States, MDMA currently is listed in Schedule I of the Controlled Substances Act (CSA), title II of the Comprehensive Drug Abuse Prevention and Control Act of 1970 (United States Code, title 21, chapter 13, section 813). The CSA places all substances that are regulated under existing federal law into one of five schedules. This placement is based upon the substance's medicinal value, harmfulness, and potential for abuse or addiction. Schedule I is reserved for the most dangerous drugs that have no recognized medical use, and Schedule V is the classification used for the least dangerous drugs.

Schedule I

(A) The drug or other substance has a high potential for abuse.

(B) The drug or other substance has no currently accepted medical use in treatment in the United States.

(C) There is a lack of accepted safety for use of the drug or other substance under medical supervision.

Schedule II

(A) The drug or other substance has a high potential for abuse.

(B) The drug or other substance has a currently accepted medical use in treatment in the United States or a currently accepted medical use with severe restrictions.

(C) Abuse of the drug or other substances may lead to severe psychological or physical dependence.

Schedule III

(A) The drug or other substance has a potential for abuse less than the drugs or other substances on schedules I and II.

(B) The drug or other substance has a currently accepted medical use in treatment in the United States.

(C) Abuse of the drug or other substance may lead to moderate or minimal physical dependence or high psychological dependence.

Schedule IV

(A) The drug or other substance has a low potential for abuse relative to the drugs or other substances on schedule III.

(B) The drug or other substance has a currently accepted medical use in the United States.

(C) Abuse of the drug or other substance may lead to limited physical dependence or psychological dependence relative to the drugs or other substances in Schedule III.

Schedule V

(A) The drug or other substance has a low potential for abuse relative to the drugs or other substances in Schedule IV.

(B) The drug or other substance has a currently accepted medical use in the United States.

(C) Abuse of the drug or other substance may lead to limited physical dependence or psychological dependence relative to the drugs or other substances in Schedule IV.

The act also provides a way for substances to be controlled, added to a schedule, removed from control, and rescheduled. Proceedings to add, delete, or change the schedule of a drug or other substance may be initiated by the Drug Enforcement Administration (DEA), by the Department of Health and Human Services (HHS), or by petition from any interested party, including the manufacturer of a drug, a medical society or association, a pharmacy association, a public interest group concerned with drug abuse, a state or local government agency, or an individual citizen. When a petition is received by the DEA, the agency begins its own investigation.

The DEA also may begin an investigation of a drug at any time based upon information received from law enforcement laboratories, state and local law enforcement and regulatory agencies, or other sources of information. Once the DEA has collected the necessary data, the DEA administrator, by authority of the U.S. Attorney General, requests from the HHS a scientific and medical evaluation and recommendation as to whether the drug or other substance should be controlled or removed from control. This request is sent to the assistant secretary of health of the HHS. Then the HHS solicits information from the Commissioner of the Food and Drug Administration (FDA) and evaluations and recommendations from the National Institute on Drug Abuse.

Once the DEA has received the scientific and medical evaluation from HHS, the administrator will evaluate all available data and make a final decision about whether to propose that a drug or other substance be controlled and into which schedule it should be placed. The medical and scientific evaluations are binding to the DEA with respect to scientific and medical matters. The recommendation on scheduling is binding only to the extent that if HHS recommends that the substance not be controlled, the DEA may not control the substance.

The History of the Scheduling of MDMA

In October of 1984, Congress enacted a ruling (Emergency Scheduling Act, 50 *Federal Register* entry [FR] 23118) to give the U.S Attorney General the power to schedule a drug for one year on an emergency basis and to bypass the typical process of lengthy hearings in cases where the public health is at risk. Furthermore, the Attorney General has the option of delegating this task to the DEA.

On July 1, 1985, the DEA placed MDMA in Schedule I on a temporary emergency basis for one year. After one year, the placement was extended by six months (51 *FR* 21911). It should be noted that when the DEA scheduled MDMA, they had not been delegated the task by the Attorney General and had basically jumped the gun. Because of this loophole, several MDMA distributors were able to escape their sentences in the mid-1980s.

On May 22, 1986, once the three hearings of the previous year were completed [see "The History of MDMA"] the administrative law judge Francis Young announced his recommendation: "The record now assembled contains much more material about MDMA than the Agency was aware of when it initiated this proceeding. The evidence of record does not establish that MDMA has a high potential for abuse. It cannot be placed in Schedule I because it does have a currently accepted medical use in treatment and it does have accepted safety for use under medical supervision. Based on this record it is the recommended decision of the administrative law judge that MDMA should be placed in Schedule III." [For a full transcript of the opinion and recommended ruling, see docket 84-48 at www.erowid.org/chemicals/mdma/mdma_law2.shtml.]

On November 13, 1986, MDMA was placed permanently in Schedule I (51 *FR* 36552). This ruling was appealed by Lester Grinspoon, M.D. The United States Court of Appeals for the First Circuit agreed with the petitioner that the method of deciding currently accepted medical use (saying it was not an FDA-accepted medication) was inappropriate and ordered the DEA to remove the drug from Schedule I on September 18, 1987. The drug was removed from Schedule I effective January 27, 1988 (53 *FR* 2225). On February 22, 1988, the DEA administrator again placed MDMA in Schedule I, effective on March 23, 1988 (53 FR 5156), and this action was not appealed.

An interesting piece of legislation that passed after MDMA was made illegal, in an effort to stem the tide of so-called designer drugs, was the Controlled Substances Analogue Enforcement Act of 1986. Drugs intended for human consumption that were substantially similar in structure and effect to drugs that were already in Schedule I or II were treated as if they were the scheduled drug itself and considered to be automatically placed into the same schedule as that drug. Thus, MDE (methylenedioxyethylamphetamine, or Eve) was placed in Schedule I by virtue of its similarity to MDMA. [For more details on scheduling, see "The History of MDMA." For Congress and Senate bills and laws, see also www.thomas.loc.gov, www.senate.gov, www.house.gov, and www.alchemind.org]

Recent MDMA Legal Maneuvers

The Anti-Ecstasy Proliferation Act

Senate bill 2612, proposed by Senator Robert Graham (D) of Florida and Senator Charles Grassley (R) of Iowa which was modified and rolled into the Children's Health Act of 2000 (Public Law 106-310), called for the United States Sentencing Commission to amend the federal sentencing guidelines to provide for higher penalties associated with the manufacture, distribution, and use of Ecstasy. Those penalties would be comparable to the base levels for offenses involving any methamphetamine mixture. Furthermore, the bill calls for greater emphasis on the education of young adults, the education and training of state and local law enforcement officials, and adequate funding for research by the National Institute on Drug Abuse.

The Methamphetamine and Club Drug Anti-Proliferation Act of 2000

Congressman Christopher Cannon's (R-Utah) methamphetamine bill, HR 2987, incorporates the major provisions of the Club Drug Anti-Proliferation Act (HR 4553) sponsored by Republican Congresswoman Judy Biggert of Illinois. HR 2987 calls for the United States Sentencing Commission to amend the federal sentencing guidelines to provide for higher penalties associated with the manufacture, distribution, and use of Ecstasy. Furthermore, the bill calls for five million dollars in funding to the public health service for school and community-based abuse and addiction prevention programs aimed at Ecstasy, PMA (paramethoxyamphetamine), and related club drugs.

The Club Drug Anti-Proliferation Act also contained an information ban section. It is described as illegal "to teach or demonstrate to any person the manufacture of a controlled substance, or to distribute to any person, by any means, information pertaining to, in whole or in part, the manufacture, acquisition, or use of a controlled substance, knowing or having reason to know that such person intends to use the teaching, demonstration, or information for, or in furtherance of, an activity that constitutes an offense."

This would have made it a crime to distribute information about the manufacture, acquisition, or use of a controlled substance. Specifically, the word "teaching" appeared in the original draft of HR 4553, which would have made the publication of this book a criminal offense. On July 25, 2000, the House Judiciary Committee struck the information ban from the bill but left unchanged the punishment provisions equating Ecstasy with methamphetamine.

On September 27, 2000, the Methamphetamine and Club Drug Anti-Proliferation Act of 2000 was incorporated into the Children's Health Act of 2000 (HR 4365), and this version passed in the House and Senate. The sentencing provision that would have equated MDMA with methamphetamine was removed. Instead the new law instructed the Sentencing Commission to use its own discretion in setting the penalty for Ecstasy and other club drug offenses and stated that Congress had a sense that the punishment for "high-level traffickers" of Ecstasy was not stringent enough and penalties should be increased.

In January 2001, under the Ecstasy Anti-Proliferation Act of 2000 (section 3664 of Public Law 106-310), Congress instructed the U.S. Sentencing Commission to increase the penalties for the manufacture, importation, exportation, or trafficking of MDMA. Federal sentencing guidelines are based on marijuana equivalents. For example, 1 g of powder cocaine equals 200 g of marijuana, 1 g of heroin equals 1 kg of marijuana, and 1 g of mescaline equals 10 g of marijuana. Under the old guidelines, 1 g of MDMA was equivalent to 35 g of marijuana. The new proposal, to equate 1 gram of MDMA with 1 kg (1,000 grams) of marijuana, was argued against at a public hearing on March 19 in Washington, D.C.; Drs. David Nichols, Charles Grob, Rick Doblin, Julie Holland, and Richard Glen Boire, among others, advised the sentencing commission as to the inadvisability of equating MDMA with heroin in terms of penalties.

In 1999 there were 4,705 deaths recorded attributed to heroin intoxication; 9 people died secondary to Ecstasy use. Compare this mortality ratio of more than 500 to 1 to a penalty ratio of 1 to 1. Further, although the proposal was to equate MDMA with heroin, gram for gram, their dosage units differ markedly. An average dose of heroin, 5 to 10 milligrams, is substantially less than 125 mg of MDMA. When adulterants and fillers are factored in, on a per dose basis, the penalties for Ecstasy are five times more serious than for heroin. On March 20, the U.S. Sentencing Commission voted unanimously to equate 1 gram of MDMA with 500 grams of marijuana. The commission, an independent federal agency that sets national sentencing policy, submitted this permanent rule to Congress, which went into effect May 1, 2001.

Penalties for Possession and Sale of MDMA in the United States

The average newspaper article about MDMA prior to 2001 frequently quoted "up to fifteen years in prison or a $125,000 fine" as the penalty for MDMA possession. This penalty has been cited repeatedly in articles about MDMA since its initial emergency scheduling in 1985. The penalties for MDMA possession or intent to distribute are complex. No mandatory minimum sentence exists for MDMA, as it does for some other drugs, such as crack cocaine. The maximum penalties are found in the statutes, but they are rarely enforced. The actual sentence is determined by federal sentencing guidelines, which are complicated by many aggravating and mitigating factors. It is basically a point system, which takes into account the weight of the drug, the criminal history of the defendant, and whether children, pregnant women, weapons, or serious injury or death were involved. Everyone with the same amount of MDMA will not have the same sentence. Pleading guilty and avoiding a trial allows for a reduction in points, as does cooperating with the authorities in making other cases for them. Moreover, intent to distribute often can be based on the amount of drug in the defendant's possession, rather than the behavior of the defendant. With a federal arrest and prosecution, the charge of trafficking and conspiracy is more likely than with a state charge.

The new sentencing guidelines to be followed by federal judges will increase the likely prison term for the sale of 200 grams of Ecstasy from fifteen months to more than five years. Under the old guidelines, a five-year prison sentence (level 26), would involve 2,857 grams of Ecstasy, anywhere from 11,500 to 46,000 pills, based on a pill weight of 250 mg to 350 mg. Under the new amendment, offenses involving 100 grams of Ecstasy, or 400 to 1,600 pills, would meet the criteria for a level 26 offense.

Before the new sentencing guidelines, the average prison sentence for MDMA possession was thirty-three months. The new law will increase the average penalty to ten years.

Although there is a statutory maximum limit of twenty years for a first offense, there are currently no federal mandatory minimum sentences involving Ecstasy. However, there is a sentencing guideline minimum: if intent to distribute is the charge, the offense level begins at 12, so a first-time offender can spend ten to sixteen months in prison regardless of the weight seized.

In New Orleans, a local DJ and a concert hall manager face up to twenty years in prison and $500,000 in fines for staging a rave. The prosecution by the Drug Enforcement Administration involves using the federal "crack house law." Passed by Congress in 1986 to combat crack cocaine, this law was designed to punish the owners or operators of houses used for the manufacture, storage, distribution, or use of illegal drugs. At the time of publication the case was not yet settled.

Examples of State Penalties

California

MDMA is not mentioned specifically, and state prosecutions are pursued under the Controlled Substances Analogue Enforcement Act of 1986. A person convicted of possessing a personal use amount of MDMA in California faces a maximum of one year in the county jail or state prison. "Diversion" is the more likely sentence, which is drug education or rehabilitation instead of prison. Punishment for possession of MDMA with intent to distribute carries a state prison term of sixteen months or two years or three years, depending on the offense level. Diversion is not an option.

As of April 2001 the California legislature was considering a bill (AB 1416) that threatens to (1) make MDMA a Schedule I controlled substance in California, and (2) make it a crime to be "under the influence" of MDMA in California. Those convicted of being under the influence of MDMA would be punished by a mandatory minimum of ninety-days in county jail and up to a maximum of one year in jail.

Delaware

A law is being proposed to increase the punishments for MDMA in this state. Possession of fifty or more doses would be considered trafficking and would receive a mandatory minimum term of imprisonment of three years and a fine of $50,000. Possession of one hundred or more doses would receive a mandatory minimum term of imprisonment of five years and a fine of $100,000. Possession of five hundred doses or more would receive a mandatory minimum term of imprisonment of fifteen years and a fine of $400,000.

New Jersey

Possession of MDMA carries a sentence of three to five years in prison, but a first-time offender could serve less than a year in county jail, regardless of the amount of drug seized.

Texas

Punishment for possession of MDMA in Texas depends on the drug weight: Less than 1 g is considered a state felony, with a mandatory minimum of 180 days in county jail, up to two years, and a fine of up to $10,000. Possession of 1 g but less than 4 g is a third-grade felony, with a mandatory two-year minimum sentence, up to ten years, and a fine of up to $10,000. Possession of 4 g but less than 400 g is a second-degree felony, with a mandatory two-year minimum sentence, up to twenty years, and fine of up to $10,000. Possession of 400 g or more receives a mandatory five-year minimum sentence, up to a possible life sentence.

The penalties for distribution or manufacture of MDMA or for possession with the intent to distribute are determined by weight of the MDMA seized. Less than 1 g is a state felony that carries a mandatory minimum sentence of 180 days in county jail, up to two years, and a fine of up to $10,000. Between 1 and 4 g is a second-degree felony with a mandatory two-year minimum, up to twenty years, and fine of up to $10,000. Between 4 g and 400 g is a first-degree felony, carrying a mandatory five-year minimum, up to possible life imprisonment and maximum $10,000 fine. For 400 g or more, a person gets a mandatory ten-year minimum sentence, with possible life imprisonment.

International Law Regarding MDMA

The World Health Organization and the United Nations Commission on Narcotic Drugs placed MDMA in Schedule I internationally on February 11, 1986.

Australia

MDMA is classified as a Schedule II "dangerous drug" as part of the Drugs Misuse Act 1990. Commonwealth penalties for possession are two years plus a $2,000 (approximately $1,000 U.S.) fine for a small quantity (less than half a gram). Possession of half a gram receives twenty-five years and a $100,000 (approximately $50,000 U.S.) fine. A "traffickable" quantity is between half a gram and 500 g. Possession of 500 g gets a life sentence. A commercial quantity is over 500 g.

Brazil

MDMA arrived in Brazil in the early 1990s. Its cost at that time ($30–60 per pill in U.S. currency) restricted its use to the elite. The drug was picked up on the law enforcement radar screen beginning in 1995, when large seizures began to occur.

The law that regulates illegal drugs in Brazil (Law No. 6368) went into effect on October 21, 1976. It does not mention any particular drug, but refers to narcotics and substances that create physical or psychological dependence. Article 6 of that law charges the Ministry of Health with determining which substances are to be controlled. MDMA is listed as a psychotropic substance that is prohibited in Brazil in accordance with Resolution RDC No. 62 of July 3, 2000. The penalties are a prison term of six months to two years for users, and three to fifteen years for traffickers. The resolution does not mention any quantities. A range of fines are specified, which are tied to an index defined by the judge according to currency fluctuations and inflation. A new law is currently being discussed.

Canada

The legislation that governs MDMA, the Controlled Drugs and Substances Act, passed on May 14, 1997. MDMA is listed in Schedule III. Importing or trafficking in MDMA is a crime liable to imprisonment for a term not exceeding ten years. It is punished less harshly than cannabis (Schedule II) or cocaine (Schedule I).

China

The minimum penalty for possession is a sentence of less than three years in prison plus a fine. The maximum sentence is seven years to life in prison plus a fine. The minimum penalty for trafficking is seven years in prison plus a fine. The maximum sentence is fifteen years to life in prison or even death, plus confiscation of property. MDMA was added to the existing drug law (which was written largely about opium) on March 14, 1997. The slang term for MDMA in China is "head-rocking pills."

Greece

Ecstasy has been classified as a Schedule I drug since 1987 (Law 1729). Its use is illegal, even for psychiatrists, without a special order from the Ministry of Health. Possession for personal use brings a penalty of up to six months' imprisonment. For manufacture, sale, distribution, importing or exporting, the penalty is up to ten years.

Hong Kong

The penalty for possession is a fine of 100,000–1,000,000 Hong Kong dollars (approximately US$1 = HK$7.8) and imprisonment for three to seven years. The penalty for trafficking is a fine of HK$500,000–5,000,000 and imprisonment for three years to life. These laws were enacted on June 30, 1997, the last day of British rule.

India

The Narcotics and Psychotropics Substances Act (1985) has two schedules, which supposedly are updated regularly. According to the 1999 version, however, Ecstasy/MDMA was not listed. It is unclear whether there has been an update or if there have been any prosecuted cases involving Ecstasy. All judgments related to drug use depend on the quantity (personal use vs. trafficking). Anyone found with narcotics on their person is subject to up to ten years' imprisonment. Prosecution for possession of less than 5 g is up to the judge's discretion.

Israel

MDMA has been considered an illegal drug since 1991. In 1998 a few derivatives were declared illegal, including MDA and MMDA (3 methoxy 4,5 methylenedioxyamphetamine). The penalty for possession for personal use is up to three years' incarceration. Selling to minors carries a penalty of up to twenty-five years' imprisonment and trafficking up to twenty years' imprisonment.

Italy

There is no law that specifically covers MDMA. The penalties for sale or possession are those for Schedule I drugs in that country. It seems as though the authorities are much more interested in heavy trafficking, especially on an international basis; possession of small amounts of MDMA is rarely prosecuted. The penalties for sale or manufacture, or import/export are incarceration from eight to twenty years and a fine of 50,000,000 to 500,000,000 lire (approximately $2,500 to $25,000 U.S.). For possession of a smaller quantity (not considered trafficking), the penalty is one to six years and a fine of 5,000,000 to 50,000,000 lire (approximately $250 to $2,500).

Singapore

Ecstasy was cited as a "class A controlled drug" in the Misuse of Drugs Act in 1992. The penalty for possession and consumption of MDMA is a fine of up to 20,000 Singapore dollars (approximately US$1 = S$1.7) or ten years imprisonment or both. The penalty for trafficking (possession of more than 10 g of the drug) is up to twenty years' imprisonment and fifteen strokes of the cane. Illegal import or export carries a penalty of up to thirty years in prison and fifteen strokes of the cane.

Spain

In Spanish legislation, MDMA is considered to "cause serious damage to the health." Nevertheless, since May 30, 1986, the possession of MDMA for personal use (less than twenty tablets) has not been punished. In terms of larger amounts, the penalties for those who cultivate, manufacture, traffic in, or otherwise promote, favor, or facilitate illegal use or who possess MDMA with those aims are a prison sentence of three to nine years and a fine of three times the price of the amount of drug seized (Spanish Penal Code, article 368).

Switzerland

Switzerland's Supreme Court ruled in June 1999 that dealing in Ecstasy is not a serious crime. MDMA remains illegal there but is considered a "soft drug." The Federal Tribunal ruled that while Ecstasy is in no way a harmless substance, there is no evidence that it poses a serious health risk. The drug is used mostly by "socially integrated people" and does not generally lead to criminal behavior, said the court. Swiss drug legislation allows the use of MDMA for medical or research purposes, depending on case-by-case permission from the Swiss Federal Health Office.

United Kingdom

MDMA was added to the 1971 Misuse of Drugs Act in 1977. The penalty for possession is up to seven years in prison and an unlimited fine. The penalty for trafficking is up to life in prison and an unlimited fine. In 1977, Great Britain amended its Misuse of Drugs Act to label all ring-substituted amphetamines (including MDMA, MDA, MDE—anything with an amphetamine basic structure upon which chemical substitutions have been made) as class A drugs. MDMA was included in the list of drugs specified in Schedule I of the Misuse of Drugs regulations of 1985, that is, it is considered to have no acknowledged therapeutic use. An amendment of the Misuse of Drugs Act to include another thirty-six identified substances is under discussion. It is interesting that these drugs are discussed in terms of their similarity to MDMA rather than their basic chemical structure (www.homeoffice.gov.uk/drugslet.htm).

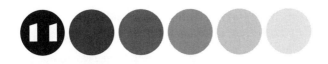

MINIMIZING RISK IN THE DANCE COMMUNITY

An Interview with Emanuel Sferios

JH: What does DanceSafe do, and what is your role there?

ES: DanceSafe is a drug abuse prevention program, and I am the founder and executive director. We utilize a harm reduction and popular education philosophy that also can be referred to as a peer-based education model. We have chapters in about fifteen cities now, which are made up of young people within the rave and nightclub community, many of whom are users of dance drugs themselves, though some are not. We train these volunteers to be drug abuse prevention counselors, harm reduction workers, and health and safety educators within their own communities. Our main activity is setting up booths at events where Ecstasy, ketamine, and GHB (gammahydroxybutyrate) are used. We provide harm reduction literature, and our volunteers engage their peers in discussions about drug use by employing "pop ed" or peer counseling techniques. These methods avoid the use of the imperative (should, shouldn't, do, don't) and ask open-ended questions. Our goal is to empower users to reflect on their own drug use and the reasons they may be using or abusing drugs so that they can make more informed decisions about their health and safety.

JH: Can you tell me about your pill-testing program?

ES: We provide adulterant screening services, also known as pill testing.

There are three branches of this program. One is onsite pill testing, which has gained us a lot of media attention. It is a very effective outreach tool as well as a harm reduction service. We screen supposed Ecstasy tablets for adulterants by using a chemical reagent. The user will approach the booth and usually hand the pill over to one of the trained harm reduction workers. The volunteer will measure the pill, scrape some material from the pill onto a white ceramic plate, and hand the pill back to the user. We put a drop of a chemical reagent onto the scrapings; depending on the color change, we can tell whether there is an Ecstasy-like substance in the pill. By "Ecstasy-like," we mean MDMA, MDA, or MDE, though MDE is very rare. It is a test for the presence of an Ecstasy-like substance in the tablet; it is not a test for purity or strength. There could be something else in the pill, but it is a useful test despite its inability to detect purity because most of the pills on the U.S. market today that contain MDMA or MDA do not contain anything else. Conversely, most of the pills that contain something else do not contain MDMA, so they won't change the appropriate color under the Marquis reagent—the chemical in the test kit—which is available on our Web site [www.Dancesafe.org].

JH: How do you know that some tablets on the U.S. market contain adulterants and some don't?

ES: We have another program for adulterant screening besides the onsite testing and the testing kits. We offer a laboratory pill analysis program. We have contracted with a Drug Enforcement Administration (DEA)–licensed laboratory in Sacramento, California, that is allowed to handle controlled substances. We have set up an Internet-based program where users or anyone else can send an unknown tablet to the lab, directly and anonymously, and the lab will test the pill using gas chromatography and mass spectrometry. They provide us with a picture of the pill, the results of the analysis, and information concerning where the pill was obtained and the date it was acquired. We post all of this information on our web site, usually in less than two weeks. This way the user, and anyone else, can see the actual ingredients of the tablet and be able to avoid tablets that have potentially more dangerous compounds, like PMA.

JH: Let's talk about PMA.

ES: PMA (paramethoxyamphetamine) is a hallucinogenic amphetamine, unlike MDMA. Approximately eight years ago a large batch of PMA tablets was introduced into the Ecstasy market in Europe, manufactured by someone who most likely was trying to avoid the penalties associated with MDMA. Another reason why PMA may have been introduced on the market is that precursor chemicals used to make it are more readily available and not as strictly controlled, so that the expense and risk of purchasing precursors to MDMA are avoided. The problem is that PMA is an extremely dangerous compound. It was experimented with in the 1970s, when people were looking at various psychoactive compounds, but it never became a popular recreational drug, because some people died. The dose level that appears to be somewhat safe is below 50 mg, but at doses even slightly higher than that, heart rate and blood pressure can rise dramatically.

JH: And temperature?

ES: And body temperature as well. So an Ecstasy user is unlikely to die or experience serotonin syndrome or a heatstroke reaction [hyperthermia] if they take only one pill that contains PMA. If they take three or four, however, they are very likely to have a severe adverse reaction. There have been probably more than two dozen deaths resulting from PMA overdoses.

JH: Is that in the last eight years? Were they clustered around certain dates?

ES: We know that there have been nine deaths in the United States since April 2000. First, there were three in the spring in the Chicago area and then six in Florida during the summer. And then there was one, or perhaps two, in the Toronto area in the fall. In the spring of 2000, there were half a dozen deaths in Australia from the same batch, and before that, there were deaths in Europe and England. It seems that the pills will cause one high-profile death or more in a country. These pills are very distinctively marked. They are the Mitsubishi tablets—they have the three-diamond logo of the company stamped on the pill, which is a popular Ecstasy brand. [While it is common for Ecstasy pills to have corporate logos such as the Nike swoosh, the Calvin Klein CK, or Mitsubishi's three diamonds, it should be made clear that these companies are in no way involved with the manufacture or distribution of Ecstasy. Clandestine labs that stamp Ecstasy pills have co-opted these logos as a way to "brand" and differentiate their tablets.—Ed.]

JH: There was an article in New York *magazine about three years ago naming Mitsubishi as a particularly good brand of Ecstasy. I imagine that they capitalized on the popularity of that logo when making PMA.*

ES: Yes, and that is a fairly irresponsible article, because there have always been copycat pills available. A brand name absolutely does not have any bearing on the ingredients of a tablet. The impetus for the information in this article probably came from England. Back in the mid-1990s in England, a very large batch of Mitsubishi tablets was introduced that were about 150 mg of MDMA; this reinvigorated the Ecstasy market because before that fake and adulterated tablets were prevalent.

JH: I seem to remember hearing that there was a lot more methamphetamine in England for a period of time, that it was hard to get MDMA.

ES: Right. There will always be a balance between the fake pills and appropriate therapeutic/recreational dose pills, as long as there continues to be prohibition and an unregulated market. And that is because it will optimize the profit potential of the manufacturers. Basically, you need to keep people coming back and risking fake pills, because enough of the time they will get a real one. When people stopped using Ecstasy in the early nineties, or slowed down their use, the manufacturers realized that they had better put out some good pills to get the customers back. These happened to be Mitsubishis. As soon as they became popular, there were tons of Mitsubishi copycats, including these PMA tablets.

JH: What do you make of the DEA's report that less than 1 percent of the Ecstasy tablets in the United States contain adulterants. Why would they say something that irresponsible?

ES: There are probably two reasons. It could very well be that the pills that they confiscate are ones that have been "sniffed out" by dogs that are trained to identify MDMA. It also could be that the tactics used by the DEA or other federal agents are generally geared to apprehend low-level dealers and persuade them to turn on the higher-level dealers and then work their way up. I'm only speculating about this.

JH: My take on it is that the DEA wants to portray MDMA as more dangerous than it is. So if another drug (or drugs) is responsible for some of the casualties, they would rather have it look as though MDMA were involved.

ES: That would be my second reason, which is that they are simply being disingenuous. Perhaps they feel that the testing kits are a threat to their ideology, because they provide users with a safer way to consume the drug, and they see anything that promotes safer use or reduces harm as counter to the abstention-only model. The drug war and the drug-prevention strategy that comes out of it tend to use simple scare tactics. The notion that there may be other drugs besides Ecstasy on the market that are producing deaths and adverse reactions runs counter to their ideology, so they're making this ridiculous claim. If you look at our laboratory pill analysis program as well as the government-funded pill testing programs in other countries like Holland and Switzerland, you see very clearly that a large percentage of the pills being sold as Ecstasy—and made to look just like Ecstasy tablets, with the logos and colors—do not contain MDMA. You see many other compounds, such as methamphetamine (speed) phencyclidine [PCP (angel dust)], ketamine, dextromethorphan (DXM), caffeine, ephedrine, and so on. We had one pill that was cocaine. We never found a heroin tablet, though. That is largely a rumor.

JH: Let's talk about DXM for a minute, because I think that deserves separate mention.

ES: When we first started our adulterant screening program both in the lab and onsite, we correlated the majority of the heatstroke emergencies in the Oakland, California, rave community with the use of dextromethorphan.

JH: These were the green pills shaped like a triangle?

ES: Yes. Early on, when we were going to Oakland massives—"massive" is the term used within the rave culture to refer to a very large commercial rave, five thousand to thirty thousand people—we would test about two hundred pills an evening onsite. Early on it might have been that about twenty pills of two hundred were fake. Some of them would have a very strange reaction, so that it appeared that it might be an Ecstasy-like compound, but we weren't sure.

JH: What color should the test substance turn if it's MDMA?

ES: MDMA or MDA will turn black right away. DXM eventually turns black, but it's a slower reaction. There's a five- to ten-second delay at the beginning, and then it turns slowly gray; after about thirty seconds, it's black. It's the time sequence that really indicates the difference between an Ecstasy-like compound and DXM. There were some green triangles going around that gave this strange reaction, and we hadn't seen them before. When one showed up at our laboratory that contained dextromethorphan, we became aware.

JH: And was it a particularly high dose?

ES: Well, we didn't quantitatively test it then. At the next rave, in September of 1999, of two hundred pills we tested there were forty fake pills, and the vast majority of them were the green triangle DXM pills. Typically, we might see perhaps five to ten people go to the medical room at these massives in Oakland.

JH: Is there some kind of first aid tent at the massives?

ES: It depends on the promoter, but these promoters were responsible. They had trained medical staff with oxygen and a first aid room. Typically, there are no emergencies where a person has to be hospitalized. Maybe once every three or four events, there will be a heatstroke emergency. Five to ten people might go to the medical room because they are "freaking out" or a little bit overheated or dehydrated, so they can get fluids and cool off and relax. At this particular event there were dozens of people going to the medical room, and there were nine people who had to be hospitalized. We work closely with medical staff.

JH: So you were obviously concerned about these bigger numbers.

ES: Yes. We are there when people are seeking medical assistance, and we would ask them what they had taken. Their friends would say, "Ecstasy." And we would say, "No. What did the pill look like?" And they would answer, "It was a green triangle." We were able to correlate the ingestion of DXM pills with the majority of the heatstroke emergencies. Eight of the nine people hospitalized that evening had taken the green triangles. Some of them had combined it with other brands of Ecstasy, and others had not.

This led us to investigate why dextromethorphan could be contributing to heatstroke emergencies at raves. There are examples in the medical literature of cases of dextromethorphan-induced serotonin syndrome in patients taking normal doses of DXM with other medications that are contraindicated. DXM is a mild serotonin releaser and reuptake inhibitor, so it has the same kind of thermal deregulation as MDMA. It is also a CYP2D6 inhibitor, like MDMA. [See "How MDMA Works in the Brain" and "Medical Problems Associated with MDMA Use" for details on this enzyme required to metabolize MDMA.] If combined with MDMA, it could interfere with its metabolism.

JH: It also is an NMDA [N-methyl-D-aspartate receptor] antagonist, similar in action to PCP, at higher doses. At lower doses it is a cough suppressant, but at higher doses it is a dissociative anesthetic.

ES: The problem is that high-dose DXM tablets are being sold to people as if they were MDMA. These users expecting and looking for mood elevation, empathy, and the warm, loving experience of MDMA are getting a very trippy, out-of-body, dissociative effect with loss of motor control and disorientation. If they combine it with MDMA, which exacerbates the DXM effect, it contributes greatly to the number of medical emergencies at raves. We will soon be marketing two new testing kits: a secondary amine test that can distinguish between MDMA and MDA if used in conjunction with the first Marquis kit, and a third reagent that clarifies any ambiguity between DXM and the Ecstasy-like compounds.

JH: Is there a way to test specifically for PMA?

ES: Our reagent will not change color if the substance you're testing is PMA. This has been an issue that our detractors have brought up, that the kit isn't useful because it cannot positively identify PMA, the most dangerous adulterant.

JH: But if it doesn't turn a color, then it has at least identified a bogus pill.

ES: That's exactly right. The kit is useful because it screens out all the pills that do not contain MDMA. And all the pills that have been found to contain PMA have not contained MDMA. This was unknown by the DEA early on; they were not networking with health organizations in other countries as we have, and they thought that people were producing PMA in this country and potentially mixing it with MDMA and releasing it. That's simply not the case. The PMA tablets have come from the same initial batch or two. They look the same, they are Mitsubishi tablets of the same size, they are white or slightly off-white, and they seem to be circling the globe leaving behind a trail of dead Ecstasy users. When they cause high-profile deaths in one country, the dealers who have bought a few hundred thousand of them can't sell them anymore. Everyone in that country knows not to buy the Misubishis, because the media have publicized these deaths. So they lay low for a few months and sell the pills to someone in another country, because they want to recoup their losses.

JH: This has been going on for eight years now.

ES: Eight years, the same pills. The good news is that we are not seeing a bunch of new people producing PMA and selling it. It's as if it was one mistake from which we are still seeing repercussions. After this batch runs out, we hope that we won't see another one. The bad news is there are probably a lot of them still on the market, and they will be cropping up for years to come.

It's also been very irresponsible of the media, law enforcement, the DEA, the drug czar Jim McDonough in Florida, and the Florida department of law enforcement to be describing PMA as if it were simply another recreational drug. They will issue statements calling it "another dangerous variant of Ecstasy" or "just the newest designer drug in a line of deadly threats to your children," leading many to believe that PMA has a demand and a recreational market. This could very well lead people to start manufacturing and selling it, unaware that it's not a very pleasant experience and most people don't like the feeling. They will be unaware that it is very dangerous.

JH: As opposed to harm reduction, in what other ways do you think the government is creating more harm than they're preventing?

ES: The Just Say No model, the abstention model of drug abuse prevention, which took off under Nancy Reagan, has been a miserable failure. It's counterproductive in many ways. The use of such simplistic messages "Drugs Kill" or "Winners Don't Use Drugs" and the reliance upon these slogans and scare tactics, as opposed to providing accurate information on pharmacology and harm reduction techniques, basically turns off young people. They don't trust the information, because they recognize immediately that they are being lied to, that they are hearing only one side of the story. Even if the information is not an outright lie, if you only provide information on the dangers and not the benefits or the desirable effects of the drug, you will have a problem. If you don't answer the primary questions that people have when they hear about a drug—Why are so many people using this? What is the appeal?—then instinctively and immediately people know that you have a moral agenda and that you are not giving them all the information. Then they won't believe the information you do give them on the risks and dangers. They will dismiss it as just more propaganda. For example, if you go to the National Institute on Drug Abuse (NIDA) Web site and you read their information on Ecstasy, it's like reading a list of the potential side effects of hundreds of drugs in the *Physician's Desk Reference*: nausea, paranoia, seizures, panic attacks, depression, and so on.

JH: There's not one desirable effect of the drug listed.

ES: Right. The mother or father of the user, or someone who has never used Ecstasy, is left wondering, "Well, why would anyone want to repeat this experience?" In fact, they're not left with that, because they know people *are* repeating this experience. Instead they're left thinking that this is misinformation. Obviously, this drug affects people differently than NIDA says. So they look elsewhere. They come to the DanceSafe Web site, for example, where we first list the desired effects that explain why people are using this drug, thus winning their trust. Then they go on to read information on the risks and harms. The statistics on the web site confirm that they do go on to read more. We receive approximately 250,000 hits a day, with about ten thousand unique visitors a day. The most interesting statistic is that the average length of stay for someone on our Web site is sixteen minutes.

JH: Your site is getting a quarter million hits a day. That's amazing. It sounds as if there are a lot of people who want to know about the risks and benefits of Ecstasy use.

ES: People come back to the site to look for new laboratory test results on the adulterant screening program or to order testing kits, as well as to get educated about Ecstasy and other club drugs. All of the Ecstasy promoting that the government is doing right now in their media campaign has generated immense interest in the drug over the past year. Since April, when the anti–club drugs campaign started, our hits have increased tenfold. The point of the sixteen-minute visit is that people are reading the information that we provide, because our Web site is very information-based. There are not a lot of pictures. It's also a testament to the success of the harm reduction approach and why the Just Say No model does not work with teenagers.

I would like to qualify my criticism of the Just Say No model. I think it does work very well for grade-school children. The problem is that we are trying to apply a prevention model designed for grade-schoolers to teenagers. And teenagers are a completely different animal. When children get into middle school and high school, they start becoming responsible; they start becoming inquisitive. While the majority of young people are not going to experiment with illicit drugs, a great many teenagers do. We have novelty-seeking genes in our gene pool, and many people are simply curious. These people need to have accurate information and harm reduction services in order to make informed decisions.

JH: One reason that you need to have an adulterant-screening program is that we have prohibition in this country. Because of our drug policy and because these drugs are illegal and therefore are sold on the "black market," no one is regulating them and screening for impurities. I heard that the government is trying to prosecute people for murder if they have sold Ecstasy to someone who dies of an adverse reaction.

ES: Right. There's a law that allows a state to prosecute dealers, and by dealers they mean anyone who might have supplied a drug to anyone else, regardless of whether any money changed hands. If you supply someone with an illicit substance and that person happens to die after they consume it, this law states that you can be prosecuted for murder. There was a case in Florida recently where a young woman died after taking PMA. Her boyfriend had consumed the PMA tablets as well; he was the one who supplied the pills to her. He survived, but she died. The state wanted to prosecute him for murder, but they changed the charges to manslaughter, in part because her parents would not support the murder charges against their daughter's boyfriend.

JH: The problem is that people are going to be even less likely to take their friends to the hospital or to get medical attention for someone if they're worried about being prosecuted for murder. Once again the government is creating more harm than they're reducing.

ES: The drug war ideology tends to scapegoat not just users and dealers but also the drug itself. As a society, we are all responsible for the public health. We have drug policies that maximize the harm to users of psychoactive drugs. We need to accept responsibility and change our policy to one of harm reduction. To avoid accepting that responsibility, the drug warriors are looking to scapegoat anyone they can, to blame this death on the boyfriend of the girl who died, when he himself almost died. Their rationale is that this is going to make someone think twice before they sell someone else a drug. This is bad social science. Economics 101: demand creates a market. With an unregulated market, there is always going to be someone willing to sell Ecstasy or GHB or heroin to anyone who is willing to buy it, and drugs have a high demand. So this is a ridiculous notion. It is not going to slow down the spread of Ecstasy. It's not going to make someone think twice about selling Ecstasy to his or her friends. Instead, it will make someone think twice before calling an ambulance when the friend starts having an adverse reaction, like collapsing on the dance floor from heatstroke. People might get the gas chamber or spend the rest of their lives in jail if it comes out that it was they who supplied the pill, because they can be prosecuted for murder. There needs to be amnesty for any 911 call for any situation.

JH: I certainly agree with that.

ES: And, again, the fear that is generated by prohibitionist drug policies is not conducive to health and safety. This is a very stark example.

JH: That brings us to what we neglected to do at the beginning of this conversation, which is to define harm reduction.

ES: Most basically, harm reduction is an alternative approach to dealing with societal drug use or other criminalized behavior, like prostitution. It works with people to help them manage their behavior and minimize the harm that might result. Harm reduction provides an alternative to the "abstention only" model. While abstention is the only way to avoid all the harms associated with drug use, many people choose not to abstain. As long as that's the case, regardless of our moral stance on recreational drug use, it presents an immediate need to minimize these harms. Harm reduction programs provide accurate and useful information on drugs, information that drug users can utilize to minimize the risks and the potential harms from their use. Along with information, harm reduction programs provide similar services. Needle exchange is the most widely known example of a harm reduction service, to limit the spread of human immunodeficiency virus (HIV), hepatitis, and other diseases.

JH: Another example is giving out condoms to teenagers. Another way of looking at harm reduction is to see things like seatbelts or motorcycle helmets as examples. People are going to engage in risky behaviors. Harm reduction is about educating people in how to make any potentially dangerous behavior less risky. It doesn't have to be about drugs.

ES: You're right. Harm reduction is an approach used in many areas of society. Seatbelts and condoms are perfect examples. For a long time people felt that distributing condoms encouraged premarital sex. I think that now people are more educated and realize that is not the case. No one feels horny after seeing a condom machine.

JH: But I think there still is the idea that needle exchange promotes intravenous drug use, which is also silly. You either shoot your drugs, or you don't. People are forced to share dirty needles because they are so difficult to come by, which increases the transmission of HIV, not just among drug users but also among their sex partners. There has been a recent shift in the drug policy, allowing needle exchange programs to exist and doctors to prescribe needles. I think our government is coming around a little bit, slowly, in some ways, about harm reduction. Why would there be a need for harm reduction in the Ecstasy-using community and specifically in the rave community?

ES: Well, let's talk about the risks of Ecstasy use. The most common risk of using Ecstasy is not getting what you think you're getting. There are many substances sold as Ecstasy that can be more dangerous. Another risk is heatstroke. MDMA, along with many other drugs, inhibits the body's thermoregulatory system. In a cold environment, users report feeling really cold; in a hot environment, the body can overheat. The heatstroke emergencies, however, are not the result of MDMA alone. They are the result of a confluence of factors that are more closely correlated with the behavior of users and the environment that they're in. The majority of deaths after taking Ecstasy have been from heatstroke, and the majority of heatstroke cases have occurred at raves. At raves, the dance floor may be extremely hot, the promoters may overcrowd their venues trying to make more money, and the user may be dancing for many hours without replenishing lost body fluids. So when you're in a hot environment, engaging in intense aerobic activity, not replenishing your body fluids, and taking a stimulant-type drug that can inhibit your thermoregulatory ability, you can get heatstroke. In fact, you can remove the drug from the equation and still have heatstroke. We have seen people collapse on the dance floor from heatstroke when they haven't taken any drug. You see long distance runners do the same thing.

JH: I noticed you use the word "heatstroke" instead of hyperthermia. Why is that?

ES: I think that it gets the point across that this is a common occurrence in society apart from drug use. I used to call it "serotonin syndrome" on the Web site, but I got the feeling the kids were not understanding it. Calling these heatstroke emergencies "Ecstasy overdoses" or otherwise simply blaming heatstroke on the drug does not allow us to effect change to prevent this from occurring in the future. If we don't look at the confounding factors that contribute to these deaths, we will have no way to prevent them. It is misleading and irresponsible to call these deaths Ecstasy overdoses for one very important reason: in trying to blame the drug rather than the circumstances and behavior, the drug warriors are giving young people the impression that as long as they take only one tablet, they will be okay. They won't overdose. These are not deaths from overdose; these are heatstroke deaths. Moreover, people have died after having taken only one tablet of Ecstasy.

JH: It is not the drug, it's the behavior. In clinical MDMA research, when the subjects are given pure MDMA in a relaxed environment, there are no cases of hyperthermia. At the most, the body temperature goes up by 1 degree, and even that hasn't been seen uniformly. So it isn't so much the drug as the rave setting. Charlie Grob has gone so far as to say that one of the worst settings to take MDMA would be the rave setting. It really isn't smart to be dancing for eight to ten hours in a place where you can't get access to cold water and you don't take a break. I think one of the things that the harm reduction movement has done is to educate people that they need to take breaks. They need to go to the "chill-out room" and drink water. Have you addressed the issue of overhydration? Speaking of taking only one tablet of Ecstasy, one of the most famous Ecstasy deaths is thought to be a case of overhydration. I am thinking of Leah Betts—she took only one Ecstasy tablet.

ES: A few people have died, and there have been many medical emergencies related to overhydration and hyponatremia [low blood sodium]. People who drink too much water, or who sweat out all their electrolytes and replace them with water instead of an isotonic sports drink that has water and salt, are all at risk. Drinking too much water can cause your tissues to swell. When your brain swells, you can have seizures or go into a coma and die. This has happened on a number of occasions. One of the challenges has been that early on, when people started collapsing from heatstroke, the harm reduction message was "drink water, drink water, drink water." This led some people to believe that if they were having a bad experience they should drink lots and lots of water to come down.

JH: I think people misinterpreted this message, thinking water was an antidote or a way to flush it out of your system, which is inaccurate.

ES: Right. After Leah Betts died and became the poster child for the anti-Ecstasy movement in the United Kingdom, "Ecstasy makes your brain explode" was the tabloid cover story. But it isn't true. Drinking too much water makes your brain swell, which can kill you. After Leah died, the harm reduction message became drink water but not too much water, and isotonic sports beverages are better. Two to four cups an hour is about right if you're sweating. This leads into the whole safe-setting campaign that we started, following the model of other countries. You can educate users on their behavior, but you also need to educate promoters and club owners and, in fact, regulate the rave industry. There are promoters who will turn off the cold-water taps in the bathroom and sell bottled water at the bar for up to six dollars for eight ounces, as we've seen.

JH: My understanding is that there is now a law in Manchester, in the United Kingdom, requiring promoters to have water available free of charge in the clubs.

ES: We also have worked with the health department in San Francisco and passed a free water ordinance; now club owners have to provide some form of access to cold drinking water. They were resistant to this legislation, because they felt it would cut into their profits. Then we told them that if they put on their promotional literature that they're providing free water, they could increase the cover charge. People will still come, because patrons will appreciate what they're doing. It should be illegal everywhere to charge people for water in a hot environment, where they need it for survival.

JH: Can you think of some other risks prevalent in the rave community that require harm reduction?

ES: Depression is a big risk. The overuse of Ecstasy can cause or exacerbate symptoms of depression in some people. MDMA is not a daily antidepressant to be taken over the long term. It is an acute antidepressant. As a serotonin releaser, it also depletes serotonin, and so it can produce symptoms of depression between uses. I am convinced that many compulsive Ecstasy users are unconsciously self-medicating their preexisting depression.

JH: I think so too.

ES: There's a stigma in our society about depression. Many people are not comfortable admitting that they are taking an antidepressant, but there is not a stigma in many youth cultures about taking Ecstasy. It's interesting to me that I see a lot of first-time Ecstasy users who say exactly the same thing that people who are taking Prozac or Paxil say. "I feel better than I've ever felt in my life." And they want to repeat the experience.

In our peer counseling practice, we have educated users on the pharmacological effects of MDMA. We tell them that it is a serotonin releaser and that SSRIs [serotonin reuptake inhibitors, such as Prozac and Zoloft] also will increase serotonin. We say that if they're using MDMA a bit too often, they should consider the possibility that they are self-medicating depression. Perhaps they would benefit from proper diagnosis and treatment. In fact, we've seen many users subsequently seek appropriate treatment, start taking an SSRI, and stop taking Ecstasy. It is also common for someone to come up to our booth and report, with some concern, "My friends all took the same pills that I took, and they're all rolling really hard. I even took two, and I don't feel anything. I used to feel Ecstasy, and now it doesn't work. Is there something wrong with me?" And I'll ask them, "Have you started taking an antidepressant?" Usually, they're very surprised, because they hadn't told anyone. They'll ask, "How did you know?" And I'll explain to them that SSRIs prevent the Ecstasy from working by blocking the serotonin reuptake site where MDMA binds. And then I'll ask them, "Do you think you will stop taking your medication in order to experience your Ecstasy highs again?" And not one of them has said yes. They've all valued their antidepressant medication and the positive impact it has had on their lives more than their monthly or weekly Ecstasy experience.

JH: Are there any other harm reduction tips you want to impart?

ES: The international slogan for Ecstasy harm reduction is "Less Is More." We are making T-shirts that have this slogan on the front and the Dancesafe logo on the back. Pharmacologically, with any psychoactive drug, that is the truth. You will enhance the benefits and minimize the harm by using lower doses less often. You do not build up as big a tolerance as quickly, and you reduce the risk of neurotoxicity, the "cracked out" feeling that comes afterward (as users call it), and the potential for depression. As John Cloud said in his *Time* magazine cover story [2000], it may not be a good thing to reproduce the best experience of your life too often.

This leads into the notion of benefit enhancement. One of the reasons I think there is so much abuse among young people is that they are not presented with any socially sanctioned ways and reasons to use the drug. The drug becomes simply a "party drug." The therapeutic history of MDMA is lost on a lot of young people. They have no idea about it, and they lack respect for the drug. Our society tells them that wanting to feel good or recreate with illicit drugs makes them bad people. Using drugs becomes simply a rebellious act. Taking five or ten pills and getting as "high" as they can is a large part of the culture.

I sometimes call my harm reduction lectures "respecting Ecstasy," because I think that when young people are taught responsible use information, they are given respect for appropriate ways to enjoy the drug. To do that, you need to acknowledge the potential benefits of using the drug in moderation. You can use MDMA in such a way that you're not being self-destructive. Our current drug policy, and the drug culture promoted by the drug warriors, denies young people that model.

A perfect example is the differences in alcohol abuse by young people in America compared with Europe. America has a huge problem with binge drinking, especially on college campuses. In European countries, where teenagers are allowed to drink and where they have a glass of wine at the dinner table with their parents, they learn socially sanctioned ways to drink. There is simply not the problem of teenage binge drinking in those countries. Likewise, in the United States, we utilize responsible drinking messages, because we recognize and provide, at least to adults, socially sanctioned recreational uses of alcohol. We call it social drinking. It's a way to relax after a hard day at the office and so on. We don't tell people that if they choose to drink, they should drink as safely as possible. This is the way that harm reduction frames its messages. The DanceSafe motto is "If you choose to use, use as safely as possible."

Ultimately, we are going to change the description of our organization from a harm reduction organization to a responsible use organization. From the very beginning, we have clearly defined ourselves as harm reduction for the nonaddicted user, for the recreational drug user. Like alcohol, people can use MDMA socially and responsibly. We are trying to educate the broader society as well, and we haven't started to use responsible use messages yet. Nonetheless, we need to model our message on successful responsible drinking campaigns. I see DanceSafe not merely as an educational organization trying to educate individual users, but also as a marketing organization using social marketing techniques to affect social behavior and create a responsible drug culture.

That may seem radical to many people, but if all it took were education to change social behavior, you would not see advertising today. Marketing is used to increase and channel consumption by the population. We need to use the same marketing techniques to limit self-abusive behaviors among recreational drug users. That means changing the culture. Instead of saying "I'm rebellious, and I'm bad because I'm using this drug, and so I might as well take as many drugs as I can and get wasted out of my mind," a person could say, "These drugs have legitimate therapeutic and recreational uses, and these are the appropriate, responsible ways to use them."

MDMA-ASSISTED
PSYCHOTHERAPY

Introduction

Self-love. Joy. Forgiveness. Acceptance. Peace. These are the goals of long-term psychotherapy. These are the rewards of years of difficult soul-searching and pouring over the most painful details of one's life with a stranger, who slowly becomes a partner in making sense of it all. These are also the feelings experienced by many when they take MDMA for the first time. The drug gives the user access to these emotions, because it helps remove their blockade. Fear. Think of MDMA as an immediately acting "anti-neurotic" drug. All the defenses that typically get in the way of self-discovery and disclosure melt away, replaced by courage to take a thorough inventory and share what is found.

There is little debate that good psychotherapy works. Working in partnership with a therapist, digging in the dirt to find the places where you got hurt, to paraphrase the musician Peter Gabriel, is bound to reveal the important pieces of your life's puzzle. Take the time to explore your innermost feelings, confront your demons, tackle your core issues, and you will be healthier, happier, lighter, cleaner. Good psychotherapy, like a fine wine, takes time to ripen. The alliance you build with your therapist matures gradually. People are often fearful of opening up, protective of their old wounds and of their current behavior patterns. Typical psychotherapy progresses in fits and starts; there is progress, and then there are plateaus. Some of the deepest, most painful material, which can be causing significant problems for the patient, takes the longest to unearth. The layers of defenses have built up over the years.

On hearing about MDMA's history of psychotherapeutic use, my psychotherapy supervisor was intrigued. "People are always looking for ways to make therapy faster," she said encouragingly. In New York City, where I live and practice psychiatry, it is quite common to see a therapist. Many adults are in therapy, usually once or twice a week, and it is not unusual for their therapy to last for years. Diverse New Yorkers have one common desire: whatever it is they want, they want it *now*, without waiting. MDMA is a chemical catalyst for growth and change. It hastens the therapeutic process, digs deep, and brings about impressive results more easily. The idea of increasing the efficiency of psychotherapy appeals to me tremendously, but I imagine it also would appeal to those who have to undergo therapy and especially those who pay for those services.

Consider the effect of a thorough spring cleaning on an individual who has been going through life sweeping his or her own psychic dirt under the carpet. This pronounced effect does not go unnoticed by therapist and patient alike. A group of Swiss psychiatrists, including Juraj Styk, Marianne Bloch, and Samuel Widmer, conducted psychotherapy with MDMA from 1988 to 1993. Peter Gasser surveyed these psychotherapy patients and reported the following results (Gasser 1994–95). In all, 121 patients underwent a total of 818 sessions. The average duration of therapy was three years. At the time of the evaluation, more than 90 percent of the patients described themselves as "significantly improved" (65 percent) or "slightly improved" (26 percent). Typical reported benefits were improved self-acceptance, enhanced feelings of self-esteem, and reduced levels of fear and psychosomatic complaints.

The impact of the psycholytic sessions was greatest on the patients' emotional lives: 65 percent of patients said the sessions were very important emotionally, 56 percent cited the importance to their interpersonal relationships, and 49 percent stated that it produced important biographical insights. Rated as very important to most people was the experience of unity and complete love, which was reported by 71 percent of the respondents. Fully 84 percent of the patients noted an improved quality of life, and only 3 percent cited a worsened quality of life. Better self-acceptance was reported by 82 percent of respondents. Eighty-one percent of patients reported improved relationships with family, and 3 percent reported worsened relationships. About six in ten people felt less fear of death, and 2 percent felt more fear. Virtually no patients reported an increased use of drugs after therapy. Nicotine was used more frequently by 3 percent, cannabis by 2 percent, and alcohol by 2 percent. On the other hand, a substantial number of patients reported less use of drugs. Nicotine was used less frequently by 21 percent, cannabis by 7 percent, and alcohol by 20 percent. During the course of psycholytic therapy there were no severe adverse incidents, no suicides, and no psychiatric hospitalizations.

MDMA acts as a catalyst to the psychotherapeutic process in four ways:

Connection
MDMA enhances the therapeutic alliance, which is the basis of any doctor-patient relationship. Studies of psychotherapy have pinpointed that it is this empathic rapport that coincides with success (Hartley 1985). It is important for patients to trust the therapist, to believe that they can open up fully and explore safely. MDMA is not just a mind-expanding drug, it is a heart-opening one as well; it has been proposed as a pharmacological facilitator of empathy. The freedom to let go and to love, to invite people into your world and to want to explore theirs, blossoms.

Recall
There are some reports that people under the influence of MDMA have been able to recall childhood events and traumatic episodes with tremendous clarity. Memories that were once laden with anxiety and hidden from view make themselves available for review. What was once cloudy or too painful to explore is like an old house with all its lights on and all its doors open. It is up to the therapist and patient to choose which rooms to examine, which repressed memories to pull out of the closet. In addition to enhanced remote memory, the memory of the entire MDMA experience is intact, so that whatever insights are garnered during the session are retained.

Insight
It is not enough to remember well and to be able to communicate easily. For therapy to be effective, conclusions must be drawn and decisions reached. MDMA is an excellent tool for assisting insight-oriented therapy. The combination of sharpened faculties, enhanced concentration, and a heightened sense of self assists both the patient and therapist in putting the pieces together and drawing profound conclusions from the material brought forth during the session.

Acceptance
The ultimate goal of psychotherapy is to develop compassion and forgiveness for others, so that the burden of hatred, fear, and resentment is lifted.

Acceptance of life circumstances, of previous traumas and "trespasses," helps us lighten our load and grow as happier, freer individuals. In successful psychotherapy, it is most important to forgive yourself. Lasting behavioral change comes out of self-love, not self-hatred. For people to want to tend their own gardens, to dig in the dirt and pull out the weeds, they must believe that they deserve to blossom. The greatest gift of the MDMA experience is the self-esteem, acceptance, and self-love that helps catalyze lasting changes in self-defeating behavior.

Enhanced memory combined with confidence refines the ability to explore difficult psychological issues. Heightened insight assists in learning, and acceptance can bring a sense of peace. All of these qualities add up to a uniquely transformative experience that often brings about significant changes in the life of the patient. The MDMA-assisted psychotherapy session lasts just four hours, but the discoveries and decisions made during that time can last a lifetime.

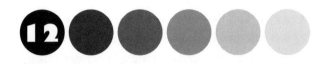

USING MDMA IN HEALING, PSYCHOTHERAPY, AND SPIRITUAL PRACTICE*

Ralph Metzner, Ph.D., and Sophia Adamson

In this chapter, we describe observations from individual and group experiences with MDMA (and other empathogenic substances†) relating to their application in self-healing, psychotherapy, and spiritual practice. We also offer some guidelines, distilled from the experience of about two dozen therapists and practitioners, for the most effective use of these substances. Traditional societies, such as those of the Native Americans, do not separate the three areas; thus, their ceremonies, including peyote rituals or sweat lodges, are at the same time worship, curing, and problem solving. In modern West-

*This material was originally published in *ReVision: The Journal of Consciousness Change* (spring 1988): 10, no. 4, 59–72, under the title "The Nature of the MDMA Experience and Its Role in Healing, Psychotherapy, and Spiritual Practice."

†The term "empathogenic," meaning "generating a state of empathy," was independently proposed for these substances in 1983–84 by Ralph Metzner, a psychologist and psychopharmacologist, and David Nichols, a professor of medicinal chemistry at Purdue University. Nichols subsequently rejected the term and now prefers "entactogenic," meaning "touching within," for MDMA. We continue to use the term "empathogenic." The substances we include in this category, known to us at present, are the phenethylamines MDA, MDMA, MMDA, and 2-CB. Empathogens are a subcategory of psychedelic ("mind-manifesting") drugs, such as LSD and psilocybin. See also the *MAPS Bulletin*, vol. 4, no. 2, pages 47–9, for an extended discussion on the nomenclature of MDMA.

ern societies these three endeavors function along the lines of professional guilds, and their special interest groups may be one of the reasons why Western societies, except for the Native Americans, have found it so difficult to deal with psychedelics in a rational, socially beneficial manner.*

It is the primary thesis of this chapter that the empathogenic substances induce an experience that has the potential for dissolving the defensive intrapsychic separation between spirit, mind, and body and that therefore physical healing, psychological problem solving, and spiritual awareness can, and usually do, occur at the same time in the same experience. In traditional peoples' healing ceremonies, when curing or therapy takes place, it happens in the context of a ritual shared by a group, which also is regarded as a sacred experience. This is very different from the conventional Western medical model, which treats healing drugs as something to be administered on a daily schedule and not as an experience to be shared between doctor and patient. The records of the sessions with empathogenic and psychedelic substances indicate that the experiences fit naturally within the integrative worldviews of indigenous, shamanic cultures.

The changes that occur in a person's consciousness during such experiences are likely to be changes in attitude toward the body, which facilitate the body's own healing and regenerative processes. The psychological problem solving that occurs is also most frequently a shift in perspective, a reframing of a belief that also may be healing and have spiritual implications. When a person has a realization of the spiritual core of being, there are often healing and therapeutic changes, almost as by-products. In all three areas, the integrity and responsibility of the individual is affirmed, and the person is empowered; dependence on the doctor, or the medicine, is reduced. These attitudes and changes can be, and often are, carried over into a person's ordinary life afterward.

The research with psychedelic drugs carried out during the 1960s led to the hypothesis, widely accepted by workers in the field, that psychedelics are nonspecific psychic amplifiers and that the content of a psychedelic experience

---

*For an elaboration of this argument see the article by Ralph Metzner entitled "Molecular Mysticism: The Role of Psychoactive Substances in the Transformation of Consciousness," in *Shaman's Drum*, Spring 1988. The article also appears in *Das Tor zum inneren Raum: Festschrift für Albert Hofmann*, edited by Christian Ratsch.

is primarily a function of set (expectations, intention, attitude, and personality) and setting (physical and social context and presence and attitude of others, including the guide). This set-and-setting hypothesis is a useful model for understanding the experiences with MDMA as well: the specific insights, feelings, and resolutions of problems that occur are unique to the individual. Nevertheless, a certain commonality exists in the kinds of feeling states usually named: ecstasy, empathy, openness, compassion, peace, acceptance, forgiveness, healing, oneness, and caring. People are able, if their intention in taking the substance is serious and therapeutic, to use the state to resolve long-standing intrapsychic conflicts or interpersonal problems in relationships.

Teachers and practitioners of meditation and other forms of spiritual work describe the experience as being fundamentally an opening of the heart center. The heart center (or chakra) is considered to be related to healing and involved in all interpersonal relationships, especially familial and intimate ones. In many systems, because of its location midway between the abdominal and pelvic lower centers and the throat and brain higher centers, the heart center is regarded as the bridge between the mental and spiritual aspects above and the bodily and instinctual nature below. Thus, the opening (even partially) of this center is seen as the foundation for all further psychospiritual growth and practice. As an example, one woman observed, in her first experience with MDMA, a kind of knot in her heart center. As she focused warmth and caring attention on it, it seemed literally to loosen and unravel; simultaneously, she was aware that several of her personal relationships were somehow being healed. At the end, she felt better about each of these relationships.

One meditation teacher has suggested that the MDMA experience facilitates the dissolving of barriers between body, mind, and spirit—the same separation within the individual that is seen in society, as noted earlier. Mind and body can be coordinated: mind, including feelings, has a positive empathic attitude toward the body, which, in turn, feels accepted and protected. Thus, instinctual awareness as well as mental, emotional, and sensory awareness can all function together, rather than one being the focus at the expense of the other. Similarly, spirit or self is no longer felt as a remote abstract concept, "above" somewhere; instead one senses the presence of spirit infusing the structures of the body and the images and attitudes of the mind. Awareness is expanded to include all parts of the body, all aspects of the mind, and the higher reaches of spirit. This permits a kind of reconnecting, a re-membering of the totality of our experience, an access to forgotten truth.

In other research on altered states of consciousness, the catalyst or trigger of a mind-opening experience can be rhythmic drumming, hypnosis, fasting, solitude, meditation practice, a particular piece of music, or other factors. In the case of these experiences, the chemical catalyst triggers a change of feeling state in which insights and perceptions (though often appearing ordinary and commonplace when they are afterward described to others) are felt with a depth and poignancy of emotion that was for most people unheard of in their lives up to the time of that first experience.

This is not to say that similar or identical changes of consciousness cannot be produced or arrived at without the use of these empathogenic substances. Obviously, many people have had and continue to have empathic and heart-opening experiences without the use of any external aid, pharmaceutical or other. Those people who are able to attain such insights and solutions without external catalysts are to be commended. For most people the heightened and deepened state of awareness facilitated by the drug serves as a kind of preview, as it were, a taste of the possibilities that exist for much greater emotional openness and relatedness than they had imagined. They are aware, too, that the drug experience is a temporary state and one that can be converted into the ongoing reality of everyday consciousness only with continuing therapeutic and spiritual practice—and not with the continued use of the drug. Most people do not want to repeat the experience very often—it is thought to be too intense, too sacred. Although the possibility of becoming psychologically dependent on this or any other drug cannot be ruled out, there is a fairly high degree of consensus that it is not addicting. Cases of tolerance and dependence with larger or more frequent dosing have been reported.

The folklore and terminology that have arisen with respect to these substances give one a good indication of the basic nature of the experience. As a name, Ecstasy points to the warmth, well-being, euphoria, pleasure, joy, and sensuality almost universally reported. The empathy so often cited has a distinctly different feel to it than "sympathy"; the latter is seen as an unconscious reaction of feeling the same as someone else. Empathy is sympathy with understanding, with consciousness; you do not forget who you are, even though you can "feel within" (*em-patheia* in Greek) the other. People feel that they have true compassion, forgiveness, and understanding for those with whom they have important relationships. Most important, in terms of the therapeutic implications, they have empathy and compassion for themselves, for their ordinary, neurotic, childish, struggling persona or ego. The relative absence or attenuation of normal anxiety and fear in these states is perhaps the single most important feature with regard to their therapeutic value. People report being able to think about, talk about, and deal with inner or outer issues that are otherwise avoided because of the anxiety levels normally associated with those issues.

Perhaps the most interesting code name for MDMA, which seems to have originated with a group of therapists on the West Coast, is the term Adam, by which is meant not Adam as a man but rather Adam-and-Eve as the androgynous ancestor. The figure of Adam is an important symbolic figure in gnostic and hermetic writings, and C. G. Jung wrote extensively about it. He represents "primordial man," the "original being," the "man of the Earth," the condition of primal innocence and unity with all life, as described in the Bible's account of the Garden of Eden. Feelings of being returned to a natural state of innocence before guilt, shame, and unworthiness arose are common in these Adam-like ecstasies, and so are feelings of connectedness and bonding with fellow human beings, animals, plants, and all the forms and energies of the natural world. Since gnosis is direct experiential knowledge of divine reality, it would not be inappropriate to call psychedelics "gnostic catalysts."

To illustrate the role of MDMA and other empathogens in the three areas of psychotherapy, healing, and spiritual insight, we take quotes from the first-person accounts published in *Through the Gateway of the Heart* (Adamson 1985). The general finding is that breakthroughs in any of these areas occur, depending on the individual's set, or intention. The psychocatalytic action of the empathogenic drug operates only within the context of a prepared and attentive attitude. Those who take the drug "for recreation" or "just to experience the high" are likely to get just that: a pleasant, even pleasurable, few hours, with little or no intellectual insight. The following account, edited from a verbatim transcript recorded during an MDMA session, exemplifies the process of attaining a new and enlarged perspective on the role of ego. The subject is a thirty-five-year-old woman who is a graduate student and programmer:

> The ego wants everything. It's like an octopus grabbing and grabbing. Ego wants to control, and it gets threatened. The reason my ego is so threatened is that I've lived so much of my life not here. The ego knows it has a very tenuous hold. Meditation threatens my ego. All my spiritual work threatens my ego. So my ego tries to take hold of it as its own. "I'll be more perfect and spiritual"—that's my ego. What the ego has to know is that the change in me is that I want to integrate, to incarnate. I want to be here; ego does not have to be threatened. I realize for the first time that I want to be here. . . . I'm not my ego. . . . My ego is part of who I am, but I'm not my ego.

What is being described here is a shift in identification—from being fully identified with the ego to becoming the larger Self, the larger consciousness, from which the ego perspective is seen as limited and fearful. This subject went on to have a truly intense experience of mystical enlightenment in that same session. The following account by a different subject, written several days after an MDMA session, describes the aftereffects, or results, of an anamnestic review of childhood trauma during the session:

> Material about a sexual molestation incident — first reported during a hypnosis session several weeks ago — has had much more meaning for me since I heard the tape of the Adam session. In it I sounded as if I were seven years old. The impact comes from the deep recognition of how many ways the event molded my response to the world around me, in part because of the distrust of my parents that was focused by the incident. Reliving this incident helped to free up my energy and emotions in a number of ways. It feels as though this process will be ongoing for some time. In general, my journey with Adam affirmed who I am, what I am doing, where I am going. The affirmation was experienced through an opening of the heart rather than a deep intellectual understanding. . . . In this set and setting, with empathy for all aspects of life, learning took place the content of which was easily and deeply received. . . . I am able to perceive, receive, and respond to love in a much more open way than I did a few weeks ago.

A third example of therapeutic breakthrough comes from the experience of a compulsive sexual masochist, who, after tasting the pleasure of the MDMA experience, had some apprehension that he might become addicted to it. He also derived insight into the nature of his compulsion:

> I didn't really think that I could become addicted to the experience in the sense of being addicted to alcohol or to sexual excess with prostitutes. I perceive those as addictions precisely because of their compulsive quality, the quality of never actually obtaining a satisfying, whole, pleasant experience. With the experience of MDMA, on the other hand, I feel none of that compulsion. It really has an entirely different quality, as if it's in some way outside all the time, outside my life and my neuroses, literally a taste of the infinite bliss of being a conscious entity. In a very fundamental sense, it is the kind of experience that every conscious being really wants and needs. We get a sense of our true selves and how they are perfect, beautiful, whole, and complete. It fulfilled all of my childhood dreams, all of the unfulfilled longings, and all of the feelings of limitation and loss have been swept away by the sense of who I really am.

The book *Through the Gateway of the Heart* contains two accounts of MDMA therapy of rape victims, who were helped considerably. One woman, a therapist herself, experienced complete amnesia of her attack, as well as dissociated panic attacks and recurrent nightmares for a year. She then was able to move through the trauma in a series of four MDMA sessions over a period of twelve months. She wrote:

> Adam broke through the repressive/defensive network and took me back into the experience of the attack that was too much for my psyche to bear. During the experience with Adam, I moved in and out of the attack: being plunged into the horror, then moving into a transitional phase of regression, into what was reported to me to be almost infantile, even fetal, states. . . . At times I would come around with what was reported as exceptional presence—a vibrancy and change of color, an expansive quality rather than a fearful, contracted quality—and with a beaming sort of aura. I felt expansive, physically exhausted but full of love and a deep feeling of peace. It has seemed that Adam has allowed me to move into the fragments of the attack, to re-experience what I needed to re-experience, and to desensitize myself to my surroundings. The dissociative episodes have ended, and I now can move through trauma and come out of it in an open and loving way, rather than with more memory of the assault.

The successful therapeutic outcome of this and similar situations has important implications for the future applications of empathogenic substances in the treatment of the aftereffects of trauma. The condition post-traumatic stress disorder, which affects the victims of physical and sexual assault, soldiers suffering from breakdown in war zones, and torture victims, has not found an effective therapeutic approach as yet. MDMA therapy may be the sought-after method, because of its ability to access memories blocked out by repression. The only limitation on its use would be in the cases of persons who were tortured by the administration of psychiatric drugs or toxins, whose negative set would preclude them from participating in a drug-induced therapeutic experience. The following account illustrates a healing experience, a change of attitude that involved post-session changes in lifestyle and health habits:

> I remind myself that I am becoming a home to the indwelling Spirit; it will see out my eyes, and it likes to see beauty, proportion, and harmony. . . . I proceed to ask for guidance and support for integrating these changes into my life. I intend to become a perfect temple for this God-consciousness. . . . I had always felt unconscious and therefore cut off from my body. . . . During the course of a single Adam session, I experienced a deep, natural healing within myself. I re-owned my body. In the two weeks that have followed, I have observed the following behavioral changes. I choose lighter, healthful foods and no longer desire heavy, fatty foods. There has been a definite increase in the grace with which I move, an instinctive desire for water and a marked increase in daily fluid intake, and no desire for caffeine or alcohol. And for the first time in my life, I can feel myself consciously and lovingly aware of the body in which I live.

Another subject, a forty-four-year-old woman with breast cancer, reported an experience of "dissolving into tiny cells that were part of everything." She repeatedly told herself to "let go, just let go, and as I let go, I could feel the cells in my body moving toward healing." Placing her hands on various parts of her body in need of healing, she said, "I was the healing and I witnessed the healing." Her physician subsequently reported an improvement in her condition.

One man who suffered long-term debilitating pain from spinal arthritis reported an unusually dramatic healing. During the MDMA sessions, he experienced "arthritis crystals breaking up" as he moved his body. Subsequently, he discovered that hitting himself with repetitive small flailing movements of the hands and, later, a broom, in what he described as "physical self-flagellation," seemed also to loosen up the crystals and relieve the pain. The flagellation was the treatment for his condition as well as a symbolic expression of the meaning of his disease. In a later MDMA session, he confronted and released his fear of death and went through a rebirth experience, after which, he said, "For the first time I felt pain as an ally, not as an enemy. I can use it for insight and understanding and not for self-destruction. Using the pain with love and understanding instead of constantly fighting it with deep animosity will enable me to end it." In other words, the development of empathy for himself, his body, and his pain was the crucial turning point in his approach to the disease—which was permanently successful.

Experiences of spiritual enlightenment and of discovery are commonplace in the accounts of MDMA experiences. Depending on a person's background and intention, these experiences may occur as the result of a focused choice or totally unexpectedly. The following account is a description of the union of personality and Self, human and divine:

> I allow, invite, surrender God into my own body. God consciousness aches for and eagerly awaits this moment to enter me, as it longs to enter each of us, at any and every moment. . . . Painlessly, in silent ecstasy, that which has lived as my guest, my visitor, my "higher" self becomes part of my consciousness. We merge. No longer higher, it is now inner, merging with that which I chose. The chooser becomes the chosen. . . . This phase ends here with the glad marriage of myself and my Self.

Another subject, a woman who had grown afraid to meditate because shadowy "guides" would appear, found in the Adam session that her fear of the guides, and hence of meditation, dissipated. And her guides instead gave her instructions on meditation that she was able to accept. "There were about ten of them, dressed in draped gray garments, and I could tell by feeling that some of them were male and some female. They felt like my real family. They spoke to me not in words, but in mind-to-mind communication, about the importance of meditation for my growth."

Vivid experiences of kundalini [the potential creative energy at the base of the spine—Ed.] energy phenomena are not at all uncommon in MDMA sessions, especially when the person is one who has studied and practiced yoga consciously. One subject who was a migraine sufferer first found herself out of her body, forgiving herself for past and present misdeeds. Then she let the energy move through her body: "My body danced and leaped with the kundalini energy. I just let it dance and loved it." Later she felt reaffirmed and strengthened in her work as a therapist and in her spiritual studies of the Kabbalah. This kind of experience, of gaining a fresh perspective on a teaching one has already studied or a fresh motivation to pursue a practice one has neglected, is frequently reported. It is much less likely that someone will be inspired to pursue a path with which he or she is totally unfamiliar.

Many subjects report feelings of light, sometimes (though rarely) accompanied by visual sensations of lights, auras, or images. More often, it is the emotional and the physical, kinesthetic awareness that is activated and suffused by a spiritual presence. As one subject wrote after the session: "I now feel and know that I am the eyes, ears, feelings of the spirit. I feel so safe, so protected. The Holy Spirit is myself. There is no mystery any more. We are here to do, to feel exuberant." Others feel fiery energy and radiance coursing through their bodies and minds, dissolving pain or solving mental, fear-created hang-ups. There are also experiences one might call "cosmic consciousness," involving a sense of no longer being confined to this planet, or at some universal center. These kinds of experiences are, however, much less common with empathogens than with psychedelics, such as LSD or magic mushrooms (*teonanacatl* or psilocybin). One subject wrote this:

An awareness of being here, beyond here. Both. Very deep, very far, galaxies, very far out there. Spacious, open, dark. Thin lines of bright colors, rapidly changing. Mostly floating like a baby through the universe. Floating through existence. Infinite, the whole universe. . . . I remember what Augustine said. Something about the heart always restless until it finds rest in God. I felt that complete rest, no searching, finally home.

In all these experiences, it is clear that the physical healing, the psychological therapy, and the spiritual realization usually are interwoven and connected in an inextricable way. Our categories are merely reflections of our academic and professional preconceptions and are not retained in the flowing process of experience. MDMA and other empathy-generating medicines simply seem to facilitate the opening of the heart center, or the intelligence of the heart, and from this open point of freedom and awareness choices can be made and knots of past karma disentangled that have repercussions on many levels of consciousness.

Guidelines for the Sacramental Use of Empathogenic Substances

The following guidelines have been compiled from the collective experience of twenty to thirty therapists who have used these substances in their work and who have based their methods on observation of hundreds of individual sessions. Although there is by no means uniformity of approach among the different practitioners, the guidelines offered represent a distillation of methods that have proven efficacy. Their description here should not be construed as encouragement of the use of illegal substances. Rather they are applicable to any state of heightened empathic awareness, regardless of how it is generated.

We use the term "sacramental" to describe the approach used by most of the practitioners and therapists whom we have interviewed. To a great extent all of them share the integrative attitude that we attributed earlier to the Native American and other indigenous cultures—an attitude that sees healing of the body, psychological problem solving, and spiritual awareness as interrelated aspects of a unified process. Even those therapists who would not espouse any formal religious element in their work with these substances nevertheless tend to see the MDMA experience from a spiritual perspective and to support those perspectives when they arise in the client or patient. It is for this reason that we have chosen the term "sacramental" to refer to the whole complex of drug use plus set and setting with healing, therapeutic, and spiritual aspects.

Although the use of MDMA and other drugs of this family occurs statistically most frequently in what might be called a hedonistic or recreational context, with no particular therapeutic or spiritual purpose in mind, these types of sessions will not be discussed here. It is our belief that such recreational use, though probably harmless (certainly less harmful than alcohol or tobacco), does not have the intrinsic interest and healing potential that guided, intentional, therapeutic, and sacramental use has. [See the section "Risks of MDMA Use," for a fuller appraisal of the risks inherent in recreational MDMA use.]

Preparation and Set

The single most important foundation for a beneficial experience is intention or purpose. One should ask oneself, and discuss with the therapist or guide, What is my purpose in entering into this altered state of awareness? Typically, people approach the experience with fundamental existential and spiritual questions. These questions might include the following: Who am I? What is my purpose in life? What is the next step in my spiritual path?

These are questions that all seekers have, and it is natural to want to ask them in the course of an encounter with one's sources of inner wisdom. In addition, there may be more personal and therapeutic questions, including questions concerning physical illness; traumatic or conflicted experiences from the past, such as early childhood and birth; and unbalanced or unsatisfactory relationships with others, particularly parents, spouses, lovers, children, family, and friends. It is not uncommon for people to spend major portions of the experience reviewing and healing interpersonal relationships. Other kinds of questions people have addressed concern work and career, creative expression or blocks in that area, and sometimes international and global issues. Some therapists and guides encourage the person to make a written list of questions, which then can be reviewed just before the session or perhaps recorded during the session.

Some people prefer to declare an intention to explore certain areas or topics, rather than posing questions. In either approach it is good practice to release the questions or intentions to one's own higher self, or inner guide, just before ingestion of MDMA. In this way, a person is not too intent merely on problem solving, which, on occasion, can tend to limit one's experience. When an intention has been declared and released in this fashion, whatever experience unfolds then is likely to answer one's questions, including those implied but not asked. If the experience is a person's first one with psychedelic medicines, it is important to review any fears or other expectations one may have with the guide or sitter. If there has been extensive previous experience with psychedelics, but not MDMA, it is equally important to review them, so that the nature of one's expectations based on past experience can be understood.

The question of sexual feelings and expression between the two people should be raised. If their relationship is professional, the principle of no sexual contact should be discussed and affirmed. If the two people are friends who are not lovers, their feelings for each other should be stated and clarified. They are going to be in a state of extraordinarily heightened emotional intimacy for several hours. This state allows an unusual degree of access to fears, concerns, and frustrations in the area of intimacy. But it is not advisable to use that state for the initiation of an ordinary sexual encounter. Even if the guide and the voyager are married or lovers, it is probably best to postpone actual sexual contact to the latter part of the experience, because it would tend otherwise to distract from the exploration of other areas.

If two people who are lovers and who are experienced with empathogenic substances wish to use a conjoint session to explore deeper levels of emotional, sexual, and spiritual intimacy, this is certainly a state in which Tantric and Taoist eroticism (which is nonstriving, noncraving, and nonpossessive) can be experienced. Many accounts testify to the extraordinary tactile sensitivity and sensuousness of the Adam state. (It should be added here that a high percentage of subjects report a partial numbing of genital sensations and a consequent lack of erection in the male. It is this fact that is responsible for the finding that, for some people, the Adam experience is the first time they experience sensuality or sensuousness without genital arousal.) For the more usual kind of session, where someone is being initiated into an experience with empathogenic medicines for the first time for purposes of psychospiritual awakening, an agreement or understanding of no sexual contact is preferable. As part of this discussion, it is important also to agree that the physical touch of a hand on the heart, the shoulder, the head, or the hand can be an important source of support and encouragement and signals empathy or compassion but not sexual interest.

Another important part of the preparation for the session, as part of the discussion of intention and purpose, is to practice a meditation with which one is familiar or a basic relaxation procedure. The purpose is to enter into the experience from a baseline state that is already somewhat clear and centered and freed from distracting everyday concerns. Some people like to read, or have read aloud, a favorite passage from a personally meaningful text, such as a chosen prayer, a beautiful poem, or similar inspirational writings.

For others the prayer or meditation might include the specific invocation of a beloved guru or teacher and the invocation of a particular deity or guardian spirit.

Some people familiar with shamanic practices and rituals like to bring "power objects," such as crystals, feathers, or any item that has been psychically charged, to the session. Others, especially if they want to explore relationship issues, might bring photographs of parents or family to contemplate or photographs of themselves to activate childhood memories. Finally, it is recommended that a person fast for at least six hours so as not to reduce the substance's effect with a full stomach. Fasting also is part of a general psychic and physical purification. This will tend to make the journey much more productive and pleasant.

Alchemical Catalysts

Because the goal of alchemy was the transformation of consciousness, symbolized by the biochemical transformations taking place within the human body (the vessel or furnace), it is appropriate to call these chemical substances that facilitate a transformative reaction "alchemical catalysts." The discussion here is limited to the catalysts that generally are considered to have empathogenic effects. We will not cover the larger and more varied hallucinogens, such as LSD, psilocybin, or mescaline.*

The compounds of this class that have been used in therapy include MDA, MDMA, MMDA, and 2-CB. Many others have been synthesized and found to be psychoactive, but none has gained the widespread attention that these have. Chemically, they are referred to as phenethylamines. Botanically, some of these compounds are found in the volatile oils of certain plants, including nutmeg and mace. Structurally, they resemble dopamine, a neurotransmitter; mescaline, a potent hallucinogen; and amphetamine, a stimulant. The psychological effects are not unlike a blend of mescaline and amphetamine, though they are less hallucinogenic than the former and less stimulating than the latter.

MDA is 3,4-methylenedioxyamphetamine; this drug became fairly well known in the 1960s, when it was called the "love drug" among the hippies.

---

*See Metzner, "Molecular Mysticism."

It is active at doses from 50 mg to 200 mg. In his book *The Healing Journey*, Claudio Naranjo called it the "drug of analysis" and reported that it was especially useful for therapeutic regression and recollection of childhood experiences. It has a duration of action of six to eight hours and is generally more stimulating, or amphetamine-like, than MDMA. Its reputation is as an aphrodisiac, and it is used in some circles as a stimulant for dancing and sex. Because it has been illegal since the late sixties and other compounds with fewer somatic side effects have been found, it does not currently find much use in therapy, as far as is known.

MDMA is 3,4-methylenedioxymethamphetamine; the drug is active at doses of 50 mg to 250 mg, with 150 mg as an effective dose for the average adult. It differs from MDA in its duration of action, which is four to five hours, and in having fewer amphetamine-like side effects, such as muscle tremor or jaw clenching. The onset of pharmacological effects is usually within twenty to thirty minutes after ingestion, and there is a transient moderate rise in blood pressure and pulse rate. Subjectively, there is a surge in feelings of bodily heat and greatly increased attention and alertness; at the same time there is a feeling of bodily relaxation and ease. MMDA also is mentioned in Naranjo's book, where it is said to induce an experience of the "eternal now." (Both this description and the description of MDA given in that book could apply equally to MDMA.) Perhaps because of the alleged difficulty of its synthesis, it has not found much use among therapists and researchers interviewed for this chapter.

The only other chemical used in the present series is 2-CB, which is 4-bromo-2,5-dimethoxyphenethylamine. This drug is more potent than MDMA, being active in some people at 18–20 mg; 25–30 mg is the maximum dose. Energy tremors, jaw clenching, heat, and increased blood pressure are the usual side effects. There is great individual variation in sensitivity to this substance, so one should at all times proceed with caution, by beginning with a lower dose and only gradually escalating to higher amounts. Psychologically, 2-CB is empathogenic, like MDMA, though it appears to be somewhat more body-oriented; it also has mild visual effects not unlike mescaline. Some therapists and researchers have experimented with MDMA followed three to four hours later by 2-CB, which serves to extend the empathogenic experience by the same length of time.

The side effects of all of these substances occur in response to the amphetamine-like stimulant action in some people. They are very much dose-dependent. Jaw clenching and fine to gross muscular tremors are noticed most frequently. Many people have found that a calcium-magnesium supplement (330–500 mg), taken just before, during, or after MDMA, can minimize the intensity of these side effects or eliminate them altogether. There is usually complete loss of appetite during the experience and even for a few hours afterward. The person may experience fatigue the next day, perhaps partly due to the reduced food intake. It is recommended that a person take vitamin and mineral supplements before and after the experience. Plenty of water should be available at all times, because there is considerable dehydration. Contraindications for the use of these substances, which have not been extensively researched clinically, include heart disease or high blood pressure; hypoglycemia and diabetes; seizure disorders; and, of course, pregnancy. When in doubt, consult a physician.

These substances, unlike any other known psychiatric medication, produce an intense but transient altered state of awareness. Even though one's perception of everyday reality is not altered appreciably with these empathogens (unlike the hallucinogens such as LSD), one's emotional response to reality is greatly different. Although a person may be able to walk around, converse, or even drive an automobile during these states, it is obviously not desirable to do so. The heightened state of emotional sensitivity could slow down one's reactions. Moreover, engaging in these activities would take one away from the interior exploration of the psyche, which is the main point of the experience.

Setting and Context

Generally, the preferred setting for sessions in the therapeutic-sacramental mode is a serene, simple, comfortable room in which the person can recline or lie down and the therapist or guide can sit nearby. Clothes should be loose and comfortable, and a blanket should be available in case of transient episodes of chilling. It is best if there is access or proximity to the elements of nature. A fire in the fireplace serves as a reminder of the alchemical fires of inner purification and the life-preserving fire of Spirit. Fresh water to drink and proximity to a stream or ocean reminds us of the watery origins of our life. Ideally, earth and its natural forms—soil, plants, trees, rocks, and wood—would be close to the touch. Trees or plants in or near the room of the session make wonderful companions. Crystals or other stones may be brought and contemplated.

A somewhat different, though also profound, experience may be had if the setting is outdoors, in nature. It is probably best that such sessions, if they involve walking or possible interaction with people, be undertaken using lower doses (50 to 100 mg MDMA); alternatively, such excursions can be taken in the latter, milder portion of the session. For those who have had previous experience with full-intensity indoor sessions, such outdoor experiences can be extremely rewarding. Characteristically, one may experience a kind of deep emotional, almost visceral bonding with the land, the plants, the rocks, the animals, and the environment in general. Perceptual changes with empathogens are usually minimal, but a deep feeling of appreciation for and connectedness with all life-forms is often reported in such sessions.

The music—usually selected and played by the guide or sitter—can have a profound effect on consciousness, as with the psychedelics. Entire therapeutic processes or shamanic journeys can be undertaken during certain musical selections. Typically, therapists and persons working with MDMA and other empathogens have found the serene, peaceful, meditative music sometimes referred to as "inner space" music most valuable in these experiences. Fast, rhythmic, or highly complex music seems too difficult to follow. Simple gongs, bells, chimes, and drums are also pleasing and centering during such experiences, whether one plays them or merely listens to them.

The attitude and behavior of the guide or sitter during the session is extremely influential. This role should be played with integrity and sensitivity. If the guide is the person's therapist, he or she should have a therapeutic agreement to explore any areas of concern. If the sitter is a friend or even a partner, it is best to have agreement and understanding before the session as to the role of the guide. Most people prefer and are perfectly able to do their own best therapy in these states. They want the sitter merely to be there, listening to and recording the remarks of the voyager and providing encouragement and reassurance if needed. Intense exploration of certain issues—for example, relationships, sexuality, or birth trauma—should be undertaken only by previous arrangement or at the request of the voyager.

In the state of emotional openness of these experiences, it is extremely easy for the voyager to become caught up in an analytical, verbal mode of discussion with the guide that would take him or her away from the experience of heart center awareness. Even if the interpersonal interaction between the two is warm, affectionate, and trusting, it still can be a distraction from the deeper intrapsychic awareness that is possible when attention is focused inward. These shifts in attention are subtle and elusive. The wise guide will watch for signs that the voyager is losing connection to the deep source within and will refocus attention toward that source. Sometimes simply asking voyagers whether they are "coming from" the heart or the head in the discourse is sufficient to center the attention once again.

Process and Method in Individual Sessions

This is not the place to enter into a full discussion of the processes and methods of individual therapy assisted by empathogens. Psychotherapists interested in this topic are encouraged to consult the comprehensive guide by Dr. Stanislav Grof entitled *LSD Psychotherapy*. Although the book deals mainly with LSD, the information is generally applicable to all psychedelics and empathogens. In the remainder of this chapter, we merely give a few suggestions, primarily for the person who is undergoing the experience.

There are two general principles long accepted in psychedelic research that could be proposed as ethical guidelines for this kind of work. First, no one should be given the drug, or be persuaded to take it, against his or her wishes or without full disclosure of the possible risks and benefits. Second, no one—therapist or layperson—should consider administering or guiding a session with these substances if he or she has not had personal experience with them. The questions, purposes, or agenda brought to the session, as discussed earlier, set the tone of the experience. Whatever unfolds during the experience seems to be, in a sense, an answer to those questions—even though this may not become apparent until much later. Most therapists suggest to voyagers that they go first as far and deeply within as they can, to the core or ground of being, to the High Self—or similar directions. From this totally centered place, full of compassion and insight, one can review and analyze the usual problems and questions of one's life. It is not uncommon for people to feel and report to the therapist that all their questions and problems have been dissolved in the all-embracing love and compassion that they are feeling. Even in such an initial state of total unity and transcendence, it is often helpful later to ask the questions and perhaps record one's answers or comments on tape for post-session review.

Because the MDMA experience usually involves almost total attenuation of the usual fear or anxiety reactions, it is ideal, in one sense, for exploring traumatic memories or phobic reactions. On the other hand, the fear reaction itself sometimes cannot be explored in the usual manner. Subjects typically say, "I can't get in touch with the fear." One therapist noted that when such a situation arose, he instructed the patient to think of a fear-arousing situation and to associate the present Adam state of ecstatic well-being with it. Two or three weeks later, in regular psychotherapy, when the patient again brought up the conflict, he suggested that she evoke the memory of the Adam state. The patient then was able to merge the fear complex with the ecstatic empathy feeling, which led to the dissolving of that entire reaction pattern.

Just as affirmations or statements of intention are used to bridge one's ordinary state of consciousness with these heightened states, so can intentional affirmations made during the Adam state apply to the ordinary state of consciousness that is subsequently reestablished. Individuals have made statements of intention with regard to questions of emotional attitude, communication in relationships, and creative expression. Even changes in diet, exercise, or lifestyle have been decided and later applied. The empathy characteristic of these states is such that one can think clearly about the various available options without the usual distortions caused by emotional attractions or aversions. A person can assess the probable emotional impact of things one might choose to say to a partner or friend and modify one's expression so as to minimize the defensive or hostile reactions. A person can hear things without becoming hurt or angry and can say things without fear or timidity. The Adam state might be described as one of *release from emotional identification patterns*, or "dis-identification."

If these statements sound too good to be true, we can respond only by saying that they are based on repeated experiences and observations of many hundreds of intelligent, articulate people. The profound simplicity of the Adam state is striking. People often express this in the form of apparently banal statements—such as that one only needs love and all else falls into place or that coming from the heart center or from the source, all other choices are easy and right. What these observations and experiences imply is that perhaps the greatest value and potential of this substance lies in the training of psychotherapists. The ability to experience and articulate empathy toward the patient often is regarded as the most important criterion of effective psychotherapy. Psychotherapists who have worked with MDMA affirm that besides their own learning, they frequently also have insights into their client's problems.

Various practices of meditation, yoga, guided imagery, shamanic journeys, and rebirthing breathing can be performed while in this state. Most people who have attempted them have found it most effective to practice such methods either with low-dose MDMA (50–100 mg) or toward the latter half of a session (after two or three hours). Many people report that such methods—which are essentially self-initiated and self-guided explorations of consciousness—are enormously facilitated and amplified in these states. Most forms of meditation, however, require a motionless sitting posture, and such immobility may be hard to maintain for very long in the ultrarelaxed Adam state, especially for a beginner. On a positive note, the kind of detached, yet compassionate attitude called for in most meditation systems can be attained and maintained effortlessly with empathogens—this attitude then serves as a kind of foundation for deeper and deeper states of meditative absorption.

Most therapists and guides familiar with these substances probably would recommend that a person remain quiet and receptive during the session, to obtain the maximum potential benefit from the experience. On the other hand, for a small percentage of people (perhaps 20–30 percent), it is an important part of the therapeutic process to express themselves verbally and/or physically, sometimes loudly and repeatedly. These are the people who are ordinarily excessively shy, timid, or introverted and who do not express their feelings readily. The MDMA session may be the first time in their lives that they accept and openly affirm that they love someone, or several people, perhaps including themselves. Usually, such people need to be free to express their feelings in only one session. After that, they can and do monitor their expression, perhaps because they have incorporated changes in expressive behavior into their everyday lives.

Various forms of bodywork—such as Trager or massage—also can be amplified in range and depth if the recipient's awareness has been sensitized by empathogens (at low doses). The usual report from such experiences is that the recipient of the bodywork who has taken MDMA is in a very relaxed state in which every bodily movement or response is carried out with a much greater range and less resistance. The effects of finger pressure on the shoulder, for example, might be felt in a flow of connectedness all the way to the feet. Body therapists who have taken a small amount of MDMA and then practiced their art report that their sensitivity, their ability to tune in to the client's bodily and emotional state is heightened greatly.

Process and Ritual for Group Session

In the most common type of group session with MDMA or other empathogens, a group of friends simply partake of the medicine and continue their interpersonal interactions. The interactions might include sensual activities, such as touching, caressing, or massaging, and there is usually a heightened feeling of affection and amiability among the participants and toward others. We call such usage of the medicine "recreational," and though it seems generally harmless and probably benign, it does not appear to facilitate the kinds of deep emotionally transformative experiences that are possible with guided individual or structured group sessions.

There appear to have evolved two basic approaches to group work. In one kind, the participants have no interaction with one another during the session—although before and after there is significant sharing of intentions and experiences. Each person explores his or her own "trip," listening to music with earphones and communicating if necessary only with the guides or sitters. In the other kind of group, there is communication during the session, but in a scrupulously ritual fashion.

Some groups have experimented with nighttime sessions, following the example of Central and South American shamanic cultures that use mushrooms or ayahuasca [a psychedelic brew]. Because the onset of normal fatigue can appreciably shorten a session begun in the evening, however, many people have resorted to daytime sessions. Typically, a group assembles on a Friday evening, talks and shares their intentions with one another, and sleeps that night in the same building. Starting the session in the morning, they continue until the evening, sleep another night, and then meet for the final sharing and celebration on the following (Sunday) morning.

The particular substances used also vary from group to group. In some, different participants may take different substances, including LSD, mushrooms, MDMA, or ketamine. In others, only MDMA is used or MDMA followed three to four hours later by 2-CB to prolong the empathogenic state. Our research shows that even though the use of different drugs by participants in the first kind of group—the noninteractive group—is fairly common and not problematic, in the second, ritualistic kind of group, it is best for participants to be on the same wavelength in terms of sharing the same (or very similar) medicine. Most therapists and group leaders seem to agree that it is not advisable for someone who has not had previous individual experience to participate in a group experience with a particular substance. The first time a person takes any substance, including MDMA, he or she may engage in intense and loud processing of previously repressed feeling states, either orally or through physical movements. This kind of behavior, which can be extremely distracting to the others, usually cannot be stopped on one's first trip, and the group ceremony requires participants to be able to modulate and control the expression of feelings.

In the kinds of group ritual in which talking is permitted, the ritual that is used is the talking staff, or talking stick. This method is adapted from the practices of several Native American tribes; these tribes follow a similar format in peyote sessions of the Native American Church as well as in nondrug healing circles and in political decision-making councils. The group sits in a circle that is not interrupted. (Participants may lie down during some phases of the experience, in which case they lie with their heads toward the center, making a star pattern.) One talks or sings the song one has learned only when one has the staff. One speaks or sings from the heart, and the other group members attend respectfully. The combination of channeling powerful inner experiences and the contemplative attention of the group is a powerful, almost magnetic attracting force that can draw a person's expression through in a surprising manner. Sometimes when they have the staff, group members choose not to talk or sing but simply to share a silent meditation. In these kinds of groups, a typical session might consist of forty minutes of individual inner exploration while listening to music, followed by a round of songs and statements with the talking staff. A kind of rhythm develops in which internalized experience alternates with externalized expression.

An agreement of strict confidentiality in these groups is made: anything that anyone says, does, or ingests does not pass outside the circle of the group. This not only protects the individuals from unwanted gossip or possible legal consequences but also serves to build trust. As a result, truly extraordinary revelations sometimes occur in these groups. Similar agreements are used in other Native American groups, such as the sweat lodge ceremony—so that the people participating can feel completely confident that what they share will not be divulged. It is the group leader's responsibility to ensure that this level of trust exists in the group.

Besides the agreement concerning the confidentiality of communication, touch and sexual behavior in the group are best discouraged. Even in the case of couples who are participating together, engaging in intimate behavior would be seen by the rest of the group as exclusive and as dissipating the energy. It should be understood, though, that sometimes the simple touch of a hand from one's neighbor can be the most profoundly reassuring and comforting gesture. One needs to find a balance. Inexperienced participants sometimes make the mistake of assuming that someone who is crying, sobbing, moaning, or groaning is in need of help or comfort. Whereas the comforter seeks to make a painful experience go away—to placate—the person concerned is much more likely to want, need, and cherish the opportunity to experience deeply buried feelings for the first time. Just a simple touch, indicating presence and support if needed, is probably the most effective therapeutic aid in such situations.

Some therapists have used guided imagery sequences or verbalized meditations in groups. The state of fluid empathy and emotional resonance characteristic of the MDMA experience seems to facilitate and deepen the response to such ritualized inner journeys. Among the sequences we have observed are retracing of the path from before conception to just after birth, which connects one to spiritual and intrauterine levels of memory; following an evolutionary sequence from single-cell organism through invertebrates, vertebrates, amphibians, reptiles, mammals, and hominids, which celebrates our evolutionary ancestry; and gaining an awareness by tuning into the four alchemical elements, which are basic principles of nature and consciousness, archetypal symbols that function in an integrative manner within the psyche. There is not space within this essay to describe these rituals in more detail.

Some groups have adapted other kinds of rituals from shamanic tribal cultures. These rituals include finding an outdoor "power spot" and meditating there in silence before and after the session; having a blanket with ritual power objects that people bring into the center of the circle and letting these objects become "charged" during the session; and offering prayers to the four directions, the nature spirits, the ancestors, and the allies. Group rebirthing breathing work or movement patterns, such as tai chi, also have been incorporated into a group ritual. As stated earlier, these kinds of ritual activities usually work best in low-dose sessions; at higher doses, participants may have difficulty complying with complex verbal instruction.

Follow-up and Aftereffects

An interesting question for many people concerns the extent to which the insights and changes of such experiences with empathogens are permanent. Is it possible to transfer the learning, the new attitudes, and feelings into one's everyday reality? To put this question another way, what kind of behavior or personality changes occur in people after the deeply charged states of consciousness of the kind described in *Through the Gateway of the Heart?*

From reviewing the work of therapists and guides who have witnessed sessions with MDMA and other empathogens, one is led to the conclusion that there are two main kinds of outcomes. For one group of people, there are no discernible outward changes in behavior. The significant changes are seen in attitude and in emotional responses to situations. They discover, perhaps, that what they are doing is in line with their true spiritual purpose. They feel confirmation in their commitment; they have more compassion and true understanding. The second group is made of people who, in the MDMA experience, see things in their lives that they want to change. They proceed in a more or less systematic manner to bring about those changes. Patterns that people have altered have ranged from physical symptoms, dietary habits, work habits, and attitudes to basic changes in worldview, religious or spiritual practice, or fundamental career choices.

Some people have only one experience with Adam and make major life changes as a result of such an experience. Others find that they need perhaps three, four, or five sessions to clear out basic problems (usually interpersonal or relationship knots). Afterward, they may find that the experience doesn't "take" anymore. There is almost a kind of psychic tolerance or a feeling that the space of the MDMA experience can be entered at will, without ingesting the substance, and does not require the major reorganizing that it did the first time. The intention, or set, of the individual in taking the substance is also crucial in terms of the aftereffects. The intention before the session affects experiences during the session, and the intentions acknowledged and affirmed during the experience affect the long-term outcomes. Intention seems to function as a kind of bridge between states of consciousness.

It is also the impression of many therapists and observers that the empathogens, more than other psychedelics or hallucinogens, leave one with the ability to recall the state of consciousness—to have a kind of voluntary, purposive flashback. One therapist, for example, reported that clients could be asked to remember how they felt during an Adam session and then use that feeling of compassion and well-being to look at and deal with a troublesome issue in their present life. Some have used physical anchoring techniques, such as listening to the music they heard during the session, to trigger a momentary reliving of their experience. It is almost as if the doorway of the heart center, once opened, stays open or can be opened very easily again by choice.

There is a feeling of being empowered to make conscious choices about the direction of one's life and one's relationships or work or creativity and that one can empathically sense the emotional consequences of one's choices. A person can choose his or her direction of attention and focus of awareness. One woman reported feeling that there were paths that went out from the heart center and that she could choose which one was most appropriate for her—and not just take the one she always took, the traditional, expected path. Many possibilities lie open for those who have found themselves in this great gateway to the inner realms. This sense of the heart center as a crossroads from which major directions are chosen is expressed in the following poem, which came out of experiences with MDMA and with which we will close these remarks on the sacramental uses of empathogenic substances:

Sixfold are the paths at the crossroads of the heart
Forward and backward, left and right, upward and downward
The path forward leads to the future and is called
"Imagination, or the Children."
The path backward leads to the past and is called
"Remembrance, or the Ancestors."
The left-hand way is that of the female and is called
"Eve, the beautiful, the receptive."
The right-hand way is that of the male and is called
"Adam, the strong, the dynamic."
The upward path leads to the world of Spirit and is called
"Transcendence, or Liberation."
The downward path leads to the world of Matter, and is called
"Embodiment, or Involvement."

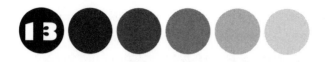

EXPERIENCE WITH THE INTERPERSONAL PSYCHEDELICS

Claudio Naranjo, M.D.

Introduction

In response to Julie Holland's invitation to contribute to this volume, I have proposed that she publish my talk on the "feeling enhancers" presented at the 1993 Psychedelic Summit at the Unitarian Church in San Francisco, where I was honored to be the opening speaker.

As one who came to the United States in the mid-1960s from a country where there was neither a psychedelic movement nor psychedelic prohibition, I was particularly aware of how the American war between the government and psychedelic enthusiasts interfered with research and the utilization of psychedelics in psychotherapy.

It seemed to me that the refractoriness of the American establishment was not only a response to its unfamiliarity with the psychedelic experience but also an expression of this implicitly anti-Dionysian culture. And the intensity of psychedelic prohibition is not simply the offspring of an ingrained, overly controlling tendency in the American character; there is also the issue that the psychedelic movement has vehemently insulted the institutions that traditionally control drugs and through which LSD might have otherwise found an official distribution channel. Take, for example, Tim Leary's romantic plea for total deregulation in the early 1960s plus his own disdain for the psychiatric world. One could sympathize with him in view of how slow mental health professionals were to realize the therapeutic potential of LSD and the fact that some early medical investigators of LSD were sponsored by the Central Intelligence Agency. Yet I have always thought that his all too heroic rebelliousness and his messianic eagerness to liberate the world has paradoxically resulted in an interference in the adoption of LSD by the establishment.

The American war for and against drugs was the background for my book *The Healing Journey*, published in the late sixties. I wanted to draw attention to psychotropic substances that had not been labeled dangerous or been criminalized and were not likely to be, for they constituted what were considered "tamer" psychedelics that did not elicit disturbances in thinking or psychotic-type reactions. Also, I focused on the specifically therapeutic use of these substances, which I classified into two groups: the "feeling enhancers" and the "fantasy enhancers."

Before I turn to the specific matter of feeling enhancers I want to share my overall impression that the therapeutic aspects of psychedelic experiences are of more significant impact in personal evaluation than the wondrous spiritual ones. Whereas psychedelic-induced spiritual states are transient, therapeutic gains have considerably more stability. Moreover, the therapeutic process, which entails cleansing the psyche of dysfunctional imprints from childhood and recovering the ability to love, opens people up in a more stable manner and brings them closer to the depth of their spiritual potential. I think that the feeling enhancers hold the greatest promise. I consider myself very fortunate that I had the opportunity to open the field of therapeutic application some two decades ago. Here I give an overview of what I have learned.

On Feeling Enhancement and the Facilitation of Psychotherapy

In 1962 I met Sasha Shulgin, the most inventive of the psychedelic chemists, who introduced me to the potential that lay in investigating the substituted phenylisopropylamines. I was on my way to the Amazon, where I was to carry out my first psychedelic research project. I was interested then in the jungle brew known as *yagé*, or ayahuasca, the effects of which I came to interpret as an awakening of the reptilian brain and a bestowal of sacredness on the body and in our "animal within."

If all psychedelics contribute to the undoing of the ego—the Little Mind that obstructs the Big Mind—it could be said that the effect of the LSD-like psychedelics is most strikingly an undoing of the cognitive structure that constitutes the underpinning of the ego. The "ego death" they bring about is in the nature of a "blowing of the mind," and thus they may be appropriately called "head" drugs. By contrast, the harmala alkaloids such as ayahuasca seemed to be "gut" drugs—catalysts facilitating the flow of instinctual self-regulation, even at a physical level. It is against this background that I embarked on the exploration of MDA, a drug that turned out to be a psychotropic of a new species: a "heart" drug.

MDA: The Drug of Analysis

It was obvious from the very beginning that this substituted amphetamine had to do with the heart and not so much with the gut or the head. With the expression "feeling enhancer" I wanted to convey that its primary effects were on the emotional sphere, and that these effects were not those of a simple stimulant. One facet of this enhancement seemed to be increased feeling awareness, and another was an enhanced inclination to express feelings, but this was not all. Today I would call it a "feeling optimizer" for the optimal feeling, which is love.

Our psychological heart's blood is love, but in academic life, love is an expression that is avoided as not being scientific. Since the subject cannot be avoided, however, it is regarded as more tasteful to talk about empathy or positive emotional reinforcement. "Feeling enhancement" seemed proper in terms of the academic speech ethos. It seemed appropriate to suggest not only the elicitation of warm feelings but also the happy feelings that frequently derive from the outflowing of the heart. This quality was later emphasized by the name Ecstasy given to MDMA. Yet more deeply—as a precondition or foundation for love—I think that there lies another optimization, an optimization in our attitude toward pain. I believe that all our emotional problems have to do with a wrong attitude toward pain, a form of defensiveness to early experiences of pain that we were not ready to face that has become ingrained. Consequently, much of our learning to live right—the "gate to happiness," we might say—lies in finding another attitude toward pain, another way of being face to face with pain. This I consider to be the most significant aspect of the feeling enhancers. Before sharing further thoughts on the characteristics of MDA, I turn to a story.

Sasha Shulgin had told me of some observations in Gordon Alles's laboratory notes. Alles, the discoverer of amphetamine, thought that MDA might be useful as a vasodilator (a medicine that lowers blood pressure), and he tried it on himself with a platismograph around one of his fingers to test this hypothesis. After some time he found himself becoming more talkative than usual. At a certain point he saw a yellowish smoke ring in the room, but nobody was smoking. That was suggestive of a hallucinogenic property, particularly in view of the fact that the structure of the MDA molecule is a sort of hybrid between amphetamine and mescaline.

I was at the right place at the right time, an eager seeker hoping to find more medicine for my soul, and so it fell upon me to explore the substance further. I was a psychiatrist working for the Center for Studies in Medical Anthropology at the University of Chile Medical School, which was ready to support me in such ventures. Since there was neither a drug scene nor a drug scandal in Chile, I found myself in a position very much like that of Dr. Stanislav Grof, who was able to investigate LSD during the same years in Czechoslovakia. Instead of concentrating on LSD, I went in other directions. One was the domain of the phenylisopropylamines, and another was the exploration of a South American shamanistic concoction (yagé, or ayahuasca) and the alkaloids of the African psychotropic plant iboga.

From early testing on myself and on a few acquaintances, it was clear that MDA was a drug, unlike LSD, that elicited an expansion of emotional awareness without interfering with thinking. Its effect did not take the subject away from the ordinary world of objects and persons, but rather seemed specific for the processing of unfinished businesses in the interpersonal world. In retrospect, I can say that I was exceedingly lucky to hit on MDA, for its effects are similar to the now more well-known drug MDMA, Ecstasy. The discovery of this different kind of psychedelic was published in a succinct report, co-authored with Shulgin and Sargent (1967), evaluating MDA as an adjunct to psychotherapy. Afterward, I became involved in MDA-assisted psychotherapy, such as I have described in *The Healing Journey*.

I reported in that book what was found in working with people at the university clinic in Santiago. These patients given MDA would travel right back to early childhood and to early traumatic memories, particularly incestuous rape. Freud discovered this same realm of experience at the beginning of his career but then created a theory to explain it away. (I believe that he took the side of parents, not being ready to believe that they could do such things.) The undoing of childhood amnesia could involve other kinds of memory as well. In one MDA session, for example, a middle-aged woman remembered that as a child she had been locked in a room and had witnessed through a window the murder of her father by her mother's lover. I could not prove that this event was true, but I believed it. The understanding of herself and her life that resulted from this memory brought about a remarkable healing.

In *The Healing Journey* I referred to MDA as the "drug of analysis," because of the spontaneous age regression it induces and the interest it stimulates in reformulating—almost redigesting—the past. Descriptively appropriate as that may be, a still more essential characteristic of MDA would be conveyed by calling it a truth drug, in view of the nondefensive openness it (as well as some other phenylisopropylamines) catalyzes. Unlike the truth serum of fiction, this is not a drug that leads to the disclosure of information against one's will. Instead, there is a concern for truth and a facilitation of authenticity.

Because authenticity is the chief vehicle of therapies geared to self-knowledge, MDA and the other feeling optimizers are impressive psychotherapy enhancers. Just as other psychedelics have specialized therapeutic applications, such as the induction of mystical experiences, work on dreams, or the experience of perinatal states, the feeling enhancers open up what might be termed a "way of love." This is a spontaneous willingness to keep the flame of love alive in the face of pain—rather than becoming defensive and manipulative and, in consequence, blind. The gift of the feeling optimizers is the ability to remain a healthy and loving child of Paradise in spite of the contamination of the past and pollution of the interpersonal world. This ability is supported by a radically different stance in the face of pain, a nondefensive attitude that allows for the transmutation of pain into bliss.

Suffering is inextricably bound to earthly existence, but it may be a narcotic or an awakener, according to our willingness to take it in and use it for our growth. Our pain can be a stimulus to defensiveness and selfishness or to compassion and love. The difference is like that between a contrary wind that obstructs our progress and one that, through skillful use of the sail, permits us to advance somewhat against it. Such willingness may be the fruit of an austerity developed along our psychospiritual journey, yet it is also the transient gift of the feeling optimizers. They may take users directly to the realm of Adam and Eve (as if in reward for openheartedness) or they may take them not to hell, as in the case of LSD-like psychedelics, but to a worldly place of pain, to the other side of earthly Paradise, which is purgatory. This is the realm of psychotherapy par excellence.

I think that the name Adam, with which Leo Zeff baptized MDMA, was a very fortunate one. I was never happy with the overly academic and euphemistic term "entactogen" (which sounds like Latin and Greek and suggests the inner sense of contact more appropriately called "relationship"). I always liked Adam, because it indicates earthly paradise. And if psychedelic heavens can be related to the prenatal condition of life in the womb, earthly paradise echoes the postnatal condition of the newborn.

At the time of writing *The Healing Journey*, I thought it likely that since it is the more sick people who have the greater need to deal with the pain of the past, it would follow that the potentially addicted ones would tend to have "bad trips" and little enticement for the use of MDA as an escape into pleasure. When MDMA (with effects only subtly different from MDA) became available, I had occasion to see that I was wrong. There are people (with a hypomanic disposition) who manage to repress pain and experience instead euphoria and warmth in a way that seems to echo their customary denial of pain and anger. Instead of the therapeutic purgatory that they need, their hedonistic bias succeeds in directing them to a paradise, though their visits to paradise remain a sort of opium of the people, a spiritual exaltation that becomes a substitute rather than a remedy for their condition. In such cases, I think that preparatory psychotherapy and the therapeutic readiness of a person before the initial session—and therapeutic skill on the part of someone during the session—can make a great difference.

MMDA: The Eternal Now

Here I take up the thread of my story. I was ready to move into a new exploration, and this was to be MMDA. By the time Sasha Shulgin and I published its animal and human pharmacological characteristics in collaboration with

Sargent (1973), I was using it in psychotherapy. The most important quality I found in MMDA—a sense of what I call "the eternal now"—was something that I was particularly ready to appreciate, in view of an unexpected source of frustration that I had just encountered in my attempts to conduct therapy under MDA.

I was a budding Gestalt therapist in those days, having come in recent contact with Fritz Perls, and I had attempted to bring Gestalt therapy to bear on the psychedelic experience. I was frustrated in this endeavor, because while I tried to have people focus on the here and now, they insisted upon the "there and then," keenly determined to dwell on their memories. I must confess that I was a little slow to catch on to the fact that just as the more remarkable potential of MDA is its ability to bring long-repressed memories to the surface, the potential of MMDA is an increased awareness of the present.

For this reason MMDA lent itself admirably to Gestalt work, better than MDA. It not only focused on the here and now but also enhanced work involving imagery—not archetypal imagery like LSD and the fantasy enhancers but personal imagery, as in ordinary dreams. (I put iboga and harmala in the category of fantasy enhancers.) Furthermore, I found that MMDA often triggered psychosomatic symptoms and lent itself to exploration of this domain. All in all, I think that through the use of MMDA in conjunction with Gestalt therapy I helped many people. Discovering the specific excellence of MDA and MMDA in the facilitation of psychotherapy was like having twins in more than an intellectual sense, but the winds of adventure inclined me to the new.

Sasha Shulgin's skill in the synthesis of new psychoactive molecules is now becoming widely known. In those days he already had produced a number of analogs that were waiting for human testing, and this prompted me to turn to comparative research with some of these substances. Shulgin, Sargent, and I (1969) also published a summary report on the testing of various isopropylamines and closely related compounds.

MDMA: A Nontoxic Alternative to MDA

For me, the greatest news since the discovery of MDA and its healing potential has been MDMA—which differs chemically from MDA in the same way that amphetamine differs from nor-amphetamine. The effects are essentially the same as those of MDA, though it has a somewhat shorter duration of action and less of the toxicity.

While MDA is a therapy enhancer without the psychotomimetic potential of LSD, it has the serious drawback of toxicity. In my experience this was not a constant effect but one that became apparent every now and then in an unpredictable manner. In this sense it is like chloroform. In the old days, some patients would die from chloroform anesthesia, but this could not be anticipated. The reasons were unknown, and something similar seemed to be the case with MDA. I had observed at the time of writing *The Healing Journey* that once in awhile MDA brought about skin rashes and that beyond a certain dosage (about 250 mg), some people became incoherent, which could be attributed to cerebral vascular effects. I had warned my readers, urging them to test a person's reaction to MDA cautiously, starting with a very low dose. I fortunately did not have any accidents during my work in Chile. Given the fact that about thirty people took the drug , I view this as a blessing. A Chilean colleague was less lucky (and certainly less careful), for he administered 500 mg to a friend who experienced aphasia. After that, several deaths were reported in the United States.

We know that with MDMA the case is strikingly different. It has been known and used widely for many years, and despite accidents attributed to high blood pressure or inappropriate use it is remarkable for its lack of danger to healthy people. I would say that it is the champagne of the feeling enhancers. My approach to MDMA-assisted therapy (just as it was in the case of MDA) could be described as providing people with a special opportunity to talk about their past and present lives and problems, with a view to developing insight into their relationships and personalities. I emphasize this, because most people I know have used MDMA with a model borrowed from the use of LSD—that of listening to music through headphones while blindfolded. Much can be gained from that alone, but essentially the feeling enhancers have to do with the world of relationship and with the enhancement of the sense of "I" and the sense of "You" (which are interdependent). They are remarkable for the greater openness that they elicit and the ability they engender to communicate better concerning relationship problems.

I also emphasize this aspect because at one of the Esalen ARUPA

(Association for the Responsible Use of Psychedelic Agents) conferences devoted to an exchange between MDMA therapists, I found myself at odds with my colleagues in the psychedelic network. To my astonishment, everybody who spoke there professed to believe that the best way to take people on an MDMA trip is to urge them to withdraw into listening to music. I remember that Dr. Rick Ingrasci (past president of Association of Humanistic Psychology) and I were the only oddballs in that meeting: we talked to people and listened to them.

I also use music, but frequently I prefer to begin a session without it. I see verbal interaction as an invaluable vehicle for guiding people and helping them go deeper into their difficult experiences. This became apparent when I would come back into the room after a brief absence, and a patient would say, "Oh, I thought the effect had gone away, but as we talk it is all coming back." It is not the case that talking needs to be a distraction; it depends on the kind of talking and the empathic understanding one can provide.

After some time working with MDMA in individual and group situations, my main interest became its use within groups of people who had ongoing relationships with one another, such as families and communities. In this situation MDMA lends itself to occasional sessions geared to "clearing away the garbage" so as to keep relationships healthy. I have worked in this way not only with associated psychotherapists but also with people concerned with the quality of their partnerships in business and with good friends who wanted to keep their relationship free from the deterioration that most are prone to undergo in the course of time. Typically, I would work with groups of fifteen to twenty people consisting of a number of subgroups, in each of which people are involved in ongoing relationships outside therapy, for example, a family of three, four partners in a business firm, or the staff of a spiritual community.

One case report might convey some sense of the nature of an experience of group therapy in the way I have conducted it. While I have used the expression "analytical psychotherapy" in connection with my approach to individual therapy with MDA and MDMA, the kind of group therapy I have developed is one in which I have intervened little, except in the preparation of the group and in the course of a session of retrospective sharing and group feedback. I not only coordinate and share my own perceptions but also assist toward further elaboration of the experience.

An important part of my role in preparing for the MDMA session has been to create an atmosphere of surrender and spontaneity within the boundaries of a simple structure that limits movement away from the group but allows for withdrawal, protecting everyone's experience from invasion. In the case of MDMA administered to a group of optimal size and composition, I have witnessed a remarkable coincidence between the need of some participants to regress and be mothered and the availability of others to give such mothering. Since the effect of MDMA can be a peak experience or a delving into pain (or both), it is easy to see how it is possible that some persons find themselves in the garden of earthly paradise while others undergo the fires of purification—and the experience of the former is a gift to the latter. Again and again I have had the impression that as the result of the catalytic effect of MDMA upon the participants, the group becomes a spontaneously organizing system, for the good of all.

I now turn to a personal letter in which one middle-aged woman tells me of her experience at a group session, as an illustration of the kinds of things that can happen. It is not an unusual report in its content, and it is particularly illustrative of how much can happen through appropriate group preparation, without one-to-one therapeutic interactions. I think that experienced therapists will know well that this noninteraction is not a matter of simple strategy but rather a sort of art of "not doing" developed through experience and supported by a faith in group and individual organic self-regulation. All in all, it is not something that can be explained easily, nor is it something that can be prescribed mechanically, for it seems to require an educated ability to be present in the right way with sensitivity to what is happening. I have to add that this particular group had prepared for the experience with several days of psychotherapeutic exercises and meditation. The woman identified as K was a member of the group who chose to participate without taking MDMA, and J, who did take MDMA, is a sex therapist.

> After swallowing the capsule, I adopted an attitude of confidence—in myself, in life, before the unknown (which always scares me). Rachel's loving and strong presence made it easier for me. I felt strong palpitations that scared me, but I had confidence in you, who would assist me if it were necessary. I began to lose my skin sensations; I felt cold and as if I were lacking in air. This made me very afraid of death, afraid of dissolving or

that my heart would explode. I lay on my side as if folded upon myself, closed in, and within me I began to feel more peaceful and secure. A moaning came from my body, soft and trembling, as if shivering from cold. Then I realized that I was a baby, or a fetus, still unborn and sent into being to realize "Being," emerging out of nothing, solitude and cold. I was very afraid of being born.

Then somebody covered me, and I felt that somebody was by my side and caressed me. I saw that it was K, and I told her, "I am being born into this world." This was certain to me like the light of day. I was then able to let go into pain and weeping, for I felt secure before another human being, who gave me much warmth and tenderness. I sucked my fingers and her fingers, and I felt my teeth with which I could bite. When I felt more at ease, I could uncurl my body a little and talk to her. I told her, "Don't leave yet." I very much needed to talk to her and to tell her what I was going through and what I had lived through with my parents. I felt no anger toward my mother, only pain; I said this with great conviction, as if coming to own it completely. "She was not able to do more; she didn't know how to be with me." I did feel angry toward my father. I gave him hard words for so much damage that he had inflicted on me in a subtle way throughout my life.

I told K that I had written a poem to my inner child, and she wanted to hear it. When she did, I saw her tears. I recited other poems to her, but then she left me alone a little. She asked me whether I could stay alone for a little while, and she went to somebody who was calling her, assuring me that she would return. For the first time I did not feel alone. I had her jacket over me, which I could touch and smell, and the fantasy of her remained with me. I felt happy, for I was sure of her return, and I could also be with myself. I understood that it was good that she left me alone a little, for after letting her come into me and fill me, I could now assimilate it, integrating it into myself. I had much need to touch and press against the ground with different parts of my body. J came by, and I received him too as a gift from God. I told him what I was living. I felt him and told him everything from the beginning of the experience and the deep abyss—how I felt lovingly interwoven with essence, as if all my cells were constituted of Him. I was sorry that in our "normal state of mind" we did not realize this Reality that we are. And we also talked about sexuality. He assisted me with his hands toward an integration of head, heart, and sex, opening paths. He helped release my father from my body, for I felt as if I had been possessed by him thus far.

It was in this moment when you came by, and I told you I was purging myself of my father. And so you smiled, in confirmation. I would have liked you to have stayed longer, but I didn't dare to ask you. Then J told me he needed to be alone a little, that afterward he would have to help somebody else and that he would come back. I thus learned from both of them that I could find my space of aloneness when I needed it and how that was all right; it was not bad. I continued to feel happy, neither alone nor empty. I continued to feel nourished while by myself. It all seemed a gift from God that filled me with gladness—I was receiving much without having to seek it. Yes, I felt that I no longer needed the compulsive seeking of another (mothers and fathers) but only to open up and receive what came to me at the moment.

K returned, and in her company I started to look around in the room, absorbing and opening up to the surroundings, listening to groups of people who conversed and laughed. For a moment I came in touch with an admonition that had been introjected earlier in my life: "You must go with the others." But I understood that it was more important at that moment to remain with my own experience. Afterward J told me of his experience, and I could listen to him and let him in, feeling clear and free from myself, with space for the other. Then I started to dance alone, feeling all my joy, my living cells. I found my body axis and felt that energy moved along it upward and downward. I felt that I danced like a serpent, undulating my body and feeling successively an Arab, a Hindu, a gypsy—full of strength and energy.

At several points J approached, as if seduced by me. I felt afraid, as if he were going to rape me. I told him, as if to discourage him, "Hey, wait. I have just been born." I was with him in a group in which also was V, to whose peaceful face I felt attracted. With him I could verbally express my aggression toward men. When masculine singing sounded, I said, "I would have liked to dance like a woman." But he said, "Precisely because it is a man singing. Why don't you dance now, and you'll finish with your father this way." I took it as a special challenge, and I danced. It was an experience of feminine strength—and self-affirmation before my father, of separation and autonomy. I felt as if in this destructive history, I had reached further closure.

Well, Claudio, I won't tell you more anecdotes, because this letter, I think, has reflected the most meaningful things in the experience. It was profoundly therapeutic for me. I feel as if some of my archaic, primordial lack has been covered and that it couldn't have been in any other way. I have returned to this experience many times to nourish myself, and I feel that I am coming to the end of a healing process with a more lucid, organized, and creative mind, more confident, daring to teach and share the riches I have been keeping to myself. I continue to write poetry, and I enjoy life more and more.

I hope that this session report will serve to convey a general understanding of how many issues that are distinct and separate in theory commingle in a single experience. The anonymous subject says that she has just been born, and the session as a whole may be seen as a step in a birthing process. Separation and union both have a part in this birthing. In asserting her individuality, she differentiates herself from her father; at the same time the event occurs in the context of a mothering situation—one in which she allows herself to regress through the support of others (the therapist, the group, and, most specifically, her companions). Yet regression is not all there is to birthing; just as separation and union are both part of the process, so there is here a regression to progress, the allowing of a fetal state that then becomes the stepping-stone, as it were, for self-expression.

I have said that the content of the session is not particularly special, yet it is rich enough to bring up many issues. Among these issues is the importance of the attitude with which the subject embarks on the experience—and more specifically, an attitude of confidence and even a measure of acceptance in the face of "death," or a sense of impending "explosion." It is the extent of this acceptance of ongoing experience that makes the deep surrender possible that is in the background of an organic unfolding. The classic elements of an MDMA experience are all here: awareness of psychological pain, insight into life and relationships, self-expression in verbal communication and movement, and a progression from defensive accusation toward an understanding of others. It is clear from the account just how important the relationship between group members can be, in the sense of both mothering and intuition sharing or, more generally, peer therapy.

Carl Rogers has claimed that therapeutic groups may be the most beneficial invention of the twentieth century, and I have not known a more effective form of group psychotherapy than the skillful use of MDMA. I hope that this glimpse into the nature of the experience may be a stimulus for future health authorities to give more positive attention to this neglected approach, for we cannot afford to squander resources in days when emotional health has become so vital to the human destiny. MDMA is an extremely valuable resource for processing past life experience and for healing relationships in the context of dialogue. Yet the great gift that heaven seems to be offering us through scientific know-how remains unused at a time when there is an urgent need for collective mental health. Given that the regulatory and medical establishment considers these statements unproven, I believe them to be research priorities.

For a long time I thought that *The Healing Journey* had been a failure, for it had not appeared to stimulate the interest of either the medical establishment or the lay public in finding out how to put these gifts to use for the good of all. The book seemed to have been liked mostly by insiders, who needed it least. Over the years, however, I have been surprised to see scarcely a book about psychedelic therapy, and I think *The Healing Journey* continues to fill a void, to some extent, giving credibility to psychedelics as the precious therapeutic catalysts they are. I hope that it serves to support my contention that we cannot afford the luxury of wasting their potential while we linger in a deadly police-minded mentality, for they constitute precisely the kind of remedy that we need as we approach a new collective Red Sea crossing.

I believe that it is the absence of a channel for the potential beneficial use of psychedelics that is to be held responsible for our collective psychedelic disease, with its addiction and criminalization. I am convinced that abuse comes from bad use, and this has been the result of restricted opportunity for good use. Of course, the repressive quality of government with respect to drug issues is an expression of a repressive bias in the very structure of civilization and also of the prohibitionist leanings that we have inherited from our early Puritan ancestors. We are living through times, however, where it has become critical to our very survival that we go beyond the overly stable and fossilized spirit of the institutions that we have created. I trust that our government will rise from its slumber before long and reconsider its dysfunctional policy. What is needed now is not prohibition but true expertise: the training of specialists who can use psychotropic substances wisely and skillfully. I am happy to see that we seem to be coming to a time when a reconsidering of psychedelics by the establishment is under way, and I pray that enlightened government may perceive and put to use the potential of psychedelics for our individual and collective healing.

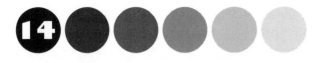

CLINICAL EXPERIENCE WITH MDMA-ASSISTED PSYCHOTHERAPY

An Interview with George Greer, M.D.

JH: I think that I would like to start by having you explain what sort of work you do.

GG: I'm a psychiatrist in private practice. I have a small outpatient psychotherapy practice, and I also work half-time in a residential treatment center for post-traumatic stress disorder (PTSD), mostly with patients who have experienced sexual or physical abuse in childhood. They also generally have depression and other mood disorders, eating disorders, attention-deficit hyperactivity disorder (ADHD), and addictions. It's a very intense patient population. They come to our program from all around the country after being in hospitals for about a month. It's a residential program designed for after-hospital care. I'm the psychiatrist there, and I evaluate patients and prescribe medications.

JH: Tell me about your involvement with the Heffter Institute.

GG: That's my third job. I'm the medical director, secretary, and treasurer of the Heffter Research Institute, and I coordinate all the operations and review of research protocols. We have an executive director who does fundraising and a business manager.

JH: And what does the Heffter Institute do?

GG: We plan, promote, and support research with psychedelic drugs in basic science areas, to learn how the brain works and how the mind works, and in clinical science, to use psychedelics to treat medical and psychiatric conditions. The research is being performed mostly in other countries at this time, but there is also some research in the United States. We've been working about eight years now, and the fund-raising is going well. The main program we're planning is at the University of Zurich with Dr. Franz Vollenweider.

JH: It sounds as if you dedicate some of your time to promoting psychedelic research. I am curious about how that interest began for you.

GG: It began for me in college. It was in my sophomore year, when my roommate said he had learned things from taking mescaline. Then I had some very profound learning experiences that changed my outlook on life more toward spirituality, and I became involved in meditation. In medical school, I learned about the work of Dr. Stanislav Grof, and I went to a six-week program at Esalen Institute in 1975 to learn more about the psychotherapeutic use of LSD. When I finished my psychiatric residency in 1979 in California, I met with Ralph Metzner [consciousness researcher and psychotherapist], who suggested that I conduct clinical sessions with ketamine, which was available to physicians. Then I learned about MDMA, which was being used by psychologists. I began to read the regulations and found that if I synthesized it myself, I could prescribe and administer it to my own patients if I had peer reviews and informed consents.

JH: When did you first hear about MDMA and from whom?

GG: I probably heard about it very vaguely in the 1970s, and in 1980 I heard more clearly from psychologists who were using it in therapy. That's when I contacted Sasha Shulgin and made a batch in his lab, because he knew how to do it. I also had some training with psychologists who had been using it for a few years. I started using it at the end of 1980. I thought it was important to do it legally, so that people could talk about it freely. I could not tolerate risking my medical license by doing underground work.

JH: What specifically had you heard from the psychologists? What were they seeing?

GG: They just said that it was very helpful for psychotherapy and personal growth. It facilitated getting over neurotic hang-ups, getting more in touch with the self in a basic way, and relating more to partners. It just sort of speeded up the therapy process by reducing defenses.

JH: Can you estimate how many therapists you think were using MDMA in the late seventies?

GG: In the late seventies, it was probably just a handful. In the early eighties, it became much more prolific. There were several therapists using it in the San Francisco Bay area, probably several more in Los Angeles, and a number on the East Coast. I would guess less than a hundred by the time it was scheduled, but that's a ballpark figure.

JH: There were East Coast therapists engaged in MDMA-assisted psychotherapy? I had never heard for sure that there were any; it seemed a purely West Coast phenomenon to me.

GG: There was at least one group using it in New York City. There may have been other groups who just didn't communicate with the people I knew.

JH: It seemed as though the real story broke when the Drug Enforcement Administration scheduled MDMA in 1985 on an emergency basis. Many psychologists and psychiatrists came forward then.

GG: My understanding is that a reporter for *People* magazine had heard about its recreational use and then learned from Marilyn Ferguson [editor of *Brain/ Mind Bulletin*, pioneer of the consciousness movement] about its therapeutic use. She sent him to see my wife, Requa Tolbert, and me, and they spent three days interviewing us and people who had had sessions with us. He wrote a story but never published it. He said the reason was that the editors wanted him to make it half-bad and half-good, and he could not find the half-bad side. Then *Newsweek* and other news magazines got wind of the story, followed by the TV stations. The fact that the drug was being sold in bars in Texas got plenty of publicity. After that, I understand Senator Lloyd Bentsen of Texas asked the DEA to do something, so they put the emergency scheduling in place in mid-1985.

JH: Were you involved in the countermovement, among the group of therapists who tried to point out to the DEA that there was a beneficial side to MDMA?

GG: Yes. The DEA planned the scheduling in late 1984, I think. Then Lester Grinspoon and some other people and I became involved in petitioning the government to place it in Schedule III. That effort started in the late summer of 1984, and then, after all the publicity broke, the emergency scheduling happened in 1985.

JH: Were you present at any of the hearings?

GG: There were three different hearings in different parts of the country. I went to the one in Kansas City and testified. The DEA lawyers examined me.

JH: What sort of things did you say when you were on the stand?

GG: I said that I had given MDMA to about eighty people and that no one had had any serious negative effects from using it, except for some anxiety or panic. The vast majority of people said that it helped them achieve their goals for the session, which was usually to learn about themselves or a particular psychological problem. It could be a wide variety of things. Most people wanted to take it once or twice and were not interested in the drug in terms of its addictive potential. That's pretty much what I laid out for them at the hearings.

JH: How did you feel when Judge Young made a recommendation to the DEA that Schedule III placement was appropriate?

GG: It was wonderful. I thought he really understood and appreciated the value of the drug. It was a great victory. It didn't have the authority to make the DEA do anything, unfortunately, but it was a great achievement that we got our word in and were understood.

JH: Were you surprised that you could go through all these legal motions and have a judge make a recommendation and then see that ruling totally ignored by the DEA?

GG: I wasn't surprised. We knew that he was an administrative law judge; he wasn't a regular federal court judge, and the statutes said his judgment was only a recommendation. It did not have the force of law per se. The way that the statute is written, the DEA does not have to follow his recommendation. We knew that, and I don't think we were surprised that the DEA didn't agree with him.

JH: I understand that there was an appeals process and that once again Schedule III was recommended, and again the DEA made a move to place MDMA permanently in Schedule I.

GG: It was a technical matter. An appeals court in Boston said that the DEA could not schedule the drug on the basis that they had. They could not equate Food and Drug Administration approval with accepted medical use; they had to use a different standard. So the DEA said they then used a different standard but still claimed that it had no medical use. It was kind of a formality, and it wasn't surprising.

JH: That wasn't particularly frustrating for you? It just seemed like a little coda?

GG: No, it was all very frustrating. The whole thing was overwhelmingly frustrating but not unexpected.

JH: What was the most frustrating aspect for you? Was it that you had found an efficient and effective tool in a field where there weren't too many tools?

GG: It was as if I had discovered how to use oil paints in my art, and then all the paints were banned because people sniffed them. All along, I knew it was a fringe thing; I was using it legally but in a huge sort of legal loophole. There was no FDA involvement at all in using the drug therapeutically, which must be very, very rare. All of us knew that it was a risk, in that sooner or later it would get onto the street, and things would change. I don't think I ever thought that this wouldn't happen or that we were home free.

JH: You did have a feeling that the work that you were doing was somewhat tempo-rary? Even though it wasn't illegal, did you have a feeling that you were going to get shut down at some point?

GG: I had heard in late 1982 that MDMA was being used recreationally at parties in New York City. At that point, I decided to start writing up the results that I had found with the people to whom I had given it. I knew that if it were being used at parties, it very likely would be scheduled. I already had asked everyone to fill out a complete pre-session questionnaire; then I designed a similar questionnaire that I could send to people after their sessions. For some people, it was a couple of years later that I got the follow-up data. I started collecting it, assembling it, and organizing it, and I worked on that part time for almost a year to get it in a format to be printed. It was self-published in late 1983, and then it was published in the *Journal of Psychoactive Drugs* in 1986, after a conference on MDMA that summer.

JH: Tell me about the conference.

GG: It was organized through the Haight-Ashbury Free Medical Clinic by Dr. David Smith and Rick Seymour, editor of the *Journal*. It was a two-day conference, in Oakland, California, for people to present information on MDMA—all sorts of information, from toxicity to therapeutic use to recreational use. People made presentations and submitted papers that were published in the *Journal of Psychoactive Drugs*. It was a good, balanced conference. Someone from the DEA was there to present their perspective as well.

JH: This took place after the scheduling?

GG: About a year after.

JH: Did people present anything about potential therapeutic benefits?

GG: My cases were mostly people who were functioning well, who had neurotic-type problems or wanted a personal-growth kind of experience and had found benefit with the drug. Dr. Phil Wolfson had used it with a young man who had episodes of psychosis, either schizophrenia or schizoaffective illness, and his family. He had done a family session and presented that. The family bonding improved quite a bit. The patient himself, I think, was better for a while, but there was no lasting improvement. Dr. Jack Downing presented information from a human physiology study of vital signs and neurological findings. He also had given MDMA to a woman, a therapist who had been raped. I remember that this story appeared on a television news broadcast. She had an MDMA session, relived aspects of the rape itself, and resolved a lot of it. Her symptoms and flashbacks essentially disappeared. She had dramatically improved after a single MDMA-assisted psychotherapy session. Then Dr. Rick Ingrasci presented information about using the drug for psychotherapy. One of his patients, who had terminal cancer, appeared with him on the *Phil Donahue Show*. MDMA had helped her greatly to come to peace with herself and not be fearful or anxious or stressed.

JH: You've mentioned two areas I want to spend more time on. The first is PTSD. You have worked specifically with people with this diagnosis, who have a history of physical or psychic trauma. Can you describe how an MDMA-assisted psychotherapy session might help people to process some of this trauma?

GG: It's purely theoretical, but my understanding of PTSD is that the emotional impact of the physical sensations of the trauma gets locked in the lower brain centers, like the limbic system, and never gets resolved by verbal or ego-integrated processes in the cerebral cortex. (Some of this is from Dr. Bessel van der Kolk's theories.) The techniques that help PTSD involve the reexperiencing and cognitive processing of the experiences. The memories can be verbalized and released, instead of cycling around in the limbic system in an emotional loop, causing flashbacks and emotional dysregulation— distress, increased arousal, affective shutdown and inhibition, panic attacks, that sort of thing. The theory behind eye-movement desensitization and reprocessing [EMDR] treatment for PTSD is that it activates a connection from the limbic system to the cortex—people start to reexperience and verbalize these memories, which is helpful.

MDMA reduces psychological defenses but probably in a different way. This makes it very hard for the person to have a fear reaction to psychological content, so I imagine that it also would remove the cortical inhibitions toward experiencing the trauma memories, which can be very unformed. They're affective memories, body sensation memories, something that the ego can't get a handle on. That's why it can't be processed. MDMA opens that door and allows that experiencing and prevents the overwhelming fear and anxiety overload that would perhaps re-traumatize the person. The nervous system comes into balance. That is the way I think it helped this woman and the way it could help others with PTSD.

JH: There's more of a sense of calm and maybe a certain amount of bravery in looking at an event that the patient either didn't have access to or just didn't feel equipped to explore.

GG: Right. The content feels less threatening to the person in the moment. If they start to think about the event without MDMA, normally they might get anxious or distract themselves or repress it entirely. With MDMA, they might start to think about it and say, "This is okay. This is not threatening me. I'm not getting anxious." So the process can continue.

JH: It's interesting that you say that MDMA helps to dampen a fear response. There is a sense that I get from people who tell me of their MDMA experiences that they feel more equipped to dig and to look at places where they've been hurt, which is what therapy is all about. It seems to be a combination of calm and not quite fearlessness, but more like a strengthened sense of self, of confidence. You see that you can handle what you're digging up; it's not going to break you.

GG: Yes. I think that the only thing it does is prevent the knee-jerk fear response. The drug only turns off this fear reaction, and everything that happens occurs out of innate abilities that the patient has. I don't believe that MDMA gives people enhanced cognitive abilities, enhanced intelligence, or other aptitudes that aren't really there already.

JH: I think it makes it easier for people to express their true selves. This comes up in couple's therapy to an extent, where the typical defenses and posturing that may arise out of fear of exposing oneself are markedly diminished. People can really share more of who they are.

GG: My first experience with my wife, Requa—we weren't married at the time—was exactly that. It was just easier to talk about things that normally we would have been afraid or skittish or uncomfortable to talk about. It just seemed easy. Afterward, it was still a lot easier.

JH: That's something that deserves to be underscored, which is that whatever you learn with an MDMA-assisted experience or whatever skills you acquire, you leave with them. You learn how to communicate and operate with less fear, and you are able to incorporate that into your life. It's not as if you forget how you felt or what you discovered.

GG: Yes, I think that's possible, but people don't always decide to do that. At higher doses, say, 200 mg, people can get carried away in the euphoria. I have heard of couples back in the eighties who would take MDMA and get very close and intimate, and afterward they still had problems in their relationship that weren't resolved and did not get resolved in everyday life. There's no guarantee; it all depends on the people and their intention, their willingness, to work it out.

JH: It's very important to integrate the skills that you uncover. I understand that you didn't give MDMA as part of your private practice.

GG: I had one patient who had heard about my use of it, so that was the only patient in my private practice who had MDMA-assisted psychotherapy sessions with me. I just felt that it was too experimental to recommend to any of my private patients. It was a separate part of my work.

JH: It was something that you were doing with acquaintances.

GG: Right, and with people who had heard about my work through the grapevine, friends of friends or people I knew.

JH: You would help lead individual or couples sessions. Did you do any group or family work?

GG: At times, there were small groups of perhaps four people who knew each other and wanted to have a deepening bonding experience. The one patient I worked with in therapy had about three MDMA sessions. She was seeing me for depression and neurotic kinds of problems—self-esteem and relationship difficulties—and it greatly speeded up the progress of our regular psychotherapy sessions. She had a very positive transference, and was more at ease in trusting me and talking about embarrassing things in our regular therapy sessions between the MDMA sessions. My perception of her progress was that MDMA facilitated the treatment alliance, the positive transference, and reduced her defenses so that she could deal with her core issues more quickly and more efficiently. I think she would say the same thing, in that she became a psychotherapist.

JH: That's very interesting. When you say three sessions, how far apart were they scheduled?

GG: They were probably four to six weeks apart—at least a month but more likely six weeks.

JH: I'm assuming that you used a dose of about 125 mg. Did you use any booster doses later in the session?

GG: We offered that, always. We started with 75 to 125 mg, and the person could tell us that they wanted a low, medium, or high dose within that range. An hour and a half to two hours later, we would offer them an additional 50 mg, and most would take it.

JH: How long would the sessions last?

GG: I often performed the sessions together with Requa, who has a master's degree in psychiatric nursing, and we would be with the person for six to eight hours. The first two to three hours the person would listen to music with headphones, lying down and wearing eyeshades. During the second three-hour period the person would start talking and interacting with us and doing something more like psychotherapy. We would talk about problems and issues and work through difficult feelings. When we thought that the person could take care of themselves and the emotional processing was complete, we would leave. We usually did the session in the person's home, so they wouldn't have to travel afterward. Occasionally it would be in our home.

JH: You mentioned that one patient had self-esteem issues. I want to get your opinion on how you think self-esteem, self-acceptance, and self-love are affected by MDMA.

GG: I think that all those are beliefs, so they have a cognitive aspect and an emotional aspect. They're concepts about the self. To the extent that those beliefs are based on a fear—such as "I'm not good enough because I have this feeling. There's something bad inside me, and I'm afraid of it and don't want to look at it. I'm too scared to look at it, and that means I'm not a worthy person. I'm not a whole person"—the person feels incomplete. People feel that there is something bad inside them that is threatening and dangerous to them and to anyone they come close to emotionally. With MDMA, they can look more closely and see what that bad thing is. They can look at whatever they feel they're ashamed of at a gut level and see through it and call its bluff. Frequently, they will discover that there really is nothing inside them that is bad or wrong. Maybe there are things that are unpleasant or obsessive or addictive, but these things are not standing between their awareness and their core being. When they can get in touch with all their feelings—good and bad—and discover that they're not afraid of them, they can just accept them as part of themselves. That self-acceptance leads to a different feeling, "I'm okay. There's nothing wrong with me."

JH: I think that this sort of feeling of self-acceptance and self-love really leads to the bliss and joy that people associate with the drug Ecstasy.

GG: When people take it recreationally, I'm sure that's true. With MDMA, there are no problems that cannot be solved.

JH: Getting back to the issue of a dissolution of fear or anxiety, how would that affect the perception of pain? I know that you had a patient with chronic pain. Was it from multiple myeloma?

GG: Yes.

JH: There's a body of research that suggests that anxiety and fear of pain can heighten the perception of pain and exacerbate the experience. I know that terminal patients can have a tremendous fear of death. The fear of ego disintegration, the fear of no longer being, can play into the perceptions of their physical symptoms. I was wondering where MDMA fits into this theory.

GG: This patient's pain came from collapsed vertebrae that had been caused by the multiple myeloma, which is a form of bone marrow cancer. He was a very intelligent man, very insightful. He had been doing visualization, as developed by Dr. Carl Simonton, who was one of his physicians. He had been visualizing the white blood cells attacking the cancer cells. He was doing all of those psychological, self-hypnosis pain control techniques, but they were not working for him. He couldn't be very physically active—couldn't go fishing, couldn't get around very well for a number of years, I think. In addition to reducing fear, MDMA has an analgesic or anesthetic effect. This has even been measured in mice or rats; there is a "tail-flick" response, or something of the sort, that is diminished. In fact, in people who have taken MDMA and pinch their own skin, the tactile response is there, but the pain is reduced.

I think for this man, it was a combination of the direct analgesic and/or anesthetic effect and the euphoria and reduction of fear. In the session, he said he was pain free for the first time in four years. I'm sure all those factors were involved, but the fact that he experienced no pain at all for an hour or two made him very euphoric in itself. He did a self-hypnosis anchoring of the pain-free state; in other words, he mentally connected his pain-free state with imagery or thoughts that he had during the session. He "anchored" that pain-free experience so that he could experience it again, which is a technique in hypnosis. For weeks afterward, when he did pain-control self-hypnosis, he was able to regain that pain-free, or relatively pain-free, state. The MDMA session more or less primed his own technique, so that he was much more pain-free and able to be active again and get a lot of his life back. After a few weeks, the pain gradually would increase, and he would have another session of anchoring. He had about three sessions. I think he had two sessions with us and then a session or two on his own, and each time he would anchor the pain-free state so that his own technique was effective for several weeks.

JH: When he would have a session, he would have an analgesic effect?

GG: Each time the session would get him back to either a total or an almost total pain-free state.

JH: I really wanted to have a chapter in this book about palliative care, about working with the dying. Unfortunately, I haven't been able to find anyone who's qualified to write it. MDMA does seem to be a potent analgesic, and I believe it also enhances a person's concentration and the capacity to have that sort of meditative, hypnotic, guided imagery experience.

GG: Yes, because at moderate doses, people's mind and ego organization are intact; they can direct the mind and attention toward a mental task and complete it relatively well.

JH: I would even venture to say that one's attention and concentration are enhanced with a moderate dose.

GG: Yes, I would agree. There's less distraction.

JH: In the same way that a low dose of amphetamine would enhance your concentration and attention.

GG: Exactly. If you think of it as a continuum of attention deficit disorder, where dopamine releasers or stimulants enhance the focusing of attention, MDMA definitely has a similar effect. Getting back to the palliative care issue, I did receive phone calls from AIDS treatment centers. They told me that some of their patients were using MDMA in a therapeutic way. It was legal at the time, but these centers were using it underground for patients who were medically much sicker than my patient. They were terminally ill, in lots of distress and pain. It was immensely valuable to help them come to peace with their lives, to relieve anxiety, to just have a much better quality of life with AIDS after their session. To my knowledge, the sickest terminally ill people who have used MDMA were these AIDS patients. Anecdotally, these centers reported that many patients were experiencing benefits and found it very worthwhile.

JH: The case reports and the anecdotal evidence about people who are dying are so encouraging and heartwarming. It is immensely helpful to have closure with the family, to be able to open up and say the things that you want to say to the people around you before you go. I think this is invaluable and really soothing.

GG: Yes, exactly. When people are dying, their lives often are not complete, and they have not caught up with everyone. It helps the family and everyone to let go and finish their unfinished business. Elisabeth Kübler-Ross has written a great deal about unfinished business with one's relations and also with oneself, which is helpful to attend to in the dying process. I think MDMA can facilitate that greatly.

JH: I do too. On many levels, I think MDMA is appropriate for use with people who are terminally ill or markedly sick. First, they get a few hours of feeling better, emotionally and physically, and having some respite from their symptoms. It's also possible that they will learn to manage their symptoms, their physical pain, better. The fringe benefits of having closure with their families and experiencing less fear about the dying process can go a long way toward relieving their pain, psychic and otherwise.

GG: I think so, but they have to decide that they want to do that. If they wish to, then I think MDMA can be helpful to them.

JH: Are there other groups of patients that we haven't talked about that you think may be appropriate to explore in terms of clinical research?

GG: I've been thinking about this, and I think the question is: What patient population would not benefit from it? Almost all mental disorders are complicated by the affected person's fear of things they perceive either inside or outside themselves. Certainly this is true of all the anxiety disorders, depressive disorders, and personality disorders. Fear and psychological, pathological defense mechanisms are involved in most every mental disorder. I've thought more recently that MDMA might help treat psychotic disorders and manic disorders, because the serotonin system is involved with those disorders and there are studies with pre-pulse inhibition that show that MDMA enhances the filtering of sensory information [see "Using MDMA in the Treatment of Schizophrenia"]. At least one study by Franz Vollenweider and Mark Geyer (Vollenweider et al. 1999b) has shown that MDMA helps people filter sensory information better than in their normal state. Schizophrenic people have weakened pre-pulse inhibition and have deficits in filtering information, but this capacity is enhanced in normal people taking MDMA. This is hypothetical, but let's say that someone is locked into a paranoid state or a delusional state. If this person were willing to take MDMA, it might reduce whatever fear is creating or resulting from the paranoid delusions and give him or her a break from it and more of an ability to think around it. It would be a very challenging and risky thing to give MDMA to someone with paranoid schizophrenia for the first time. There are a lot of procedural and ethical problems, but if the patient were willing and competent to give informed consent and all other treatments had failed, it would seem worth trying.

JH: I absolutely agree. I think the pre-pulse inhibition data look enticing, but it's also my gut feeling that there is such a lowering of fear that it would be worthwhile to explore that in someone who has schizophrenia, in terms of their paranoia. The other issue is the negative symptoms. A schizophrenic patient with negative symptoms is someone who isn't thinking or talking much. This person isn't connecting with other people and doesn't have much emotional expression or motivation. These are all things that possibly could be combated in the short term.

GG: You could start with 25 mg, because many people have taken all the antipsychotics, and they're still the way they are. I wouldn't see any problem with starting with 25 mg to make sure MDMA did not make them worse, before going to higher doses.

JH: I'm glad that you wouldn't see any problem with it. Unfortunately, every psychiatry chairman or institutional review board that I've ever discussed this with is more hesitant. Schizophrenics are such a vulnerable patient population to research. I was very interested in giving single oral dose MDMA to medicated schizophrenic patients with negative symptoms, but I was unable to find an institution to support that. It is still my long-term goal to see if it can help.

GG: If they're not in a psychotic state, they should be able to give informed consent.

JH: One of my rationales is that schizophrenics have consented to be given amphetamine, fenfluramine, and ketamine, so it's not so far off the beaten track to try this ring-substituted amphetamine. I've been in touch with four people with schizophrenia who have used MDMA, not so much to control their symptoms as to help them be better equipped to deal with their symptoms. They want to know that they are just symptoms and to have kind of an outsider's view: "That's my paranoia."

GG: They want perspective on it. These are my symptoms. This is not me; this is not reality.

JH: At least with two of these four people MDMA has helped them let their families stay in their inner circle and not be separated. That happens to many people who are psychotic. They pull away from their families, but they need that support system and those caretakers.

GG: Maybe that could be published somewhere.

JH: There are case reports in this book. It's an area that I would like to pursue. The bottom line is that there are a lot of people who could derive benefit from one or two MDMA-assisted psychotherapy sessions.

GG: Yes. Getting back to your question, I don't know of a mental disorder that I think has no potential for benefit from MDMA. Maybe some organic disorders, but then it might help the psychological distress that a person with an organic mental illness has.

JH: One possible area where MDMA would be helpful, which hasn't been spoken about too much, is substance abuse disorders. So much of diminishing substance abuse lies in examining one's behavior patterns and seeing what's working and what's not.

GG: Right. I didn't treat any serious substance abusers, but there were some people who said they were less interested in using cocaine after MDMA. Some patients said they were not interested in marijuana as much, but then others were more interested in it. In my work at the PTSD treatment center here, I have seen people who have abused ten drugs; they have horrible drug abuse histories, including Ecstasy. Their reason for using Ecstasy is to get high, for the stimulation. It has no therapeutic set or setting whatsoever. Some of these patients said they liked it a lot; they felt better. Maybe a couple said they functioned better during that time; then they ran out of it, and they went back to the cocaine or the amphetamines or whatever else they were using. I see only people who are still having severe problems, rather than people who have resolved their problems through Ecstasy use.

JH: The context is important. I think that at the average rave scene, there are some people who are probably having some psychic benefits.

GG: I would agree from what I have read about it.

JH: In general, I think that the benefits are maximized by a supervised, judicious-use situation.

GG: I think a rave scene is more positive than sitting at home drinking alcohol and taking Ecstasy, because at many rave scenes, at least there is a positive mind-set and a positively oriented setting, though you could still call it recreational. It's certainly not a medical setting. Unfortunately, there is the potential problem that rising ambient and body temperatures increases the serotonin toxicity from MDMA in animals, which could apply to people dancing at raves and taking very high doses of Ecstasy.

JH: On the other hand, recreation is certainly therapeutic, and I think that this bonding and the socialization are good. There's a group mind that can be developed and cohesion and intimacy with everyone around you, which I think is also therapeutic. Feeling "hooked in" to something—to society or to the planet—feeling as if you are really a part of it and that you're connected is very healthy. Part of the problem with chronic mental illness is the feeling of isolation. The sicker you are, the more isolated you are, and I think that adds to the illness and is very unhealthy.

GG: Right. One of the last people we gave MDMA to was a psychologist who had ADHD. He treated people with ADHD, who feel very cut off from other people because of their attention problems and lack of empathy. After his treatment, he went back home, and people commented to him that he seemed different, more emotionally accessible. He saw a great psychological benefit for people with ADHD from MDMA, which is what you're saying. People with mental illnesses are cut off from people, because they're so distracted by their symptoms and suffering.

JH: Right. I think that's also a major reason why people commit suicide—they're socially isolated. June Riedlinger has written a chapter for the book where she talks about the potential to use MDMA as sort of an "interrupter" in the process of a person's becoming more depressed and suicidal and so cut off. Did you specifically do any sort of couple's therapy?

GG: Couples came to have MDMA together, to improve their relationship. None of these couples were in the middle of a divorce or having serious or fundamental relationship problems. I think all of them said that it improved their ability to communicate in an intimate way and in a lasting way. They were able to carry over the communication that went on during the session into their lives. There was one woman who had had an abortion and felt very sexually inhibited after it for several months. After the MDMA session, she just let go of her phobia of getting pregnant again. That irrational fear was gone, and her sexual intimacy with her husband was restored.

JH: It just points to the fact that what one learns during a session, one can take home. In terms of learning a new skill, like being able to communicate with a partner, and having less fear about exposing one's self to that person, it's a learning experience. You learn that you can expose yourself without the other person ridiculing you. You have a positive experience from opening up to that level of intimacy. You try out a new skill, you learn that it has positive results, and you take it with you.

GG: That's exactly what happens. There's a theory that state-dependent learning does not carry over, but with a moderate dose of MDMA, that's just not true.

JH: I think that one of the reasons why this state-dependent learning does carry over is that it is such a subtle shift of consciousness. It's not so far from a normal waking state. It is easy for most people to approximate the feeling that they had when they were taking MDMA. You don't need to keep taking it over and over, because you can pretty much get there without the drug.

GG: Right. I know a psychologist and hypnotherapist who has conducted hypnosis on people who had MDMA so that they could re-create that altered state and engage in the kind of psychological processing they would in that state. It sounds somewhat similar to what the cancer patient did.

JH: Where do you think our current level of MDMA research is? Compare that with where you think it should be or where it should be going.

GG: At the University of Zurich, Franz Vollenweider has done receptor blockade studies, with people who have never had MDMA and with others who have taken Ecstasy. He is just learning the mechanism of how it works. There are two ongoing studies in the United States focusing on basic pharmacology, at Wayne State and at U.C. San Francisco. In August 1999, there was an international meeting in Israel of every group in the world that has used MDMA in human research. Two psychiatrists from Switzerland and I, who have used it in therapy, also participated. In Spain and Israel research groups are planning projects to use MDMA to treat PTSD; in Spain they will use it just with rape victims. I think that research certainly is picking up. The FDA reversed course from stopping human research. Initially, they had told Dr. Charles Grob of UCLA that he had to do a lot of animal studies before he could work with cancer patients. Then they said that he didn't have to do any more animal studies but that he needed concrete outcome measurements. That was a positive step.

JH: Do you see that perhaps it may become easier to do MDMA research in the United States?

GG: A year ago, it became much harder, and then, more recently, it became easier. In the United States it's now a matter of designing a trial that has outcome measures that are concrete enough to be acceptable to the FDA. I think it's possible, but I think that it will take a lot of time and research design work. As you know, in psychiatry the outcome measures are much softer than in other areas, which makes matters very tricky. My own thinking is to work with pain, the symptoms of chronic pain, among people who are terminally ill and not terminally ill. The trick there is to find someone who has chronic pain who doesn't have to take other medications all the time. Giving MDMA with narcotics or other drugs creates a drug interaction issue.

JH: It's not good research. It's not an optimal design either.

GG: My patient with myeloma was taking only acetaminophen (Tylenol) for pain, so there were no drug interactions that we were aware of. My thinking is that pain is easily measurable. You can measure how much pain medication a person uses before and after a session. There are many possible concrete measures, as opposed to the situation with depression or anxiety or substance abuse, where there are so many variables. The door has been opened at this point, and I think that when things happen in other countries, that will help matters here. I think Rick Doblin has been doing much work on this for many years; he has been networking with the FDA and forming relationships with them, which seems to be paying off.

JH: It does seem as though there are little projects sprouting up here and there—maybe not in the United States, but around the world.

GG: Yes, and if they are published and there are positive results, established university researchers will become interested.

JH: I was speaking to a schizophrenia researcher the other day, and I mentioned the pre-pulse inhibition study. She was very interested, because there are so few things that enhance pre-pulse inhibition, which is clearly disrupted in schizophrenia. That would be an easily measurable parameter of effectiveness.

GG: Exactly. It would even be double-blind.

JH: I have one last question. Are there any caveats? Where do you think the pitfalls are that we need to keep an eye on in the future—in terms of research, potential therapy, and the issue of neurotoxicity? Where do you see minefields ahead?

GG: I haven't thought about that too much, because I am not a professional researcher living in that world every day. There have been so many blockades; we haven't even been able to get on a road to experience pitfalls. I guess one pitfall would be that a patient would get worse. Whatever problem a patient has, it would get worse after taking MDMA. We also might see one of those rare hyperthermia reactions in a research subject, which would be very bad.

JH: When it comes to hyperthermia, my assumption is that in a controlled setting, where a person is not bouncing off the walls and getting hot and dehydrated, the chances of that would be pretty slim.

GG: I agree. The chances are very slim.

JH: One of the issues that I think may not be resolved yet is that some people may not have the enzyme necessary to metabolize MDMA, which could be dangerous.

GG: There also must be individual genetic difference in one of a million or so people. Their bodies and nervous systems respond in a certain way that makes them prone to hyperthermia-type responses. I think there's a risk, but there's a risk in walking out your door every day. It's extremely remote, but there's no way to prevent it or to screen for it that I can think of. You could screen for the slow metabolizers. We weren't conducting our work at a hospital, so we never gave MDMA to a person who had been incapacitated from a mental disorder. Certainly their hearts needed to be healthy.

JH: What sorts of tests did you use to screen people?

GG: We conducted psychological interviews for a couple of hours, and everyone filled out a seven-page questionnaire. There was a lot of preparation before the sessions.

JH: Would any medical conditions exclude a patient?

GG: Yes. We would exclude anyone with heart disease, high blood pressure, liver disease, seizure history, diabetes, hypoglycemia, glaucoma, or hyperthyroidism and any woman who was pregnant. Apparently, some of the recreational Ecstasy deaths were due to arrhythmias; people's hearts stopped. We didn't conduct these exams, because none of those reports existed at the time, but now I would recommend at least an electrocardiogram and a complete physical exam—the same medical assessment you would get for any research subject taking any drug.

JH: Do you envision a time when Heffter will create an institute, maybe a physical structure in the United States where clinical psychedelic research will be done?

GG: Yes, absolutely. It's just a matter of getting the funding, but now we have an outline of our plan for the sort of facilities and activities in basic and clinical science we expect to conduct.

JH: I look forward to that.

GG: I hope that it happens before I'm too old to walk.

JH: I really appreciate the work that you are doing, and I thank you for participating in this interview.

POTENTIAL CLINICAL USES FOR MDMA

Introduction

MDMA is a unique medication, unlike any other used in psychiatry. It is a potent, immediately acting antidepressant. Most antidepressants take weeks to work, sometimes months. If a person is lucky, a medicine starts to help one feel better in a few days, but there is nothing in the psychiatric medicinal inventory that works in an hour to enhance feelings of happiness and relaxation, as MDMA does. When psychiatrists are working with someone who is acutely suicidal and at risk, they cannot afford to wait four to six weeks for an antidepressant to take effect. MDMA has the potential to be used as an immediate interrupter of depression, suicidal feelings, hopelessness, and isolation.

MDMA is also a non-sedating anxiolytic, a drug that lessens, or "lyses," anxiety, like diazepam (Valium) or alprazolam (Xanax). Psychiatry has few tools at its disposal. Occasionally, patients will be given sodium amytal, a barbiturate, in an effort to relax them enough to divulge information that has not been brought up in therapy. This medication is quite sedating, however, and it is difficult to calibrate the correct dosage such that the patient is less inhibited and more verbal but not groggy. All known immediately acting anxiolytics cause drowsiness, and most also disturb memory, but MDMA is an anti-anxiety medicine that does neither. MDMA completely ablates the fear response in most people. Unlike every other anxiolytic, it is not sedating, and full memory is retained of the MDMA-assisted therapy session.

There are millions of Americans suffering from anxiety disorders, panic disorder, and social phobia. MDMA is useful because it shows the patient what it feels like to be relaxed and less defended. Patients can learn from this experience, and they can anchor themselves in that feeling and tap into it later, without the drug. With the help of MDMA taken during therapy, it is possible to understand specific triggers that cause anxious feelings and to flesh out the sources of deep-rooted fears relatively easily. Therapists who have experience with MDMA-assisted psychotherapy have noted that simple phobias, in particular, often can be extinguished in one MDMA session. Together, the therapist and patient can reach the root cause and symbolic meaning of the phobia. In the course of discussing that connection in just one session, the phobia disappears. The same thing is possible in standard psychoanalysis, but it tends to take longer.

There are powerful case reports of people with post-traumatic stress disorder (PTSD) who have been treated effectively with MDMA-assisted psychotherapy. PTSD is a particular anxiety-related diagnosis given to people who have undergone an extreme traumatic event that negatively affects their lives. Rape victims, people who have been assaulted, victims of torture and war all can be helped immensely by MDMA-assisted psychotherapy. MDMA allows people to revisit the trauma with much less anxiety than usual and to work through what has occurred in a non-threatening context, perhaps allowing for a measure of forgiveness and acceptance to occur for the event. Uncovering the repressed memories and speaking about them calmly and openly is the first step toward clinical improvement in PTSD. I am happy to report one research team in Spain currently performing clinical research in using MDMA to treat PTSD. An American group from the Medical University of South Carolina in Charleston is also planning to study the potential use of MDMA in Chronic PTSD patients. If MDMA has any chance of being transformed into an FDA-approved medication, it is likely to be with this clinical indication.

MDMA also may be useful in the treatment of eating disorders, helping people gain a less distorted impression of their bodies and more powerful feelings of self-acceptance under the drug's effects. In food and drug addiction, improving insight into self-destructive behavior is one of the first steps in changing that behavior. MDMA is a tool, like a special mirror or microscope, that can allow people to honestly examine their entire drug-taking history, their current level of functioning, and the causes for some of their behavior. There is anecdotal evidence that breakthrough sessions augmented with potent psychoactive drugs, such as LSD or ibogaine, can effect lasting changes in people's addictive behavior. MDMA can afford that life-changing glimpse into the big picture of an addict's current situation, but it is much easier to manage MDMA's effects during a psychotherapeutic session, because it is shorter acting, with less reality distortion than the stronger psychedelics.

MDMA may have potential as an acutely acting anti-psychotic medication. One of every one hundred people around the world suffers from schizophrenia, which is characterized by a waxing and waning level of psychosis. Given MDMA's ability to minimize defensiveness and suspiciousness and enhance insight into behavior and illness, it may be a useful adjunct in help-ing people who have a chronic psychotic illness like schizophrenia. This is a theory that has never been tested, but it deserves at least one clinical trial in an effort to help the millions of people with this disease.

With any major mental illness, it is generally thought that if the thera-peutic alliance between psychiatrist and patient can be enhanced, along with patients' insight into their illness, improved mental health care is the result. MDMA-assisted psychotherapy affords the opportunity for important gains concerning issues of compliance with medication and treatment and major insights into and appreciation of the severity of the illness. Moreover, the support system of the patient can be enlisted more fully in a group or family session, where empathy, openness, and acceptance are emphasized, with sub-sequent improvement in the effectiveness of outpatient care.

There are numerous potential medical uses for MDMA. I received an e-mail from a registered nurse, the mother of four, who has lived with severe pain for most of her life due to rheumatoid arthritis. She wrote to tell me that for a few hours she was finally pain free for the first time in fifteen years. She was able to hold her children and feel at ease in her body—all because she had made the decision to break the law and try this illegal drug. She and I are infinitely frustrated that no scientist anywhere in the world is conduct-ing any clinical research on the potent analgesic properties of MDMA. An-other area to explore is MDMA's effect on the immune system. It is com-monly accepted that anxiety and stress can depress immune function, and the converse may well be true (Stone et al. 1996).

There is an enhanced awareness of the body in response to MDMA; fo-cus is shifted more toward posture and deep breathing, and many people find touch and movement to be more pleasurable. This is likely why so many people enjoy dancing and cuddling when taking MDMA and also why some instructors of the Alexander technique, which focuses on posture and breath-ing, have reported good results when incorporating MDMA into their prac-tices. MDMA helps strengthen the mind/body connection; in some cases, it acts as a person's introduction to the idea that the mind can help heal the body. Many times, people's medical complaints and chronic pain syndromes have a strong psychosomatic component. To identify the psychological un-derpinnings of the symptoms with the help of MDMA would be an important step in treatment. Many people accept the idea that a person's mental state, especially one's level of anxiety, can affect health (Cousins 1983). MDMA can be considered a tool to teach patients how to be more relaxed, thus potentially improving their level of health. MDMA also could assist those who have chronic pain or illness, augmenting techniques like biofeedback, guided imagery, hypnotherapy, and any other mind/body work to help integrate the effects of a single dose. Through mental imagery, relaxation, and inner awareness, one often can affect the course of a disease (Rossman 1987).

Most important, MDMA can be used in the field of palliative care, to ease the suffering of those who are dying. Palliative care is a branch of medicine that is still in its infancy. As the baby boomers age, there will be more patients in the last stages of life. We have a long way to go, particularly in the United States, to make dying easier. In medicine, we do not have many tools at our disposal to assist us in easing this experience for patients and their families. MDMA is an effective analgesic that works in a completely different way from such drugs as morphine. There are many anecdotal reports of people with cancer or chronic pain syndromes who have taken MDMA and discovered that their pain eases for five or six hours. It does not go away forever, but for a few hours, under the influence of MDMA, they are pain free. This is sometimes the case when pain has not been treated adequately by morphine. To grant someone respite from pain is a gift. And to address the fears of dying, the unfinished business that people may have with their families, also would likely ease the process of dying not only for patients but for their families as well. The therapeutic promise of MDMA has yet to be fully explored, appreciated, or exploited.

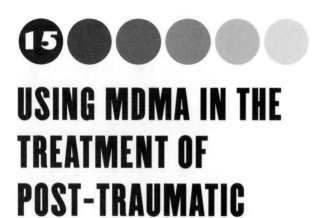

USING MDMA IN THE TREATMENT OF POST-TRAUMATIC STRESS DISORDER

José Carlos Bouso
Translated by Christopher Ryan

Introduction

The Spanish government agency in charge of the approval and control of clinical studies and medications (Agencia Española del Medicamento) has authorized the first psychotherapeutic study utilizing MDMA since its prohibition. This study will examine the possible benefits of MDMA-assisted psychotherapy among women suffering from post-traumatic stress disorder (PTSD) as a consequence of sexual assault, all of whom have failed at least one other treatment regimen. The study consists of two phases. In the first phase, several different doses will be administered, from 50 mg to 150 mg. Each subject will receive only one dose of MDMA, and the doses given will be increased by 25 mg with each group. This is a double-blind, randomized, and placebo-controlled dose-finding study. The dosage level that emerges as the most effective will be used in the subsequent therapeutic study, where it will be compared with placebo. A detailed description of the development, design, and current status of this study can be found at the MAPS Web site (www.maps.org).

Post-Traumatic Stress Disorder

The *Diagnostic and Statistical Manual of Mental Disorders*, 4th ed. (American Psychiatric Association 1994), defines PTSD as an anxiety disorder generated when a person has experienced or witnessed a stressful event that involves death, the threat of death, or serious bodily injury to the self or to another person and which causes reactions characterized by intense fear and feelings of helplessness or of terror (American Psychiatric Association 1994). PTSD is a disorder classically associated with war. The syndrome had been referred to variously as traumatic neurosis, war neurosis, or stress response syndrome (de Paúl 1995) before the current name was adopted by the American Psychiatric Association and the World Health Organization.

PTSD no longer is diagnosed only in ex-combatants. It is seen in a wide range of groups, such as casualties of traffic accidents; patients suffering from terminal illness, physical abuse, or any type of violence; and, especially, victims of sexual assault (Echeburúa and de Corral 1997). In fact, estimates of the incidence of PTSD range from 1.3 percent to 9 percent of the overall population. Approximately 13 percent of psychiatric patients suffer from the disorder (van der Kolk et al. 1995).

Clinical Characteristics

The DSM-IV sets forth the following diagnostic criteria for PTSD, characterized by the presence of three types of principal symptoms:

1. Persistent reexperiencing of the trauma through intrusive memories, recurrent nightmares, flashbacks, and intense psychological and physical distress when internal or external stimuli symbolize or in some way remind the patient of the trauma.

2. Persistent avoidance of stimuli associated with the trauma and a numbing of general responsiveness (which did not exist before the trauma). This can be seen in attempts to avoid thoughts, activities, and places that remind the patient of the trauma. It also might be reflected in an incapacity to recall some of the important details of the trauma, a sense of distance from others, limited expression of emotion, and feelings of a foreshortened future.

3. Persistent symptoms of anxiety or increased arousal that were not present before the trauma. These symptoms may include difficulty in falling or staying asleep, hypervigilance, and an exaggerated startle response.

These symptoms are accompanied by a kind of cognitive dulling (González de Rivera 1990) with associated emotional and affective numbing, which is seen in the patient's inability to express and experience affection or feelings of intimacy and tenderness (Corral et al. 1992). This leads those suffering from PTSD to lose interest in activities in which they participated before the trauma, thus leaving them socially isolated. For this reason, the social support received by the victim after the aggression plays an essential role in subsequent recovery.

In determining the cause of the syndrome, both the internal variables (the way the subject interprets the traumatic experience) and the external variables (particularly the intensity and severity of the trauma and the level of exposure) are considered. Vulnerability factors, such as drug use, history of other psychological problems, history of physical or sexual abuse, and generally stressful surroundings, may predispose one to the appearance of the disorder (González de Rivera 1990).

Post-traumatic Stress Disorder in Victims of Sexual Assault

Approximately 25 percent of the victims of any crime show symptoms of PTSD (Corral et al. 1992). This percentage rises to 45 to 50 percent among victims of domestic abuse and can go as high as 50 to 60 percent among victims of sexual assault (Corral et al. 1992). Sexual assault is the most common crime against women; it is estimated that 15 to 25 percent of all women have suffered some type of sexual assault during their lives (Koss 1983). The victim of sexual assault typically passes first through a period of generalized negative emotions, characterized by anxiety, fear, vulnerability, stress, and confusion—which tends to end after about three months. Thereafter, phobic behavior, anxiety, and other behavior alterations tend to become chronic (Kilpatrick 1992b), with no notable differences between rates of improvement after 3 to 6 months of chronic symptoms and after four years (Kilpatrick 1992a).

The probability that PTSD will develop in victims of sexual assault is particularly high, owing to the fact that in the majority of these cases, the attack occurs in a place that the victim had considered safe. Indeed, one of the most common symptoms of PTSD is anxiety generalized to places that until the attack had been considered safe by the victim. Usually, the symptoms of PTSD tend to include depression, loss of self-esteem, feelings of guilt, avoidance behavior in interpersonal relations, expression deficits, and sexual problems (Echeburúa and de Corral 1995). Fully 80 percent of victims continue to experience some of these symptoms one year after the event—in fact, these symptoms do not decline with the simple passage of time (Corral et al. 1992).

When a woman suffers a sexual attack, the most immediate and lasting feeling is fear—fear that her physical self is in danger and that there is little she can do to change the situation. Out of this sense of vulnerability, together with feelings of panic and weakness, come humiliation and shame. Having been treated like an object by the attacker who ignores her feelings, her dignity suffers. Shame gives rise to hate. Thus, the attack creates a storm of destructive emotions that did not previously exist. For many patients, the subsequent damage to self-esteem erodes their ability to exercise control over their own lives. Depressive symptoms, of course, are common as well.

The way a woman attempts to defend herself from these emotions is by separating—dissociating—from them or by limiting their effects through repressing the associated memories. But wherever she runs, the memories follow. A whole cascade of avoidance can begin—from avoiding situations that are associated with the traumatic episode to refusing to discuss the event to numbing its effects with drug and alcohol abuse. Keeping the traumatic episode at arm's length requires expending energy, which in turn produces increased anxiety and other psychological symptoms: phobias, hyperactivation (increased arousal, anxiety, pacing, and insomnia), depression, irritability, nervousness, and so on. The symptoms are the result of the low level of integration of the experience through dissociation and repression. By modifying this level of integration, we can modify the symptoms. Focusing on the experience itself will have direct effects on the symptoms.

Treatment of Post-traumatic Stress Disorder in Victims of Sexual Assault

The main objectives in treating PTSD are to confront the trauma and help the victim regain self-esteem and a sense of security (Echeburúa et al. 1990). Corral and co-workers (1995b) found better results with a treatment composed of exposure and cognitive reevaluation when compared with a treatment of placebo and relaxation therapy. It has been stated that victims of sexual assault rarely seek psychological assistance. This is due, at least in part, to the fact that these victims tend not to see themselves as "patients" (Foa et al. 1991). The avoidance symptoms also interfere with the victim's ability to seek help because of her fear of recalling and discussing the traumatic event. One of the most common treatments is to provoke a reliving of the event in a safe context, where the patient can experience the trauma again, this time with a higher level of control. In this way she also can acquire a greater amount of control over her memory of the trauma. Those victims who are capable of reliving the trauma in such a context have more chance of achieving a positive long-term outcome (Meichenbaum 1994), because reliving it in an emotionally safe and supportive environment can alleviate fear in the victims (Echeburúa and de Corral 1995). This reexperiencing of trauma can be facilitated more easily in altered states of consciousness, such as through hypnosis or the administration of some psychoactive drugs (González de Rivera 1994).

MDMA and Post-traumatic Stress Disorder

Much has been written about the therapeutic uses of MDMA, specifically concerning its potential for people who have suffered some type of traumatic experience. Greer and Tolbert, pioneers in therapeutic work with MDMA, published reports of their patients' positive experiences with the substance. They write, "Results from eighty patients indicate that MDMA seems to decrease the fear response to a perceived threat to a patient's emotional integrity, leading to a corrective emotional experience that probably diminishes the pathological effects of previous traumatic experiences" (Greer and Tolbert 1990). Moreover, "clients found it comfortable to be aware of, to communicate, and to remember thoughts and feelings that are usually accompanied by fear and anxiety" (Greer and Tolbert 1998). In a symposium held at Esalen Institute in 1985, where the state of knowledge concerning MDMA was reviewed, one of the conclusions was that "victims of child abuse and sexual attack experienced the most dramatic benefits" (Greer 1985). Grinspoon and Bakalar (1986) stated, "MDMA might also help in working through loss and trauma." Peter Stafford, in his *Psychedelics Encyclopedia*, also speaks of the effectiveness of MDMA in treating, "rape, childhood abuse, and post-war stress syndromes" and discusses specific cases of people finding beneficial results from MDMA-assisted psychotherapy (Stafford 1992). Eisner (1989) discusses the potential benefits for female victims of sexual assault who undergo MDMA-assisted psychotherapy as well as his personal understanding of how these benefits accrue. In addition, some first-person accounts of PTSD sufferers have described how they benefited from treatment that included MDMA (Adamson 1985).

MDMA has a unique ability to facilitate and accelerate the therapeutic process (Grinspoon and Bakalar 1990). MDMA is both a facilitator of psychotherapy and a type of therapy in and of itself. That is, it has therapeutic effects that make the other aspects of the therapy even more effective. When taken within a psychotherapeutic context, accompanied by trained, competent therapists, MDMA brings about a subjective state of well-being in which psychological defenses ease or disappear entirely, provoking intense experiences of openness. This makes it much easier for the patient to communicate deeply held feelings. The introspective capacity needed for analyzing and becoming consciously aware of these deep feelings also is enhanced. The absence of fear allows for the reexperiencing of the traumatic event without the anxiety and negative feelings that normally accompany any memory of the event. This increased capacity for accessing and expressing deep feelings may break through the emotional numbing that is characteristic of PTSD patients. The development of the therapeutic alliance, the variable that is most predictive of clinical change, thus is accelerated (Feixas and Miró 1993; Poch and Ávila 1998). Because MDMA assists in the consolidation of the therapeutic alliance as well as in the controlled reexperiencing of the traumatic episode, it will probably have positive long-term influence over the most incapacitating symptoms of victims of sexual assault who have PTSD: avoidance (with the subsequent reduction in phobic behavior) and hyperactivation (with the subsequent reduction in anxiety).

⚡ MDMA has two main effects in humans. First, it creates an enhanced capacity for gaining access to, understanding, and communicating deeply held feelings, sometimes feelings that were never before experienced. These effects have been called "entactogenic" (Nichols 1986). The capacity to gain and communicate insight likewise is heightened, which is a good predictor of therapeutic success (Kernberg et al. 1972).

⚡ MDMA also generates feelings of well-being and trust, which lead to empathy. It is this sense of being at peace with one's self that enables a client, formerly lost in fear, to communicate. The more that one accepts and is comfortable with one's self, the more one will accept and trust others. This effect is described as "empathogenic" (Adamson and Metzner 1988). It is commonly understood that the ability of the client to trust and feel supported by a therapist is fundamental in establishing a therapeutic alliance (Alexander and Luborsky 1986). These two types of effects are produced within a mildly altered state of consciousness unlike those states produced by the classic psychedelics. In this state the patient experiences a greater sense of self-control. From the descriptions given here, we see that MDMA can be enormously helpful in bringing about psychological healing.

One way of conducting MDMA-assisted psychotherapy is to center the treatment exclusively on the trauma. Another way is to focus on the MDMA experience itself. In this approach, the substance is not used as an adjunct to a more or less standard psychotherapeutic technique but rather as a way of provoking a "peak experience" that may be beneficial in and of itself. It consists of three phases. First, the preparation phase of therapy is oriented toward psychologically preparing patients for the effects of MDMA, addressing the thoughts, emotions, expectations, and fears they may have concerning the substance and the types of effects that they expect the substance to produce. This work is very important and may determine the success of the treatment, in that the fears that the women have about the MDMA experience may well be reflections of their anxieties and symptoms related to the traumatic episode. We can say, then, that the preparation phase is a way of working indirectly with the pain associated with the trauma.

The second phase corresponds to the administration of MDMA with the purpose of facilitating the reliving of the traumatic episode and working with the resulting experiences.

During the third phase, after administration of the substance, therapists and clients focus on integrating the MDMA experience and the insights gained into the daily life of the patient. It is crucial to keep in mind that these women have greater difficulties in speaking about their traumatic experiences than do victims of other types of trauma. They have deep feelings of shame and low self-esteem, and they also experience a feeling of being stigmatized (a phenomenon that has not been well studied but is well known in the clinic). A brief treatment that tries to confront the traumatic experience quickly risks being rejected by the client. It is very important to build trust between client and therapist during the preparation phase, without necessarily mentioning the trauma itself, so that when MDMA is administered, patients feel sufficiently comfortable to face the episode. This is perhaps the most distinct factor in treating victims of sexual assault, as opposed to people with other types of PTSD or patients with other disorders.

It is crucial that the therapist's orientation is person-centered, rather than directive, so that the work of the therapist is congruent with the type of experiences generated by MDMA. If MDMA tends to cause experiences pertaining to the internal world of the patient, the therapeutic focus most congruent with this sort of experience would be the facilitation of verbalization of this internal world. After all, verbalization is nothing other than bringing the interpersonal (objective) world into contact with the internal (subjective) world; when the subject's experience is clearer to her, she will be more capable of expressing this experience in the interpersonal world. Additionally, as this experience is expressed more clearly, the opportunity for insight, or self-understanding, grows as well. The following section gives a more detailed description of each of the three phases that make up the proposed form of MDMA-assisted psychotherapy. This description is based solely on the author's sense of what may occur during treatment and the possible subjective experiences that patients may have.

Phase One

The first phase of this type of MDMA-assisted treatment is oriented toward preparing patients to face the experience they will have with MDMA. To approach the traumatic episode directly in brief treatment can be too invasive for many patients, especially when there has not been enough time to establish a solid therapeutic alliance. Exploring patients' expectations and fears concerning the upcoming experience with MDMA helps them enter into their internal world, which will give important clues as to the ways in which the trauma affected them. This phase serves as a sort of training for patients to gain access to and communicate the traumatic experiences so that they will be more at ease in this potentially painful internal realm when they are under the influence of MDMA. Moreover, the therapist is deepening the relationship with the patient, learning to better understand the ways in which the traumatic experience has affected her, and gaining an idea of how the patient might respond when under the effects of the substance. All of this will result in a more effective therapeutic intervention.

When she sees that her internal experiences are communicable and comprehensible, the patient will be more motivated to deepen her participation and gain greater insight. When these unknown negative elements are faced under controlled conditions, they usually become less powerful, and the person has less difficulty in accepting them. As the patient actualizes the more positive parts and integrates the negative aspects, the interior world becomes more authentic and richer, allowing her more ease in negotiating the exterior world. The more the patients understands her process of self-knowing and the greater her capacity to communicate this knowledge, the more she will feel accepted and understood and the more she will gain in self-acceptance and self-knowledge. She will obtain more positive results under the effects of the MDMA precisely because MDMA is a catalyst for self-acceptance and self-understanding.

Phase Two

During the reliving of the traumatic episode under the effects of MDMA, patients first will note that they feel themselves to be calm and peaceful, a state in which it is likely that none of their anxious symptoms will appear. Many intense cathartic experiences will take place, with both positive and negative associated feelings. But the freedom from fear will help the patient face, accept, and better experience these emotions. The patient will see changes in feelings of guilt, humiliation, hate, and shame. That which has been denied can now be owned: to reexperience the traumatic episode in the absence of fear is to change completely the frame of reference of the episode.

If the resultant feelings can be better internalized, healing is well under way. We can say that in some way, the patient has walked the same emotional path again. This time, rather than being in the company of fear, weakness, and vulnerability, she is accompanied by feelings of peace, control, and strength. If patients can gain control over their feelings, it is possible that they can generalize this control to their daily lives.

Research into PTSD has shown that persons who are capable of reexperiencing traumatic episodes during the course of psychological treatment will have better long-term therapeutic results. The hypothesis is that reexperiencing the event within the psychotherapeutic context—where the patient is in a relaxed and trusting atmosphere—deactivates the fear associated with the trauma, allowing for acceptance of the trauma. MDMA facilitates the reliving of trauma in three ways:

1. MDMA creates a state of relaxation in a person, eliminating symptoms of anxiety and producing a sense of well-being and of being at peace with oneself.

2. MDMA facilitates introspection and access to traumatic memories and painful feelings, making their communication easier. Furthermore, as the patient becomes more comfortable with herself, she will be more comfortable with others, eliminating a large part of the common communication barriers and permitting clearer and easier expression of her feelings. Psychological defenses evaporate, and the patient feels safe with her emotions, with the therapist, and with the sense of well-being in which she finds herself. This process solidifies the therapeutic alliance by deepening the sense of trust between patient and therapist. Among all the processes taking place between patient and therapist, the therapeutic alliance, or empathic rapport, is the one that best predicts therapeutic change (Alexander and Luborsky 1986).

3. During the preparatory sessions patients have a chance to enter their internal worlds, to get in touch with painful emotions as well as happy ones, and to train themselves in communicating. The patient is prepared to take advantage of MDMA and to make gaining access to these intense emotions more comfortable, more effective, and

easier. This helps make the reliving of the trauma safe, profound, and intense, thus eliminating the patient's fear and allowing better integration of the trauma as well as better long-term adaptation.

It takes thirty to forty-five minutes for MDMA to take effect. The appearance of these effects often produces some anxiety in patients as they become aware of the physical sensations. It is a good idea to speak casually with the patient, with the intention of distracting the attention from these bodily sensations. If the patient is especially anxious at this point, the therapist can guide her in a relaxation exercise.

The effects of MDMA often appear quite rapidly. Suddenly, one notices a slight shift of consciousness—normally interpreted as dizziness, similar to a mild sense of drunkenness. This effect soon is accompanied by an intense feeling of euphoria. The person then becomes quite alert and focused. She can get up and walk around the room, exploring people or objects and becoming at ease with the space. Her sense of well-being is so profound that everything she sees makes her feel content. The reaction of the patient to the people around her tends to be one of immediate acceptance and a feeling of emotional intimacy with them. She feels comfortable and in the company of friends. The more the therapist can help her accept everything (including herself) during this phase, the more comfortable she will be during the rest of the experience.

After a few minutes of intense euphoria, the effects decline slightly and stabilize. The person then feels calm and accepting—free of fear and at ease. Now she is prepared to relive the trauma at her own speed. It is likely that at the beginning, the patient will not want to talk about her suffering, since she feels so good. She probably has not felt such positive feelings for a long time, and so the therapist should not force the conversation. The patient will proceed bit by bit, always talking about her emotions, and will arrive at a point at which she will begin to touch on a painful subject. From this point, the process of reexperiencing begins. The patient must always control the speed at which the experience proceeds. She will feel intense internal emotions related to the traumatic events, but these emotions will be discovered and communicated easily. Since she is in a relaxed state, the patient can live through these emotions not only with intensity but with objectivity as well, knowing that they form a part of her life and must be accepted. During the plateau phase, the patient is able to relive the trauma, communicate it, and integrate it into her psyche. The acceptance of the trauma presages positive therapeutic results.

This process is about confronting emotions rather than fleeing from them. We suffer from the *effort* of avoiding memories. At the moment in which we decide to face these fears, they no longer exist. It is as if that which frightened us was the thought of facing the fears, more than the fears themselves. Patients also may experience negative emotions. They may feel like screaming or striking out. We must allow all these types of actions, as long as they do not damage other people or property. This is something that needs to be discussed with the patient before beginning the session. It is possible that these sensations are more likely to appear in women who experience a type of stimulant effect. During the plateau stage, collateral effects may appear, such as palpitations, jaw clenching, uncontrolled eye movements, and psychomotor symptoms (a desire to move around, for example). The therapist must give clear signs of acceptance and permission—giving the greatest possible freedom to the patient to actualize her emotions. Once this process is completed, the therapist should support the patient so that she feels liberated and returns to the state of calm and peace offered by the MDMA. The plateau phase of MDMA normally lasts between two and three hours.

Finally, during the descent, about three hours after ingestion, the effects of MDMA begin to wane. Over approximately half an hour, the patient will return to baseline. The therapist's role during this period is also very important. The therapist needs to help the patient integrate everything she's gained, to reassure her that her experiences during the session have relevance to her life. Finally, the patient returns with newly won knowledge that will lead to better acceptance of her painful memories, of herself, and of those around her. Knowing something of the inner world of the patient, the therapist will be able to help integrate the insights gained during the experience. The patient must not leave the office until all of the psychological and physiological effects of the MDMA have disappeared.

Phase Three

At six hours after ingestion, the effects produced by MDMA have probably waned, but the integration and "digestion" of these experiences continue at a distinct rhythm, generally quite a bit more slowly than the metabolism of the substance itself. The incorporation of the experience and its complete and lasting assimilation require anywhere from a few days to several weeks. The short-term integration of the experience may depend to some extent on the quality of the experience. Some women may feel empty or sad, perhaps because the return to reality was somewhat abrupt. Others feel energized and hopeful about potential change. The secondary effects that may appear at the end of the session include headache, exhaustion, and mild insomnia. When they return home, they should relax, not worry about daily problems, and try to sleep.

The strategy for sessions devoted to integrating the experience should help the patient see how her insights indicate internal changes that render the outer world less threatening. The traumatic episode now can be discussed openly. It is important to explore how the patient is modifying her feelings related to the event and how this process can be generalized to the rest of her life.Optimally, the women will experience progressively less anxiety, such that situations they have previously avoided can be tolerated with only minor discomfort. This will allow patients to feel that the world is less frightening and will lead them to rediscover pleasant situations that were enjoyable before the trauma. We can say that the patient has become more conscious of her unconscious fears and is thus more able to distinguish them from actual dangers. The traumatic event will never be forgotten, but the present experience of the trauma will be less tied to the original experience, when the event was suffered in a context of helplessness and terror. It will be associated more and more with the current feelings of well-being and greater self-control, generated by a reduction in anxiety and improved emotional competency. If this is realized, we can be certain that the MDMA-assisted psychotherapy has been effective. Finally, it is very important to leave open when treatment will end, so that patients have the opportunity to contact the therapist at any time in later life to share what has come out of the experience.

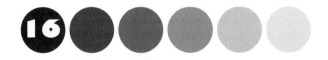

USING MDMA IN THE TREATMENT OF DEPRESSION*

June Riedlinger, R.Ph., Pharm.D.
and Michael Montagne, Ph.D.

Introduction

In this chapter we discuss the use of the substance MDMA for the treatment of depression. The first author's personal experience and work as a clinical pharmacist in psychiatry was the foundation for the hypothesis that MDMA could be a healing agent for the life-threatening illness of depression. Before discussing how MDMA may be beneficial in treating depression, a brief review of the medical criteria for the condition is warranted.

Extent and Nature of Depression

Epidemiological studies of depression have shown that the lifetime risk for major depression in the adult population ranges from 10 percent to 25 percent for women and from 5 percent to 12 percent for men (American Psychiatric Association 1994). The occurrence of depression appears to be unrelated to ethnicity, education, income, or marital status.

Major depression is twice as common in women as in men (American

---

*This chapter is based in part on a previous publication, "Psychedelic and Entactogenic Drugs in the Treatment of Depression," by Thomas and June Riedlinger, published in the *Journal of Psychoactive Drugs* [1994; 26:41–55].

Psychiatric Association 1994). Major depression tends to occur most often in the 25- to 44-year-old age group, while its rate of occurrence is lower among people older than 65. This disorder is one and a half to three times more common among first-degree relatives of persons with the disorder than in the general population, indicating that there is a genetic component to the illness. A significant number of women report worsening of the symptoms of major depression several days before the onset of menses. A higher incidence of depression also is seen during the perimenopausal and the postpartum periods, suggesting that there is a hormonal component as well.

The experience, perception, and description of the symptoms of depression can be influenced by cultural background (American Psychiatric Association 1994). In some cultures, depression may be experienced largely in physical terms rather than emotional states, such as sadness or guilt. In Latino and Mediterranean cultures people may complain of "an attack of nerves" and headaches. In Chinese and Asian cultures they may complain of weakness, fatigue, or imbalance. In Middle Eastern cultures depression is viewed as a problem of the heart, and in some Native American cultures it is expressed as being "heartbroken." Cultures also may differ in their perception of the seriousness of the condition.

Clinical Features of Depression

Symptoms of a major depressive episode usually develop over days or weeks. The primary diagnostic requirements are either a depressed mood or the loss of interest or pleasure in nearly all activities for at least two weeks. These symptoms must exist for most of the day and for nearly every day. Five or more of the following symptoms also must be present during that same two-week period of time, and they must represent a change from previous functioning:

- significant weight gain or weight loss (when not dieting) or a decrease or increase in appetite nearly every day
- insomnia or excessive sleeping nearly every day
- psychomotor retardation or agitation (a bodily slowing or restlessness that is noticeable by others)

- fatigue or loss of energy
- feelings of worthlessness or excessive or inappropriate guilt
- diminished ability to think or concentrate or indecisiveness
- recurrent thoughts of death, suicidal ideas, or a suicide attempt

Periods of sadness are inherent aspects of the human experience, and they should not be diagnosed as a major depressive episode. The symptoms that are present must cause clinically significant distress or impairment in social, occupational, or other important areas of functioning. Symptoms must not be due to the direct physiological effects of a substance, such as a drug or medicine, or to a medical condition. The symptoms are not better accounted for by bereavement after the loss of a loved one (American Psychiatric Association 1994).

The mood in a major depressive episode often is described as sad, hopeless, discouraged, or "down in the dumps." The most serious consequence of major depression is attempted or completed suicide. Up to 15 percent of people with severe major depression die by suicide. Thus, it is reasonable to consider major depression a potentially life-threatening illness. Epidemiological evidence also indicates that there is a fourfold increase in death rates in persons with major depression over the age of fifty-five.

A major depressive episode varies in duration; an untreated episode may last for six months or longer. In the majority of cases, there is complete remission of symptoms, and normal functioning returns. However, in a significant proportion of cases (perhaps 20 percent), some depressive symptoms may persist for months to years and may be associated with a substantial degree of disability or distress. In a small group of cases, the major depressive episode may last for two years or more.

Biochemical Basis of Depression

The possibility that some forms of human depression are based on central nervous system deficiencies of the neurotransmitter serotonin (5-hydroxytryptamine, or 5-HT), was first suggested by van Praag (1962) and then reinforced by the findings of other researchers (Coppen 1967; Lapin and Oxenburg 1969). Based on his later research, van Praag (1982) concluded that serotonin disorders are implicated most clearly in a subgroup of approximately 40 percent of patients afflicted with depression. He also emphasized that serotonin disorders probably play a causative, rather than a secondary, role in depression. This is suggested by the fact that serotonin-potentiating compounds, such as the precursors 5-hydroxytryptophan (5-HTP) and L-tryptophan, an essential amino acid, can have a therapeutic effect in depression (van Praag 1981).

It is significant that many of the drugs prescribed for treatment of depression have serotonergic activity. The newest class of antidepressants, the serotonin reuptake inhibitors (Prozac, Zoloft, Paxil, Celexa, and others) and, to varying degrees, the tricyclic antidepressants prevent the recycling of serotonin back into presynaptic nerve endings. Monoamine oxidase (MAO) inhibitors prevent the breakdown of serotonin by the enzyme MAO. In either case, more serotonin is available for binding to receptors (Spiegel and Aebi 1983). The specific mechanism of action of these drugs, however, is still not clear.

There is an entire class of psychoactive drugs that almost certainly derives its main effect from serotonin mediation (Freedman et al. 1970; Haigler and Aghajanian 1973; Anden et al. 1974; Winter 1975; Meltzer et al. 1978). These drugs, the psychedelics, are reported to have positive effects in the treatment of various psychological disorders, including depression. We present and discuss the value of psychedelic agents, with a focus on clinical reports and theoretical explanations for one specific drug, MDMA, that may become an efficacious treatment for depression in the future.

Psychedelic Psychotherapy

The possibility that psychedelic drugs could help facilitate the modern psychotherapeutic process was virtually ignored in the United States and Europe until about 1950. Between then and the mid-1960s, more than one thousand clinical papers describing forty thousand patients who had taken part in psychedelic therapy or other research trials were published, as well as several dozen related books; six international conferences on psychedelic drug therapy were held (Grinspoon and Bakalar 1983). Two different types of psychedelic psychotherapy were described (Grinspoon and Bakalar 1979). One emphasized a mystical or conversion experience and its after-effects (psychedelic therapy); using high doses of LSD (more than 200 mcg) was thought to be especially effective in reforming alcoholics and criminals. The other type explored the unconscious in the manner of psychoanalysis (psycholytic therapy); it focused on the treatment of neuroses and psychosomatic disorders using low doses of LSD (100–150 mcg) as well as other psychedelic drugs.

By the mid-1950s, it was recognized that psychedelics function as non-specific amplifiers, drugs that project into consciousness (amplify) memories, fears, and other subjectively varying (nonspecific) psychological material that had been repressed, or was unconscious. Among the first announcements of this highly significant finding was a report entitled "Ataractic and Hallucinogenic Drugs in Psychiatry," written by a team of international experts convened by the World Health Organization. This report challenged the prevailing idea that psychedelic drugs are psychotomimetic, that is, capable of inducing a model of temporary psychosis. Instead, the team concluded, "It may be a gross over-simplification to speak of drug-specific reactivity patterns. On the contrary, experience suggests that the same drug, in the same dose, in the same subject may produce very different effects according to the precise interpersonal and motivational situation in which it was given" (World Health Organization 1958). Thus, it was made clear that the issues of set (the users' expectations) and setting (the environment for the drug experience), which is described elsewhere in this book, must be taken into account when using psychedelics.

Another important issue to consider in a discussion of drug-assisted psychotherapy is this: at present, psychiatrists prescribe doses of mood elevators or stabilizers with which patients must comply on a daily basis. There is no currently accepted model of one-time or infrequent dosing of medications to alleviate psychic suffering. Thus, Grinspoon and Bakalar (1986) have emphasized: "It is a misunderstanding to consider psychedelic drug therapy as a form of chemotherapy, which must be regarded in the same way as prescribing lithium or phenothiazines." Instead, it is more like "a hybrid between pharmacotherapy and psychotherapy" (Grinspoon and Bakalar 1990) that incorporates features of both.

Limitations of Psychedelic Psychotherapy

Despite early reports of success in some areas of psychotherapy, both psychedelic and psycholytic therapy have certain limitations. These reports, though compelling, are open to question. In most cases these studies either are anecdotal or lack a control group in their experimental design. Anecdotal reports can be questioned for several reasons, including placebo effects and the patient and therapist's biases in judging improvement. The lack of control groups is also a problem; it is generally agreed that a good study design must include the presence of a group of subjects who undergo the entire procedure (psychotherapy) without taking the drug in question. The effects of psychedelics are so unmistakable that most researchers argue that using them effectively would rule out a blinded study design. With these few limitations acknowledged, however, it is clear that human research using psychedelic drugs turned up promising results, with implications for the treatment of depression as well as other psychiatric disorders.

Another problem is that almost all the classic psychedelics are time-consuming to use, despite claims that they accelerate psychotherapy. Even low doses have pronounced psychoactive and behavioral effects lasting five or more hours. Clients therefore should be supervised throughout this period and for several hours afterward to minimize adverse effects. According to Strassman's (1984) review of the literature on adverse psychedelic drug effects, "It appears that the incidence of adverse reactions to psychedelic drugs is low, when individuals (both normal volunteers and patients) are carefully screened, supervised, and followed up, and given judicious doses of pharmaceutical quality drug."

In addition to the time constraints, another limitation is that therapists who use the drugs with patients must themselves be well trained to effectively help guide the session. Yet training currently is limited to articles and books published between 1950 and the mid-1960s, when the drugs were used clinically, or is based on original research from that period. No internships are available to allow therapists to train experientially. That psychedelics have unique and dramatic effects in psychotherapy is probably one of the reasons that mainstream psychotherapists ignore or reject them. They believe that to incorporate these drugs into their therapy techniques would require too great a degree of adjustment and accommodation. This is more or less true for the classic psychedelics. A more viable alternative may exist, however, in a chemical subgroup referred to as "entactogens."

Psychedelic Therapy's Relevance to MDMA Therapy

Nichols and Oberlender (Nichols 1986; Nichols and Oberlender 1990) noted that MDMA is both chemically and behaviorally a different type of psychoactive drug that deserves its own nomenclature. Because its primary effect at therapeutic dose levels "seems to involve enhanced closeness and communication with others, accompanied by positive changes in feelings and attitudes" (Nichols and Oberlender 1990), Nichols proposed the term "entactogens," derived from Greek and Latin roots connoting an ability to "touch within."

Of the two major chemical types of psychedelic drugs, indole derivatives and phenylalkylamines, the latter category has a chemical subgroup called phenylisopropylamines. Although the behavioral effects of some phenylisopropylamines seem different from those of LSD, the prototype psychedelic, they reportedly have a similar chemical structure activity. This is not the case with MDMA. MDMA does have something in common with other drugs used in psychedelic and psycholytic therapies: the patient must be given MDMA under supervision of an experienced practitioner. The effects are not as intense as for a classic psychedelic drug, such as LSD, but the potential exists for individual variance, and set and setting continue to be important factors.

MDMA's Role in the Treatment of Depression

That MDMA is apparently serotonergic was first noted by Nichols and associates (1982), who introduced it in vitro to homogenized rat brains and then measured the release of serotonin from the synaptosomes (vesicles in the synapses that store neurotransmitters). Elevated levels were detected, suggesting that serotonin release may play a role in MDMA's pharmacological activity. Subsequent research described in Peroutka (1990) appears to confirm the drug's serotogenicity. As with serotonergic antidepressant drugs, however, the specific mode of action is uncertain. [See "How MDMA Works in the Brain" for a detailed discussion of what is currently understood of the mechanism of action of MDMA.]

In any case, MDMA's use in psychotherapy to stimulate positive feelings, such as openness and empathy, would seem to recommend it for a possible clinical role in treating depression. Riedlinger (1985) first proposed this in a discussion of MDMA's positive isomer activity and consequent release of serotonin in the brain. Because it is a potent releaser of serotonin into the synapse, and because of its short duration of effect, MDMA seems to be both effective and efficient as a drug for the medical treatment of depression. It works to enhance serotonergic function and mood in a matter of hours instead of weeks (as is the case for most prescription antidepressants), and it is effective when administered infrequently, perhaps in weekly or monthly dosing intervals. This compares favorably to the multiple daily dosing required for most of the currently available drugs that can be prescribed for treating depression (such as tricyclic antidepressants, MAO inhibitors, serotonin reuptake inhibitors). The other drugs often take several days or even weeks to produce antidepressant effects and frequently cause lasting troublesome side effects (appetite and sleep changes, sexual dysfunction, sweating, nausea, and headaches). Compassion for the victims of depression, in addition to the evidence of MDMA's serotonin-releasing effect, should compel further research to establish clearly whether MDMA is indeed an alternative antidepressant.

Treating Suicidal Depression with MDMA

The notion that MDMA might be useful in treating suicidal depression is based on a comparison of psychological patterns in suicidal people and MDMA's psychoactive effects. Psychological characteristics of suicidal people tend to vary between different age groups, cultures, economic classes, and gender (Hendin 1982; American Psychiatric Association 1994). Many cases seem to be manifestations of alienation. The anguish of the suicidal person is frequently that of a person in exile. He or she feels totally isolated, singled out by fate to suffer hardships and endless frustrations alone. Such people often find it hard to deal with the conflicts and demands of interpersonal relationships. They withdraw into a private, lonely world. Their justification might be that they feel unworthy of love or that others have abandoned them unfairly. In either case, the isolation typically starts to feel irreversible. There seems to be no possibility of ever establishing meaningful contact with other human beings.

According to the *Harvard Medical School Mental Health Letter* ("Suicide," 1986), "Among the immediate motives for suicide, not surprisingly, despair is most common. In one long-term study, hopelessness alone accounted for most of the association between depression and suicide, and a high level of hopelessness was the strongest signal that a person who had attempted suicide would try again. Intense guilt, psychotic delusions, and even the severity of the depression were much less adequate indicators." The study referred to in the *Mental Health Letter*, by Beck and colleagues (1985), reported that high ratings on the Beck Hopelessness Scale successfully predicted 90.9 percent of eventual cases of suicide in a sample of 165 hospitalized suicide ideators (people who initially went to the doctor with thoughts of suicide) who were followed for five to ten years after taking the test. A subsequent report regarding the study affirmed that "because hopelessness can be reduced fairly rapidly by specific therapeutic interventions . . . the assessment of hopelessness can potentially improve the prevention as well as the prediction of suicide" (Beck et al. 1989). Hopelessness itself might mediate the relationship between dysfunctional attitudes and psychopathology, especially depression.

Interpersonal attitudes related to depression, not hopelessness per se, also may be the root cause of suicide. To that extent, suicide might be considered an act of interpersonal frustration that seeks to communicate misery and break out of isolation ("Suicide," 1986). This goal may be reached, alternatively and more safely, by means of guided psychotherapy. The recalcitrance of suicidal people, however, is a problem for conventional psychotherapy. For therapy to work, a positive, dynamic interaction must take place between the patient and the therapist (Henry et al. 1990; Talley et al. 1990; Strupp 1993). The patient must be willing to communicate what is going on inside. Someone who is consumed by strong feelings of alienation and hopelessness is likely to resist interpersonal contact and open discussion. Of course, it is frequently true that patients hesitate to talk about personal problems at the start of psychotherapy and need several sessions before they warm up to the therapist. Time is often a luxury that suicidal patients cannot afford, however. They may be treatable over the long term with conventional psychotherapy, but first they must be stabilized or otherwise prevented from taking their own lives. Usually this means hospitalization, keeping a suicide watch on such patients, and even actively restraining them if necessary.

Here is where MDMA can perhaps play a viable role, based on certain effects and ramifications for guided psychotherapy succinctly described in an issue of the *Harvard Medical School Mental Health Letter* (Grinspoon and Bakalar 1985): Although MDMA has no officially approved medical or psychiatric application, a few psychiatrists and other therapists had been using it as an aid to psychotherapy for more than fifteen years, in the 1970s and '80s. It has now been taken in a therapeutic setting by hundreds, if not thousands, of people with few reported complications. It is said to fortify the therapeutic alliance by inviting self-disclosure and enhancing trust. Some patients also report changes that last several days to several weeks or longer—improved mood, greater relaxation, heightened self-esteem, and enhanced relations with others. Psychiatrists who have used MDMA with patients suggest that it might be helpful, for example, in marital counseling, in diagnostic interviews, or as a catalyst for insight in psychotherapy. Reports of therapeutic results are so far unpublished and anecdotal and cannot be properly evaluated without more systematic study.

Anecdotal reports by the hundreds of people who have taken MDMA in therapeutic settings are not irrelevant. Their testimonies indicate that certain psychological effects occur consistently across a broad spectrum of usage. This is evident in Adamson's (1985) collection of about fifty such testimonies. The forward, by Ralph Metzner, observes that these firsthand accounts include such words as "ecstasy, empathy, openness, acceptance, forgiveness, and emotional bonding" in reference to MDMA's effects. These are the opposite terms often used to describe the psychological distress of suicidal people: anguish, alienation, recalcitrance, rejection, blame, guilt, and emotional withdrawal. Eisner (1989) also describes several cases of MDMA-assisted psychotherapy in which depression is mentioned specifically as one of the symptoms that is alleviated.

The value of MDMA is that it does not make its users feel better by transporting them into a naive state of bliss. They are aware of the fact that their lives have been burdened by negative thinking, have been based on fears and anxieties. MDMA seems to lend them a different perspective for several hours by minimizing their defensiveness and fear of emotional injury (Greer 1985; Greer and Tolbert 1986, 1990). It stimulates a process by which they are able to look at their problems more objectively and thus transcend a feeling of hopeless entrapment. At the same time, they feel more in touch with their positive emotions. This sustains them as the therapeutic process takes its course. The drug gives them the courage to confront their emotional problems and the strength to work them out, often by enhancing their desire to communicate constructively. Numerous examples of this process are described in Adamson's book (1985).

The particular value of MDMA for suicidal patients and, by extension, for patients with less severe forms of depression is twofold. First, it might be useful as an interventional medicine. By providing the relief from overwhelmingly dark emotions, MDMA likely can help forestall the act of suicide or otherwise alleviate the patient's sense of hopelessness. This buys time for the drug's second major effect, facilitating psychotherapy by helping to enhance the patient's trust and by inviting self-analysis and disclosure. As previously noted, the result is a fortifying of the therapeutic alliance between patient and therapist. Furthermore, MDMA does so in a relatively short time. According to Metzner in Adamson's book (1985): "One therapist has estimated that in five hours of one Adam [MDMA] session clients could activate and process psychic material that would normally require five months of weekly sessions." Needless to say, such accelerated therapeutic healing can mean the difference between life and death for people in imminent danger of suicide.

Risks of MDMA Use

There has been concern about neurotoxicity and other possible health risks from MDMA use. Most of these adverse reactions appear to be avoidable, if samples of known purity are administered in the lowest effective therapeutic dose range and frequency, after carefully screening patients for risk factors. This is consistent with the view of Grob and colleagues (1990) that fears of MDMA neurotoxicity may have been exaggerated and that rigorous clinical trials of the drug in psychotherapy should be resumed. [Most articles that allege neurotoxicity have recruited volunteers with histories of excessive and prolonged use. No study has been published that examines infrequent, single oral dosing.—Ed.]

Animal research with MDMA seems to indicate that even its high-dose neurotoxic effects can be minimized by the concurrent administration of fluoxetine (Schmidt 1987; Schmidt et al. 1987). One report by McCann and Ricaurte (1993) suggested that fluoxetine pretreatment, at doses of 20 to 40 mg, does not compromise MDMA's therapeutic effects and, furthermore, decreases post-session insomnia and fatigue. A cautionary editorial by Price and colleagues (1990) maintains that it is premature to pursue clinical trials of MDMA in conditions that are not life-threatening. Both sides would be served by exploring the possible use of MDMA as an intervention drug for the stabilization and subsequent treatment of patients afflicted with severe and perhaps suicidal depression.

Conclusions

Central nervous system deficiency of 5-hydroxytryptamine (serotonin) has been implicated as a biochemical basis of at least some forms of depression. Existing drug treatments for depression include some with serotonergic effects. Studies suggest that psychedelic drugs are also serotonergic, which may indicate that there is a role for psychedelics in the treatment of depression. Such treatment has been attempted using psychedelic drugs in both the indoleamine and phelylalkylamine categories. Encouraging results recommend further research, with special emphasis on drugs in the group called entactogens or empathogens, which cause substantially less distortion of normative consciousness than classic psychedelics, such as LSD or mescaline. They could be assimilated more easily into existing psychotherapy approaches, where their function would be to accelerate and enhance the normal psychotherapeutic process rather than to serve as a maintenance medication. Their usefulness in such an application would be mainly at the start of psychotherapy. The goals would be to reduce the client's fear response, which often inhibits the ability to deal with repressed traumatic material; to facilitate the client's interpersonal communications with the therapist, spouse, or significant others; and to accelerate the formation of a therapeutic alliance between client and therapist.

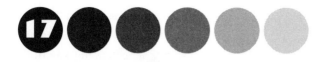

USING MDMA IN THE TREATMENT OF SCHIZOPHRENIA

Julie Holland, M.D.

The purpose of this chapter is to familiarize the reader with schizophrenia and what is currently known about its symptoms, their chemical basis, and their management. I have also included several personal reports from people with schizophrenia who have used MDMA. I am presenting this anecdotal evidence to support the idea that MDMA may help some people with schizophrenia deal with the issues that arise when confronting this disease. It is possible that the effects of MDMA can temporarily reduce some of the acute symptoms of this illness or help equip people with schizophrenia with the power to fight their illness over the long term. It is not clear whether MDMA can help a majority of people with schizophrenia. It *is* clear that good clinical research is necessary to explore the effects of single oral dose MDMA-assisted psychotherapy in these patients. Whether the results of this proposed research are miraculous or lackluster, they nevertheless will shed more light on this disease and its pharmacological management.

I have met all kinds of people with schizophrenia. This disease has fascinated me since my college days. I remember noticing people on the street, usually homeless and acting bizarrely, who I thought might be ill. The main reason I went to medical school and became a psychiatrist was to try to help these particular patients. One percent of the world's population has schizophrenia, a chronic mental illness characterized by a waxing and waning level of psychosis. Contrary to a widespread misunderstanding, a person with schizophrenia does not have multiple personalities. The schism or split be-tween thoughts and affect—between one's inner world and outer behavior—earned the disease its name. The hallmark features of schizophrenia are di-vided into two categories: positive symptoms and negative symptoms. Among the positive symptoms are auditory hallucinations (such as "hearing voices"), disorganized thoughts and speech, and paranoid delusions.

Imagine that you believe that you are being monitored by the FBI, poi-soned by your family, or perhaps that people you know have been replaced with imposters. It is common for you to have ideas of reference—thinking that everything that is happening around you has something to do with you, that everything is a clue for you to interpret or a secret code for you to trans-late. You are convinced that the purpose of a televised newscast or a song on the radio is specifically to send you a message. You may foster the belief that others can hear what you are thinking as well as the belief that you can read people's minds and they can read yours. The voices in your head may keep up a running commentary of what is going on around you, or call you de-rogatory names, or command you to do things.

Over the past fifty years, antipsychotic medications have been developed to help ease the symptoms of schizophrenia. Auditory hallucinations usually respond first to this treatment; the voices typically become quieter, though they do not always vanish. Speech then becomes more organized and less fragmented, perhaps because there is no longer competition from the voices while a person is trying to speak. Paranoid delusions usually stick around a bit longer, because they are stubborn beliefs that take some time for people to abandon. Eventually they diminish in intensity as well.

After the positive symptoms have been adequately treated, the negative symptoms often remain. Although they are less disruptive, they can be quite debilitating and are much more difficult to eradicate with typical antipsy-chotic medication. They take the form of a lack of motivation, social iso-lation, talking less, and thinking less (known in psychiatry as "poverty of speech and thought"). Also common are aberrations in attention and con-centration, usually referred to as "cognitive deficits." Some patients with schizophrenia have more negative symptoms than positive symptoms. These patients at times resemble people with autism. Emotionally withdrawn, they stay to themselves and may make rocking or other repetitive motions, seeming to be quite disconnected from the environment. Affective blunting or flattening also is typical—if emotion is felt at all, it is not conveyed in the faces or voices of these patients.

Contrast this syndrome of paranoia, social withdrawal, and decreased speech, motivation, and emotional expression with the syndrome seen during MDMA use: enhanced sociability, enthusiasm, euphoria, increased desire to speak with and connect to others, and a sense of openness and trust. It is easy to see why some people with schizophrenia have been drawn to MDMA use and why they are eager for scientific research to move forward in this area. MDMA targets the very components of behavior that are affected in schizophrenia, and it enhances the function of the two brain chemicals that are implicated in the disease. These are two compelling reasons to explore the connection between this medication and this illness. It is quite possible that we may learn more about the biological basis of schizophrenia, its symptoms, and its treatment by learning more about MDMA.

The Dopamine Theory of Schizophrenia

In the early phases of schizophrenia research, the dopamine theory dominated the scientific literature. This hypothesis stated that the disease reflects a state in the brain of too much dopamine or overactivity in the transmission of dopamine (Meltzer and Stahl 1976). To support this hypothesis, it was pointed out that the most effective antipsychotics are those that block dopamine receptors most potently (Creese et al. 1976; Seeman et al. 1976). This receptor blockade is known as "dopamine antagonism." For many years, it was felt that schizophrenia simply reflected a state of too much dopamine, and its effective treatment was to antagonize dopamine transmission. More recent theories about dopamine and schizophrenia posit that there may be an imbalance of dopaminergic activity. The positive symptoms (hallucinations and delusions) reflect a "hyperdopaminergic" state in certain parts of the brain (the subcortical regions), and negative symptoms reflect a "hypodopaminergic" state in other parts (the prefrontal or cortical region) (Deutch 1992; Dworkin and Opler 1992; Knable and Weinberger 1997).

Another theory is that the negative symptoms may reflect actual structural changes in the brain (neuropathologic changes) (Crow 1980). Supporting this theory is the observation that people with frontal lobe injuries, for example, people who have undergone frontal lobotomies or strokes, tend to have problems with initiating behaviors, showing emotion, and interacting appropriately with others (Neylan 1999). A decreased rate of blood flow to the front part of the brain also is seen in schizophrenia (Gur et al. 1989). MDMA has been shown to enhance blood flow to some of the same areas often mentioned as abnormal in patients with schizophrenia. In healthy normal volunteers given a single oral dose of MDMA (1.7 mg/kg), blood flow was increased bilaterally in various regions of the brain, including the ventromedial prefrontal cortex, the ventral anterior cingulate, the inferior temporal lobe, the medial occipital lobe, and in the entire cerebellum (Gamma et al. 2000b).

Clinical Studies: Giving Dopamine Agonists to People with Schizophrenia

It has become clear over time that while the classic antipsychotics that block dopamine receptors can quiet the voices, organize the speech, and diminish the paranoia, they do not adequately treat the deficit state or negative symptoms that remain. Some researchers have stated that despite more than twenty years of negative symptom research, there is still no proven pharmacological treatment for primary negative symptoms (Carpenter et al. 1995). And so the search continues for medications to ameliorate these negative symptoms. Medications that have been tried include dopamine agonists (enhancers), such as amphetamine. Amphetamine was used in psychiatry as early as 1936 (Meyerson 1936). Some stroke patients have been given amphetamine to enhance their motivation and hasten their recovery (Goldstein and Hulsebosch 1999). It is widely accepted that long-term use of high-dose amphetamine, sometimes called a psychostimulant, can produce paranoid psychosis in nonpsychiatric patients (Angrist 1994); at one time, this was part of the basis of the dopamine theory of schizophrenia (Snyder 1973; Ellison 1994). Amphetamine and other psychostimulants, such as methylphenidate (Ritalin) and ephedrine, have been used in schizophrenia research as "probes," or provocative tests [see Lieberman et al. 1987 for a review]. The idea behind provocative tests is to give a drug that causes an effect, any measureable effect at all in the schizophrenia population. Knowing how the probe works chemically and observing its effect on research patients yields important information about the pharmacological basis of the symptoms and their treatment.

One theory of negative symptoms posits that a failure of dopamine activation to the prefrontal cortex (an area of the brain thought to be involved in executive decision making) explains some of the cognitive deficits seen in this syndrome (Dworkin and Opler 1992). Therefore, it is believed that in small doses, psychostimulants, such as the dopamine agonist amphetamine, might be helpful in treating the deficits of schizophrenia. There have been some studies showing that amphetamine can worsen a psychotic episode in schizophrenic patients (Guttman and Sargant 1937; Angrist et al. 1980). There have been several other studies of patients with schizophrenia, however, that mentioned some decrease in negative symptoms with the administration of amphetamine (Angrist et al. 1982; Cesarec and Nyman 1985; Van Kammen and Boronow 1988; Matthew and Wilson 1989; Goldberg et al. 1991).

One study using patients with schizotypal personality disorder, who tend to show features of affective flattening and cognitive deficits similar to patients with schizophrenia, established amphetamine-associated improvement on a card-sorting test that patients with schizophrenia typically have trouble with (Siegel et al. 1996). Most amphetamine studies using patients with negative symptoms of schizophrenia qualify the statistically significant results as partial, but not complete. Although the results of these studies were not robust, one article cautions that "amphetamine may modestly improve negative symptoms in those schizohprenics in whom this symptomatology is more severe" (Sanfilipo et al. 1996). In reviewing the psychostimulant studies, a few trends are apparent: patients are less likely to become psychotic if the drugs are given orally, instead of intravenously, and if the patient is not acutely psychotic but rather is showing residual, attenuated positive symptoms of schizophrenia. Methylphenidate reportedly is more likely to bring on a psychotic episode than is amphetamine (Lieberman et al. 1987).

In considering the use of MDMA for the treatment or study of schizophrenia, it is important to bear in mind that the level of activity of the serotonergic system affects the response seen with amphetamine challenges. In animals, the results of various tests in which serotonin was depleted or cells were lesioned showed a stronger response to amphetamine challenges. Likewise, when serotonin availability was enhanced, there was attenuation in amphetamine-elicited activation (Gerson and Baldessarini 1980). When a serotonin precursor, 5-hydroxytryptophan (5-HTP), was given in conjunction with amphetamine to subjects with schizophrenia, it prevented the induction of the acute psychotic symptoms sometimes seen with amphetamine challenges (Irwin et al. 1987). MDMA immediately raises levels of serotonin and dopamine in the brain, and this may prevent an undesirable increase in psychotic symptoms in patients with schizohrenia.

Serotonin and Schizophrenia

Support for the involvement of the serotonergic system in schizophrenia has been gathering in the literature since it was first observed almost forty years ago that lysergic acid diethylamide (LSD) causes a syndrome evocative of schizophrenia in normal controls and that the structure of LSD shares similarities with serotonin (Gaddum and Hameed 1954). Although the dopamine hypothesis dominated the literature for the next three decades, further evidence to reassert serotonergic abnormalities in patients with schizophrenia came when clozapine, the first antipsychotic in forty years to show clinical superiority to chlorpromazine (Thorazine, a dopamine antagonist), was found to have potent serotonin receptor antagonism (Meltzer et al. 1989; Canton et al. 1990).

Because the serotonergic system is functionally interactive (Kelland et al. 1990) and anatomically closely connected (Tork 1991) with the dopaminergic system, there is good reason to view these two neurotransmitter systems in tandem, as opposed in isolation. The serotonin system inhibits dopaminergic function at both its origin in the midbrain and its termination in the forebrain (Kapur and Remington 1996). Thus, it may be desirable to augment the dopamine antagonist effect of classic antipsychotics with a serotonin agonist. Serotonin modulation may be beneficial in reducing the negative symptoms of schizophrenia (Leysen et al. 1993). It should be noted, however, that many of the newer antipsychotics are serotonin antagonists. This is a complex area of study. There are many different receptor subtypes of both serotonin and dopamine, and there are likely several modes of interaction between these two systems (Kapur and Remington 1996). Also confounding are the changes that take place in the brain when doses of serotonin and dopamine antagonists (for example, antipsychotics) are administered over the long term (versus the immediate effects seen with acute agonists of these same neurotransmitter systems, as is seen with MDMA).

The coexistence of illnesses known to respond to the antidepressants that are selective serotonin reuptake inhibitors (SSRIs), such as fluoxetine (Prozac), lends support to the idea that serotonin is involved in the pathophysiology of schizophrenia. The prevalence of depression in people with schizophrenia is quite high and is seen throughout the course of the disease. Approximately 25 percent of schizophrenic patients experience depression after an acute psychotic episode ("post-psychotic depression"), and as many as 60 percent experience a major depressive episode during the course of their illness (Bartels and Drake 1989). One study found the baseline incidence of depression to be 22 percent, and the incidence over a five-year follow-up period was 26 percent (Koreen et al. 1993). The suicide rate for schizophrenic patients (10 to 13 percent) is ten times the national average (1 percent), and suicide is the leading cause of premature death in these patients (Caldwell and Gottesman 1990). A general population study showed that people with schizophrenia have the highest relative risk of attempted suicide, with a risk ratio of 23:1 (Dyck et al. 1988). Mann (1987) notes that a low level of the serotonin metabolite 5-hydroxyindoleacetic acid (5-HIAA) measured in the cerebrospinal fluid correlates with suicidal behavior in depression and in schizophrenia. One cerebrospinal fluid 5-HIAA study noted low levels in schizophrenic patients, with a further reduction seen in those patients who had attempted suicide (Cooper et al. 1992). Clozapine treatment of neuroleptic-resistant patients resulted in markedly less suicidal behavior and was accompanied by improvements in depression and hopelessness (Meltzer and Okayli 1995).

Schizophrenia and obsessive-compulsive disorder show a high rate of coexistence, perhaps reflecting the involvement of the serotonergic system in both of these psychiatric diseases. One study listed the occurrence of significant obsessive-compulsive symptoms in schizophrenic patients as 25 percent (Berman et al. 1995). Schizophrenia and autism also share similar features (withdrawn behavior, self-stimulation stereotypes, inappropriate or flattened affect, poor eye contact). Some of these features of autism have been shown to respond to treatment with fenfluramine (Geller et al. 1982; Ritvo et al. 1983), a modified amphetamine with serotonin-agonist actions in behavioral models and serotonin-depleting actions in biochemical models (Clineschmidt et al. 1978) similar to MDMA.

Clinical Studies: Giving Serotonin Agonists to Schizophrenics

Several studies have used serotonin reuptake inhibitors, particularly fluoxetine, as adjunctive treatment for medicated patients with schizophrenia. Fluoxetine has been shown to improve negative symptoms significantly though blood levels of antipsychotics were elevated. (Spina et al. 1994; Goff et al. 1995); fluvoxamine (Luvox) also has been shown to ameliorate negative symptoms (Silver and Nassar 1992). In one study comparing the effects of fluvoxamine with those of maprotiline (Ludiomil, a non-serotonergic antidepressant) in medicated schizophrenic patients, the patients given fluvoxamine showed significant improvement in motor retardation, emotional withdrawal, and affective blunting compared with the group given maprotiline (Silver and Shmugliakov 1998). This effectively factors out the possibility that it is merely an antidepressant effect and suggests that it is specifically the serotonergic effect that is responsible for the improvement in negative symptoms.

In a study in which medicated schizophrenic patients received fenfluramine, three of eight subjects showed statistically significant improvement in negative symptoms, and three other patients showed significant improvement in positive symptoms (Stahl et al. 1985). Fenfluramine has properties similar to MDMA, and rats trained to discriminate between fenfluramine and placebo also tended to generalize to MDMA 90 percent of the time (Schecter 1997). Another study using long-term fenfluramine treatment, however, showed that it worsened negative symptoms in schizophrenic patients (Soper et al. 1990). An open trial (patients and doctors knew what patients were receiving) of sertraline (Zoloft) administered to patients stabilized on antipsychotics noted some amelioration of both positive and negative symptoms (Thakore et al. 1996), while a double-blind study (neither patients nor doctors knew whether patient was receiving experimental drug or placebo) found no statistically significant improvement (Lee et al. 1998).

Studies have been done using the serotonin agonist metachlorophenylpiperazine (mCPP) as a challenge test (single dose) in schizophrenic patients in an effort to test the assumption of serotonergic involvement in schizophrenia. They have produced mixed results. In normal subjects, mCPP infusion leads to an increase in body temperature, anxiety, and release of growth hormone, cortisol, ACTH, and prolactin (Murphy et al. 1986, 1991). In a 1991 Yale study of unmedicated schizophrenics, mCPP caused a larger anxiety response in patients than in controls (Krystal et al. 1991). Furthermore, it was shown to exacerbate psychotic symptoms in the patient group (Krystal et al. 1991). Iqbal and associates (1991) corroborated the finding of psychotogenesis in schizophrenic patients exposed to an mCPP challenge (0.25 mg/kg taken by mouth [PO]). Kahn (1992), however, measured an improvement in symptoms (by the Brief Psychiatric Rating Scale) of those schizophrenics undergoing an mCPP challenge (0.35 mg/kg PO).

What can be understood from all of these results? Clearly, there is no simple answer. What was once a theory of too much dopamine or serotonin is now a theory of imbalance: too much in some areas and not enough in others. A few theorists go one step further to match the levels of neurotransmitters with symptoms. Positive symptoms represent an abundance of dopamine turnover, and negative symptoms represent the opposite (Rao and Moller 1994). Because some people with schizophrenia have more positive symptoms and others have more negative symptoms, some do better with certain medications, and others respond to different medications. There are some researchers who think that schizophrenia is a syndrome, or a group of illnesses, and not simply one disease. This may mean that research conducted on large groups of subjects may not be studying the same phenomenon. Many studies now try to focus on either positive-symptom- or negative-symptom-predominant groups. Perhaps the only thing that can be generalized from all these data is that decreasing available dopamine and serotonin in the synapse seems to improve positive symptoms. It is possible, though not nearly as certain, that enhancing available serotonin and dopamine in the synapse improves negative symptoms.

Pre-Pulse Inhibition

There is one more interesting piece to the puzzle. Schizophrenic patients are known to have deficits in the way they view and respond to the outside world. Typically, people become used to a repetitive stimulus (habituation) and have less of a response to second and third presentations of the same stimulus. There is also a phenomenon known as sensory gating, which is made evident by a technique known as pre-pulse inhibition (PPI). If a smaller stimulus is introduced before a larger one—say, two tones of escalating volume— a person usually would be less startled by the second, louder tone, having been prepared by the first, quieter tone. In schizophrenia this is not the case, and it is known as a deficit in sensory gating, or a disruption in PPI. There are many medicines and drugs that make this deficit worse, but there are few substances that have been shown to enhance the inhibition of the first pulse. Nicotine is one drug that does enhance PPI, which may explain why so many schizophrenics smoke cigarettes heavily.

Swiss researchers have discovered that MDMA has the capacity to enhance PPI (Vollenweider et al. 1999b). This may be the most compelling reason to give single oral dose MDMA to people with schizophrenia. If MDMA can enhance PPI in the general population, it is possible that it can enhance PPI in schizophrenic patients. Any medicine that ameliorates any symptom or syndrome is worth studying, if for no other reason than to help us learn the pharmacological basis of that symptom, so that better medications can be created. In the past, schizophrenic research subjects have been given LSD, DMT (dimethyltryptamine), PCP (phenylcyclidine), amphetamine, methylphenidate, and ketamine, to observe the effect of these medications on the symptoms of schizophrenia (Stol 1947; Boszormenyi and Szara 1958; Itil et al. 1967; Angrist et al. 1980, 1982; Lieberman1987; Malhotra et al. 1997; Lahti et al. 1995). Many of these drugs worsened the symptoms for a short time. The rationale in performing these studies was that any observable change in symptoms yields valuable information about the illness.

Given what we know about MDMA, which is that it increases the availability of serotonin and dopamine in the synapse, that it strengthens PPI in humans, and that it appears to enhance sociality and motivation, it seems reasonable to ask the question: Can it help people with schizophrenia? The ability to connect to and communicate with others is severely impaired in negative-symptom schizophrenic patients; it is markedly enhanced among people taking MDMA. Attention, concentration, and insight all are compromised in schizophrenic patients and augmented in people under the influence of MDMA. In the same way that amphetamine and fenfluramine have been used to try to ameliorate negative symptoms, so, too, should the ring-substituted amphetamine MDMA.

Testimonials

The following testimonials are from people (their names have been changed) who have been diagnosed with schizophrenia and have found some benefit from their MDMA use. These are edited excerpts from e-mails to me describing their experiences.

Robert
Robert was diagnosed as a paranoid schizophrenic in his early twenties. He had auditory and visual hallucinations, ideas of reference, and paranoid ideation. He has been treated with olanzepine (Zyprexa).

> I strongly believe MDMA has huge potential for the treatment of schizophrenia. . . . Another commonality is a sense of well-being, not just in a personal sense but also in a communal sense, a kind of belonging that can manifest as more "connected" conversations with people or perhaps just more talking for those of few words. For me, this was a key factor in breaking down my own cycle of de-socialization. On MDMA, I found myself more able to talk with almost anyone about almost anything and felt rather freed of most (formerly unrealized or at least not admitted) neuroses/psychoses that normally plague me. Just this visceral experience of sharing thoughts and feelings with people, even if only for a few hours, had a lasting effect on my own self-view and worldview. In some sense, it gives me a role model for what sort of personality I would like to achieve without the use of external chemicals, and it gives direct proof that there is a lot of psychological flexibility in my own mind.

John
John was diagnosed with schizophrenia in his late teens. He had a history of treatment with clozapine (Clozaril) and olanzepine. Later he was "de-diagnosed" and no longer took any antipsychotic medication. (He may have been misdiagnosed; though he did have a history of referential ideation and paranoia, he never heard voices.)

I have used MDMA quite successfully in combating my psychosis. With the very first use, MDMA completely changed my life. The paranoia that I was experiencing was temporarily halted and replaced with an immense sense of love, compassion, intimacy, and closeness. Please note that MDMA only reduced my paranoia temporarily; the paranoia came back later. But the insight that I gained from these precious few hours of clarity proved to be invaluable. For one, I truly had learned how to love—the schizophrenia had taken that ability from me. I became closer to my friends and family. Second, I became a much more open, outgoing, and positive person. Again, schizophrenia had lobotomized these critical qualities in me. Finally, MDMA instilled in me an unrelenting will to live. A will to keep pushing forward on my road to recovery no matter what obstacles presented themselves. With the help of the positive MDMA effects, carefully titrated antipsychotic drugs, and a lot of people who cared about me, I slowly began to turn the tide on my disease. Over time, I gradually worked my way to the point where I could live outside a psychiatric treatment facility. In fact, it's been more than two and a half years since I left the hospital. The way I see it, I will never have to go back, ever.

James

James' first signs of schizophrenia began at about the age of fourteen or fifteen. He had a history of persistent auditory hallucinations, paranoia, delusions, ideas of reference, one suicide attempt, and a psychiatric hospitalization.

I felt as is if my mental problems had washed away. All of my paranoia, all of my reservations about people, all of the pent-up anger and frustration, the bitterness towards my family, all of it had been flushed out with a single dose. I felt like a real person. I remember reflecting on my life in disgust at how I behave on a day-to-day basis. I wanted to initiate change, to make myself more like I was when I was on "E," because I thought it was beautiful, and right. When I came down, I wasn't disappointed that it was over, and I didn't crave more, but I did remember the changes I wanted to make. My whole outlook on life changed that night. It has given me freedom from a disease that has plagued me for years, and a bit of that freedom is present even after the drug wears off. I do not think this is a cure for anything, [it offers] only a new perspective that should be used wisely.

I also had an interesting telephone conversation with a young man with schizo-phrenia whose symptoms were much more severe than were the symptoms of these other men. During a subsequent phone call, he was acutely para-noid, and he was eventually lost to follow-up. But he told me that when he took MDMA for the first time, he felt as if he were cured for a few hours, and he thought that it was important for doctors and scientists to do research on why that had happened. And I could not agree more.

USING MDMA IN ALTERNATIVE MEDICINE
An Interview with Andrew Weil, M.D.

JH: Do you think that MDMA has any place in alternative medicine?

AW: I don't know that I would put it in alternative medicine. I think it has a place in medicine. I wouldn't make a distinction there. For me, the interesting thing is that if the set and setting are properly attended to, MDMA can produce a state of great relaxation and lack of defensiveness in which the body behaves differently. You see that chronic pain can disappear and that habits can disappear. It can show people that there is a possibility that they're not obliged to have certain symptoms. The experience can motivate them to figure out other ways to maintain that symptom-free state.

JH: Let's talk about relaxation first. How do you think that MDMA can be helpful there?

AW: Many people walk around in states of chronic tension and much of their discomfort is due to that. Just to have an experience of what it feels like to be completely relaxed can show them that their experience of their bodies can be different. I think many people have never felt complete relaxation.

JH: One thing that also happens in an MDMA-induced state is that there is enhanced attention to posture and breathing, which also can be very helpful.

AW: Right.

JH: You have emphasized the importance of deep breathing. Practitioners of the Alexander technique are particularly fond of MDMA for opening up the ribs and enhancing the ability to take deeper breaths.

AW: Yes.

JH: What about the body image issues—people really looking at their bodies or taking an inventory of their bodies in a different way?

AW: MDMA can give you a chance to have a new perspective on your body, and, again, that's part of breaking old habits. For that reason it can be a very valuable experience, assuming that the experience is structured in some way. Another area that I've been very interested in is allergies. Allergies often disappear during an MDMA experience. They may come back at the end, but it shows people that there's a relationship between mental state and allergies. This can motivate them to figure out how to work on that.

JH: Do you have any anecdotes about people using MDMA in any particular instances?

AW: I have one patient that I worked with for some time, a young man who had rheumatoid arthritis that had required a couple of hand surgeries. He took MDMA about once a month and felt that it put him completely into remission. He began working with other patients who had rheumatoid arthritis. I have worked with people who have overcome allergies—cat allergies, hay fever—as a result of the MDMA experience. I have seen many people who have dealt successfully with problems like chronic back and neck pain and digestive problems as a result of using MDMA.

JH: What is your opinion about the use of MDMA in palliative care?

AW: I have less experience with that. I know of some cases of people with advanced cancer who felt it was very positive for them. It helped them come to a sort of resolution with their lives and complete emotional work that they had to do with other people.

JH: I was hoping to touch on the potential for MDMA to be used as an analgesic [painkiller].

AW: A major component of pain is the subjective experience of it. MDMA changes your perspective about what is going on in your body, so it can help people develop a new relationship with chronic pain in which it is less of a discomfort.

JH: And what about the impact of fear and anxiety on pain perception?

AW: That's a huge component of pain. If the experience is structured properly, MDMA induces an extremely low anxiety state, which can dramatically lessen that aspect of pain. Often, there is a great deal of carryover after that experience.

JH: Do you see insight as a tool to assist in physical healing? For instance, if MDMA is used in a psychotherapeutic setting, and a person comes away with a better understanding of self-defeating or self-damaging behavior in terms of lifestyle, do you think that could help someone with his or her health issues?

AW: Yes. I think that gaining insight is the easy part; the harder part is applying it.

JH: The integration?

AW: Yes. Integration may require some work and help, so that the experience doesn't just get boxed up and put into the past. But I definitely think that during the experience, one can gain insights into the nature of one's problems.

JH: Or potentially the symbolism of certain physical symptoms?

AW: Yes.

JH: What about the recreational or the pleasurable component of MDMA? Most people want to separate the recreational and the therapeutic aspects of MDMA.

AW: I don't make much of a distinction. I think recreational experiences can be therapeutic.

JH: I'm so glad you said that. I believe that as well—for instance, the therapeutic effect of play or joy.

AW: I think that's an important aspect of heath, and it's something that a lot of people in our culture don't do for themselves. I have seen many people with MDMA experiences become childlike and recover an aspect of themselves that they had lost. I think that's very valuable. But I don't have any familiarity with MDMA in the context of raves.

JH: I think that as a cultural phenomenon, it's impressive. One of the salient features of a rave setting is the sense of community. There is a theme of connection—not just to oneself or to one other person but to an entire movement or community and even to every person on the planet, the "global village."

AW: Right. Maybe fifteen years ago I was teaching a seminar that was partly on psychedelics, and we had an afternoon devoted to MDMA. I was saying to this group that the idea of taking this drug and going indoors with a huge crowd of people and blaring music seemed to me to be a waste of the potential of the substance. A woman from England said she disagreed and that many of these people were soccer toughs who would be out beating up people. It was much better to have them engaged in this kind of activity. I had never thought of it that way, and I can certainly see the value of that.

JH: One of the things that I notice among psychiatric patients, which is very sad, is how disconnected and socially isolated they are. I think it's unhealthy. The isolation feeds into the illness. Then, because they are ill, they tend to be even more cut off from society, and the effect snowballs. I believe that it can be quite therapeutic for people to have a sense of self-acceptance, or to feel accepted by a group.

AW: I agree.

JH: Self-love is also therapeutic. A lot of people's maladaptive behavior can come from self-hatred.

AW: Definitely. A common theme of the MDMA experience is that things feel "all right." People feel all right with themselves and with other people, and they drop a lot of their judgments. If that could be carried over into life, I think it could be very useful.

JH: One of the things I say about an MDMA experience is that you should take notes. Bring something out of the experience with you.

AW: Yes. Good.

JH: The quality of acceptance or forgiveness that people experience with MDMA can be valuable. Would you say that in some medical conditions, there is an element of anger or fear or guilt?

AW: Definitely. I think all of those kinds of states translate into body states.

JH: So it would probably be therapeutic to have an experience where those emotions are markedly lessened. What is your take on "psycho-neuro-immunology"?

AW: It is a field that's very well established. It's been around for three decades, and there is a vast body of research on it. The problem is that it's made very little impact on thinking and practice in conventional medicine. It's had all sorts of resonance with the general public as a result of books and TV shows. At the University of Arizona in the immunology course, for instance, the word "psycho-neuro-immunology" isn't even mentioned. There is a lack of connection between this body of research and the public's enthusiasm for it, as opposed to the actual day-to-day application in medicine.

JH: Do you see MDMA having any place in that field?

AW: Absolutely. What I mentioned to you about allergies is so striking to me. I can imagine taking an allergic patient and doing, say, ten sessions with decreasing doses of MDMA until, by the last session, the person isn't taking any. This is a way to teach patients to unlearn their allergies.

JH: Do you have any opinion about the issue of MDMA being synthetic, as opposed to natural, in terms of its use in alternative medicine?

AW: If there were a totally natural substance that had the effect of MDMA, I would use it, but there isn't one. MDMA is semi-synthetic; it's pretty close to a natural substance, but it's got a slight twist.

JH: Meaning safrole, sassafras, nutmeg . . .

AW: It's closest to safrole and myristicin and things of that sort. It's just a slight twist on a natural molecule. That, to me, is not such a big deal. I wouldn't make a major distinction there—and again, I wouldn't relegate MDMA to the world of alternative medicine. I think it can be used in medicine generally.

JH: I have heard you speak of optimism as a healing tool. For most people, the MDMA-induced state is chock full of optimism.

AW: Right. There is a psychologist at the University of Pennsylvania named Martin Seligman who studies the states of helplessness and optimism and the effect they have on health. Optimism is a behavior and an attitude that can be learned, and I think that it has many consequences in terms of how our bodies function and how our minds work. I think that just having the experience of it, seeing that there is a mental perspective from which things can look positive, is very useful—especially if you haven't had that perspective in a long time. The basic point is that mental states translate into physical states. And one of the great values of the MDMA experience is that it can show you very concretely how a shift in your mental state can produce dramatic responses in your body. Often, this has significant carryover into daily life.

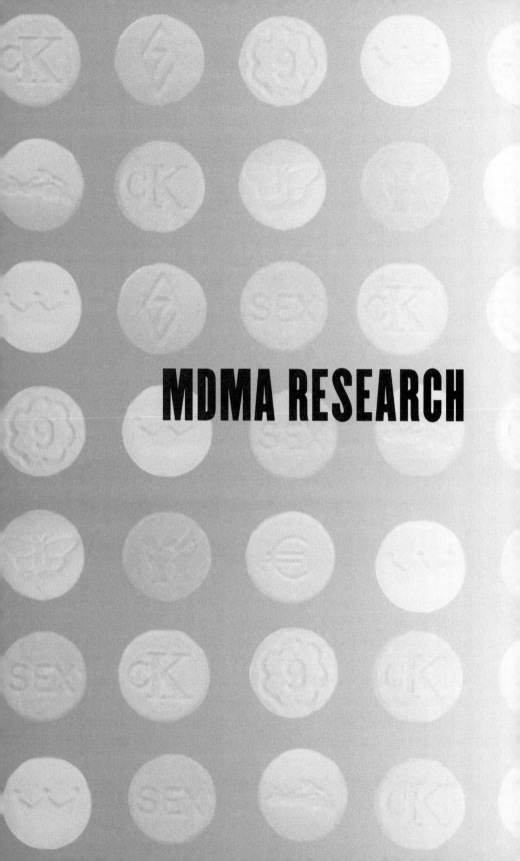

MDMA RESEARCH

Introduction

ar-ma-men-tar-i-um (noun): an arsenal; an aggregate of resources, apparatus, and so on, specifically for work in the field of medicine

The field of astronomy has the telescope; biology has the microscope. MDMA is just such a tool in the field of psychotherapy. It can be likened to a powerful mirror or scope that allows users to examine themselves more fully, thoroughly, and calmly than ever before. Contrast an MDMA-assisted therapy session with what commonly is called an "amytal interview." In this sort of interview, a psychiatrist administers a powerful tranquilizer so that the patient will have fewer inhibitions and be able to open up more completely to the therapist. The problem is that patients become nearly unconscious. They are sedated, their words are slurred, they nod off, and they have almost no memory of the entire event. MDMA lowers the defenses to allow a thorough inventory of psychological difficulties, but the patient remains an active, alert, vital participant in the process.

Another comparison to consider is with electroconvulsive therapy (ECT), better known as "shock therapy." The severely depressed patient is sedated and paralyzed prior to an electrically induced seizure in the brain. After a series of nine to twelve seizures spread out over several weeks, depressed patients typically recover to a large extent, but they have minimal memory concerning events during the several weeks over which the sessions took place. The point is that desperate and potentially dangerous methods sometimes are used to help people recover from mental illness. A single oral therapeutic dose of MDMA in a supervised setting is no more dangerous than an amytal interview or an ECT session, and certainly will yield more valuable psychic material.

Despite hundreds of anecdotal reports of impressive results in MDMA-assisted psychotherapy, there are precious few teams doing clinical trials to ascertain the benefits of the therapeutic use of MDMA. At present, only one group, led by José Carlos Bouso in Spain, is examining the potential of MDMA as a treatment for a psychiatric disorder. Bouso's research (and his chapter for this volume) focuses on women who have post-traumatic stress disorder and have been the victims of sexual assault.

In the United States, the Food and Drug Administration has advised that before therapeutic studies can begin, basic pharmacological research must be done. Before continuing, I think it best to define our terms. In clinical research, the subjects are humans and not animals. Currently, we have a plethora of neurotoxicity studies using animals who have received large doses of MDMA by injection, usually 10 to 20 mg/kg, often administered as two doses a day for four days in a row. The one clinical study looking at positron emission tomographic (PET) scans of humans given a single oral dose of MDMA was performed in Switzerland by Vollenweider's group. These researchers did not report any evidence of neurotoxicity in those human subjects. The human studies comparing polydrug users with nondrug users to make assumptions about how MDMA affects memory, birth defects, and so on should not be considered clinical studies. No MDMA was given to those people, and it remains to be proved whether these Ecstasy users ever consumed MDMA, and at what doses, since these studies were retrospective. [For further critique of this issue, see "Does MDMA Cause Brain Damage?"]

The scientific community is lagging behind the rest of society and needs to catch up quickly. Even though MDMA has been around for twenty-five years and even though millions of people have used it, widespread clinical research has yet to be performed. In the United States, there are four groups doing clinical MDMA research. In the United Kingdom, there is only one group performing clinical research. The reasons behind this appalling lack of scientific data are in part financial. The U.S. government has a long history of sponsoring research focusing on the risks of drug use. Typically, these studies are funded by NIDA, the National Institute on Drug Abuse. However, our government does not even like to support research looking at risk reduction, or harm reduction, because it is feared this may send the message to the public that the government condones drug use. Another obstacle to clinical MDMA research is the difficulty and controversy surrounding Schedule I drug research. There is no question that placement of MDMA in Schedule III, where it could be prescribed by physicians, would enhance the body of knowledge more rapidly.

When I was a psychiatric resident, the chairman of my program was less than receptive to the idea of MDMA research being conducted in his department. In his mind, there was simply too much controversy and too little justification for it. His response to my request to do clinical MDMA research in our facility was akin to a neighborhood's response to a halfway house or homeless shelter: "Not in my backyard." But what better justification could there be than to test the promise of a new medicine, an "anti-neurotic"? The answer is harm reduction. The medical community has an obligation to educate those who take Ecstasy about the potential risks of their behavior and the ways they can make it safer.

Despite hundreds of cases of Ecstasy-induced hyperthermia, physicians are still reporting cases and case series where there is no determination of the offending agent. The assumption is that MDMA is specifically to blame, but in many cases the emergency room physicians are not doing the toxicological studies necessary to prove that MDMA was consumed. Another potential area for harm reduction research is the effect of temperature on hyperthermia and neurotoxicity. Malberg and Seiden (1998) have shown that in laboratory animals, the temperature of the animals' surroundings is crucial to exacerbating or alleviating MDMA-induced neurotoxicity. No scientific team has published data on the effect of MDMA on research subjects' core temperature in terms of their surrounding temperature. Typically, therapeutic research is sponsored by the pharmaceutical industry. Millions of dollars are poured into research and development if a company believes that they have a medication that has the potential to be a moneymaker. Here we have two problems. First, MDMA was patented in 1914, and that patent has long since expired. No company could recoup its losses invested in research by being the sole provider of this medication. The second problem is that MDMA, unlike antidepressant medication, typically is given only once or twice in the lifetime of a patient. There is simply no money to be made from a medicine given that infrequently. For these reasons, funding for therapeutic studies will have to come from the private sector. To that end, I have endowed the Holland Fund for Therapeutic MDMA Research. All proceeds from the sale of this book will be donated to this fund. All donations are tax deductible and will go toward funding clinical MDMA research that seeks to add scientific data to the anecdotal data. There are also at least two organizations, the Multidisciplinary Association for Psychedelic Studies (MAPS) and the Heffter Institute, that are supporting clinical MDMA research.

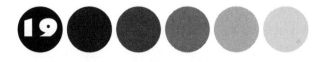

CLINICAL RESEARCH WITH MDMA: A WORLDWIDE REVIEW

Andrew M. Kleiman, M.D., and Julie Holland, M.D.

Although MDMA has been available to researchers for decades, there are few reliable clinical studies looking at its effects. Many published articles concerning MDMA cite animal data, using rats, mice, or nonhuman primates, such as squirrel monkeys or baboons. Most of the human studies take their data from people who are long-term Ecstasy users and then compare them with data from non-Ecstasy users. These retrospective studies are suspect for a number of reasons. First, we have no idea if the chemical these study participants ingested was MDMA. Second, it is likely that other chemicals (specifically ketamine, dextromethorphan, and marijuana) were ingested by these research subjects, which might explain any differences recorded between the groups. Third, many variables are at play among people who take drugs often, for example, diet, exercise, sleep habits, and preexisting psychiatric diagnoses.

In this chapter we specifically review only recent prospective clinical trials of MDMA. This means that people were given a known amount of pure MDMA and then observed for changes. These are the cleanest studies being performed at present. We are grateful to the researchers who described their studies and extend our apologies to the hardworking scientists who were not included in this chapter owing to the nature of their work. Some of their results, particularly Dr. George Ricaurte's work, are reviewed elsewhere in this book (see "Does MDMA Cause Brain Damage?"). Surveys of psychiatrists who have taken MDMA (Liester et al. 1992), psychiatrists who have given MDMA to patients (Harlow and Beck 1990), and patients who have taken MDMA in the context of therapy (Gasser 1994–95) also are found elsewhere in this book. Non-placebo-controlled prospective studies assessing the effects of MDMA in healthy humans (Downing 1986; Greer and Tolbert 1986) are covered in Gary Bravo's chapter "What Does MDMA Feel Like?"

England

Dr. John Henry's group in England was the first to report not only a case series on hyperthermia but also the discovery of MDMA-induced hyponatremia (low sodium). Discovering and publicizing the occurrence of elevated body temperature in the dancing population of Ecstasy users has saved countless lives, as has reporting the danger of drinking too much water, which leads to low sodium levels. [See the section on the risks of MDMA for more details.] Dr. Henry and colleagues, who are affiliated with the Drug Control Centre and Department of Pharmacy, King's College London, published two MDMA studies in 1998 and 1999. In the first of these investigations, Henry and coworkers administered 40 mg of MDMA to eight men in a nonblind study, to analyze MDMA's physiological effects. The study looked specifically at secreted plasma arginine vasopressin (also called ADH, or antidiurectic hormone). This substance inhibits the kidneys from making urine and so causes a dilution of the blood and an increase in blood pressure. The amount of secreted ADH in the blood is related closely in terms of physiology to the plasma sodium concentration, which is an indicator of fluid balance in the body, and to plasma levels of cortisol, which is a natural stress hormone.

The results of this analysis yielded findings of a significantly increased plasma concentration of ADH unrelated to blood MDMA concentrations. A rapid rise in ADH and fall in plasma sodium concentration, which is inappropriate within normal physiological functioning, was induced by the administration of this small dose of MDMA. The fluid imbalance can be exacerbated by other physiological consequences of the use of MDMA, such as high body temperature, sweating, and increased secretion of the body's stress hormone, cortisol. All of these factors in combination can cause potentially fatal brain swelling as well as seizures and coma.

Fallon and colleagues examined the various structures and disposition of MDMA in humans at its many stages of metabolism, or breakdown in the body, following oral administration of 40 mg MDMA to eight male volunteers. The structures of MDMA and its breakdown product, MDA, present in plasma and urine extracts were analyzed by gas chromatography and mass spectrometry (tools used to analyze the presence of certain chemical compounds). The properties of two specific structures, which are mirror images of each other, the so-called R- and the more active S-enantiomer, were determined. [R-(–)-MDMA is almost inactive at ordinary doses. S-(+)-MDMA has about twice the potency of racemic MDMA, which is a mixture of the two. See "The Chemistry of MDMA" for more on the enantiomers of MDMA.—Ed.] It was discovered in this study that a specific structural disposition of MDMA exists in humans. The R-enantiomer has a longer half-life than the S-enantiomer and differs in the concentration-versus-time product, the so-called area under the curve. Analytical methods for determining the composition of MDMA and MDA in plasma and urine were developed, which may be applicable for forensic purposes in the detection of MDMA in human beings. Thus, the manner in which the body metabolizes and disposes of two specific types of MDMA in the human body was determined and described. More studies looking at the metabolism of MDMA in humans are planned.

References

Fallon, J. K., A. T. Kicman, J. A. Henry, P. J. Milligan, D. A. Cowan, and A. J. Hutt. 1999. Stereospecific analysis and enantiomeric disposition of 3,4-methylenedioxymethamphetamine (Ecstasy) in humans. *Clin. Chem.* 45:1058–69.

Henry, J. A., J. K. Fallon, A. T. Kicman, A. J. Hutt, D. A. Cowan, and M. Forsling. 1998. Low-dose MDMA ("Ecstasy") induces vasopressin secretion. *Lancet* 351:1784.

Spain

The Pharmacology Research Unit of the Institut Municipal di Investigación Médica (IMIM) in Barcelona, Spain (Magí Farré, Rafael de la Torre, and

Jordi Camí), has carried out three studies since 1996 in the field of MDMA research. In these studies, MDMA was administered in double-blind, randomized, placebo-controlled clinical trials to different groups of healthy male volunteers who had previous experience taking Ecstasy in a recreational setting. The first study was designed to compare the pharmacological effects of a single oral dose of MDMA with the effects of placebo. Eight men participated in four separate ten-hour experimental sessions; they were given one of two doses of MDMA (75 mg or 125 mg) or amphetamine (40 mg) or placebo on different days. Both MDMA doses significantly increased blood pressure, heart rate, and the diameter of the pupil of the eye compared with placebo. Levels of plasma cortisol showed a statistically significant increase after MDMA administration. Levels of the hormone prolactin increased only after a high dose of MDMA.

Farré and coworkers reported on the metabolic pathways of MDMA in some detail; they found a nonproportional increase in MDMA concentrations in the blood after high-dose administration (125 mg and 150 mg). This is referred to as "nonlinear pharmacokinetics." In other words, the amount of MDMA found in the blood is not proportional to the amount of MDMA ingested, as that amount steadily increases. This means that if there were adverse consequences from ingesting one or two doses of MDMA, the consequences from ingesting three or four would be disproportionately graver.

Their second study, which was published only in part, was designed to study the interactions between alcohol and MDMA. A group of subjects received an oral dose of alcohol (0.8 g/kg) or MDMA (100 mg) or both substances simultaneously or placebo. The study evaluated psychomotor performance of tasks related to driving, such as reaction time and coordination, subjective feelings and emotions, and immunological status. The results showed that MDMA ingestion decreased feelings of sedation and intoxication induced by alcohol but did not change the measured performance impairment. In other words, MDMA does not mitigate the decreased reaction time and coordination rendered by alcohol, despite the fact that subjects felt more alert.

Pacifici and colleagues found that the use of MDMA reduced the number of CD4 T cells in the blood immediately after dosing. These are cells that are an important part of the body's immune system and integral to the ability to fight disease and infection effectively. Although MDMA and the human immunodeficiency virus (HIV) are physiologically unrelated, HIV decreases the body's CD4 T-cell count as well, which is part of the process that leads to the many complications of HIV in humans. This research group also found that MDMA in combination with alcohol produced the greatest suppressive effect on CD4 T-cell count compared with MDMA or alcohol alone. These results provided the first evidence that recreational use of MDMA alone or in combination with alcohol alters the immunological status of the body. It should be noted, however, that the CD4 count normalized several hours after MDMA administration.

A third study, currently under way, was designed to evaluate the pharmacological aspects of MDMA when administered in two repeated doses. This is important, since it is well known that more than half of Ecstasy users take two or more pills during recreational use. Intervals of administration in the protocol were two, four, eight, and twenty-four hours. After the second dose, the concentrations of MDMA in the blood doubled those seen after the first dose, but the pharmacological effects were similar in terms of intensity and duration. MDMA users did not report any change in the effects of MDMA after taking the second dose, and no physical effects, such as heart rate or blood pressure changes, were reported. The results of the four-hour repeated dose study showed some degree of tolerance to the pharmacological effects.

Future plans include an examination of the possible neurotoxic effects of MDMA in humans and its evolution. A group of recreational Ecstasy users will be followed over two to three years, and these subjects will be evaluated through neuropsychological, psychiatric, and psychological testing. Hormonal responses and immunological parameters will be assessed as well. These results will be compared with results from a group of non-Ecstasy users.

References

Camí, J., M. Farré, M. Mas, et al. 2000. Human pharmacology of 3,4-methylenedioxymethamphetamine ("Ecstasy"): Psychomotor performance and subjective effects. *J. Clin. Psychoparmacol.* 20:455–66.

de la Torre, R., M. Farré, J. Ortuño, et al. 2000. Non-linear pharmacokinetics of MDMA ("Ecstasy") in humans. *Br. J. Clin. Pharmacol.* 49:104–9.

de la Torre, R., M. Farré, P. N. Roset, et al. 2000. Pharmacology of MDMA in humans. *Ann. N. Y. Acad. Sci.* 914:225–37.

Farré, M., P. N. Roset, A. Tomillero, et al. 2000. Repeated administration of ecstasy to humans: Preliminary findings. *Br. J. Clin. Pharmacol.* Special issue:111.

Hernández-Lopéz, C., M. Farré, P. N. Roset, et al. 2000. MDMA and alcohol interactions: Psychomotor and subjective effects and pharmacokinetics. *Br. J. Clin. Pharmacol.* Special issue:111.

Mas, M., M. Farré, R. de la Torre, et al. 1999. Cardiovascular and neuroendocrine effects and pharmacokinetics of 3,4-methylenedioxymethamphetamine in humans. *J. Pharmacol. Exp. Ther.* 290:136–45.

Ortuño, J., N. Pizarro, M. Farré, et al. 1999. Quantification of 3,4-methylenedioxymethamphetamine and its metabolites in plasma and urine by gas chromatography with nitrogen-phosphorous detection. *J. Chromatogr. B. Biomed. Sci.* 723:221–32.

Pacifici, R., P. Zuccaro, M. Farré, et al. 1999. Immunomodulating properties of MDMA alone and in combination with alcohol: A pilot study. *Life Sci.* 65:309–16

———. 2000. Immunomodulating activity of MDMA. *Ann. N. Y. Acad. Sci.* 914:215–24.

———. 2001. Acute effects of MDMA alone and in combination with ethanol on the immunie system in humans. *J. Pharmacol. Exp. Ther.* 296:207–215.

José Carlos Bouso and colleagues (Pedro Sopelana, María Angeles Corral, Marcela Ot'alora, and Mercedes Matarranz) from the Biological Psychology and Health Department of the Universidad Autónoma de Madrid have begun to investigate the efficacy of therapeutic administration of MDMA to women suffering from chronic post-traumatic stress disorder (PTSD) as a consequence of sexual assault. The study, funded by MAPS and the Holland Fund for Therapeutic MDMA Research, has a dual focus. First, it will evaluate the therapeutic effectiveness of MDMA in a psychotherapeutic context, and second, it will determine the most effective dosage levels of MDMA, suitable evaluation methods, and the psychotherapeutic strategies appropriate to MDMA-assisted treatment. This dose-finding pilot study has a double-blind, randomized, and placebo-controlled design. The subjects are twenty-nine healthy women between eighteen and sixty years of age with a diagnosis of chronic PTSD as result of sexual abuse.

According to the study design, on the first day the subject is given a thorough explanation of the study and undergoes baseline physical and psychiatric tests. On the second day and on the third day one week later, the subject has a one-hour therapy session to reinforce the therapeutic alliance and to prepare better for the experimental session. On the fourth day the subject undergoes the experimental and therapeutic session with MDMA or placebo. During this session, the subject is randomized to ingest a capsule containing 50, 75, 100, 125, or 150 mg of MDMA or placebo. Day five consists of a psychotherapeutic session for one hour, to integrate the experiences of the day before. Follow-up sessions are conducted one, three, six, nine, and twelve months after the conclusion of the study to evaluate the stability of the treatment results.

Outcome measurements include several scales and inventories, among them the Scale of Gravity of the Symptoms of PTSD, the State-Trait Anxiety Inventory, the Beck Depression Inventory, the Adjustment-Maladjustment Scale, the Rosenberg Self-Esteem Scale, the UKU side effects rating scale, the Hallucinogen Rating Scale, the Penn Helping Alliance questionnaire, and a modified Fear Scale with a subset of phobias related to rape. A semistructured interview regarding sexual aggression is conducted before and after the experimental session. Because this study began in November 1999 and is still in process, no results are available. Mr. Bouso wishes to thank MAPS, as well as Dr. Farré, for their invaluable support and assistance.

Switzerland

Dr. Franz Vollenweider's laboratory includes the research of Drs. Alex Gamma, Matthias Liechti, Mark Geyer, and others. Their work with MDMA has been of the utmost importance in asserting that no abnormal neurological changes have been detected thus far after single oral doses in the therapeutic range. These placebo-controlled, double-blind experiments characterize the psychological and behavioral effects of MDMA and the associated neurochemical and neurophysiological changes underlying them. They use sophisticated state-of-the-art technology, including positron emission tomography (PET) scans and pre-pulse inhibition (PPI) studies to measure the effects of single oral doses of MDMA in the range of 1.35 to 1.8 mg/kg. Their research subjects are screened psychiatrically and medically and are MDMA naive. Typically, they are university students twenty to thirty years of age. Several of these researchers' studies also have assessed possible neurophysiological and psychological alterations in regular Ecstasy users.

These researchers have examined the neurochemical regulation of mood and emotion using MDMA alone or in combination with various antagonists at the presynaptic 5-hydroxytryptamine (5-HT) uptake site, the postsynaptic 5-HT2 and D_2 receptors, to study the neurophysiological and neurochemical mechanisms of action of MDMA-induced mood enhancement in healthy humans. Their completed human studies include the following:

- psychological, physiological, and short-term effects of MDMA
- brain activity via PET and LORETA [low-resolution brain electromagnetic tomography] after a single dose of MDMA
- effects of pretreatment with citalopram, ketanserin, and haloperidol on acute and subacute responses to MDMA
- effects of MDMA on PPI
- electric and perfusion brain activity and mood state in Ecstasy users

[See "Giving MDMA to Human Volunteers in Switzerland" for further details.] A future study will examine the effects of a $5\text{-}HT1_A$ antagonist on psychological and physiological responses to MDMA.

References

Frei, E., A. Gamma, R. D. Pascual-Marqui, D. Hell, and F. X. Vollenweider. 2001. Localization of MDMA-induced electrical brain activity in healthy volunteers using low resolution brain electric tomography (LORETA). Submitted.

Gamma, A., A. Buck, T. Berthold, M. E. Liechti, and F. X. Vollenweider. 2000. 3,4-Methylenedioxymethamphetamine (MDMA) modulates cortical and limbic brain activity as measured by [H2O15]-PET in healthy humans. *Neuropsychopharmacology* 23:388–96.

Liechti, M. E., C. Baumann, A. Gamma, and F. X. Vollenweider. 2000. Acute psychological effects of 3,4-methylenedioxymethamphetamine (MDMA, "Ecstasy") are attenuated by the serotonin uptake inhibitor citalopram. *Neuropsychopharmacology* 22:513–21.

Liechti, M. E., M. Saur, A. Gamma, D. Hell, and F. X. Vollenweider. 2000. Psychological and physiological effects of MDMA ("Ecstasy") after pretreatment with the 5-HT2 antagonist ketanserin in healthy humans. *Neuropsychopharmacology* 23(4):396–405.

Liechti, M. E., and F. X. Vollenweider. 2000. Acute psychological and physiological effects of MDMA ("Ecstasy") after haloperidol pretreatment in normal healthy humans. *Eur. Neuropsychopharmacol.* 22:513–21 (in press).

———. 2000. The serotonin uptake inhibitor citalopram reduces acute cardiovascular and vegetative effects of MDMA ("Ecstasy") in healthy volunteers. *J. Psychopharmacol.* 14(3):269–74.

Liechti, M. E., A. Gamma, and F. X. Vollenweider. 2001. Gender differences in the subjective effects of MDMA. *Psychopharmacology* (Berlin) 154(2):161–68.

Liechti, M. E., M. A. Geyer, D. Hell, and F. X. Vollenweider. 2001. Effects of MDMA (Ecstasy) on prepulse inhibition and habituation of startle in humans after pretreatment with citalopram, haloperidol, or ketanserin. *Neuropsychopharmacology* 24:240–52.

Vollenweider, F. X., A. Gamma, M. Liechti, and T. Huber. 1998. Psychological and cardiovascular effects and short-term sequelae of MDMA ("Ecstasy") in MDMA-naive healthy volunteers. *Neuropsychopharmacology* 19:241–51.

Vollenweider, F. X., A. Gamma, M. Liechti, and T. Huber. 1999. Is a single dose of MDMA harmless? [Letter]. *Neuropsychopharmacology* 21:598–600.

Vollenweider, F. X., S. Remensberger, D. Hell, and M. A. Geyer. 1999. Opposite effects of 3,4-methylenedioxymethamphetamine (MDMA) on sensorimotor gating in rats versus healthy humans. *Psychopharmacology* 143(4):365–72.

United States

Dr. Manuel Tancer and Chris-Ellyn Johanson from the Research Division on Substance Abuse, Department of Psychiatry and Behavioral Neurosciences, Wayne State University School of Medicine (Detroit, Michigan) have been involved in various investigations examining the subjective effects of MDMA. As part of a study program designed to gain a better understanding of the behavioral pharmacology of MDMA, they plan to compare the effects of MDMA with those of prototypical stimulants and with serotonin-releasing agents.

Metachlorophenylpiperazine (mCPP) is a serotonin releaser and semi-selective 5-HT agonist; it is a compound that releases serotonin into the synapse and produces effects like that of serotonin. mCPP has been used widely as a probe of serotonin systems in a variety of psychiatric disorders. In one study, Tancer and colleagues examined the physiological and subjective effects of MDMA and mCPP in gradually increasing doses. Five healthy volunteers participated in a three-session experiment. During the first two six-hour sessions subjects received MDMA (75 mg/70 kg, 110 mg/70 kg, 145 mg/70 kg, or 175 mg/70 kg) or mCPP (17.5 mg/70 kg, 35 mg/70 kg, or 52.5 mg/70 kg) or placebo under double-blind conditions, in a balanced order.

At baseline and hourly thereafter, several parameters of functioning and well-being were obtained. These parameters include heart rate and blood pressure; a Profile of Mood States, where participants indicate how they feel in response to seventy-two adjectives; ARCI, an inventory of forty-nine true/false questions that measure stimulant-like effects, euphoria, dysphoria, somatic complaints, and sedation; visual analogue scales, in which participants indicate how they are feeling—sedated, downcast, hungry, stimulated, high, and anxious for example; and the Hallucinogen Rating Scale (created by Rick Strassman), which measures hallucinogenic symptoms and focuses on perception, cognition, volition, and intensity of effects.

All three doses of MDMA caused a significant increase in blood pressure and heart rate compared with placebo, but there were no significant effects from any of the mCPP doses on blood pressure or heart rate. mCPP was identified as a psychoactive drug by MDMA users, and both MDMA and mCPP showed mild hallucinogenic properties, as measured by the Hallucinogen Rating Scale. Subjects who ingested mCPP had some euphoric responses, a pattern that has been reported in heavy MDMA users (McCann et al. 1999a) as well as in cocaine addicts (Buydens-Branchey et al. 1997). Overall, Tancer reported that MDMA has a unique subjective-effect profile, differing from that of mCPP, perhaps as a function of its pharmacology.

Tancer and Johanson also have many ongoing studies concerning MDMA and its subjective effects. These include a dose run-up study of 1.1 mg/kg, 1.6 mg/kg, and 2.1 mg/kg of MDMA versus placebo and a comparison of 1 mg/kg and 2 mg/kg of MDMA versus 10 mg and 20 mg of d-amphetamine and 0.5 mg/kg and 0.75 mg/kg of mCPP. These drug-discrimination studies aim to describe the specific qualities of MDMA compared with other, better-characterized drugs, to distinguish its subtle pharmacological similarities and differences, in other words, to determine whether MDMA is more like amphetamine or more like mCPP.

Studies are planned to examine the effect of MDMA on the ability of the body to regulate temperature. One study will attempt to examine the interaction between ambient temperature and core body temperature response to MDMA. This follows up on reports of hyperthermia and hyperpyrexia after MDMA ingestion at raves and also on work by Seiden and colleagues, who found that MDMA caused a loss of thermoregulation in rats. Specifically, if MDMA is administered in an ambient temperature of 20 degrees Celsius, rats' core body temperature declines. On the other hand, if MDMA is administered at 30 degrees, rats' core body temperature increases significantly. Another study will examine the effect of fluoxetine pretreatment on the subjective and physiological effects of MDMA, mCPP, and amphetamine. The hypothesis is that blockade of the 5-HT transporter will block most of the effects of mCPP, will have no effect on amphetamine, and will shift the subjective effect of MDMA to that of amphetamine.

References

Tancer, M. E., and C. E. Johanson. 1999. Subjective responses to MDMA and mCPP: A human dose run up study. Paper presented at the 61st Annual Meeting of the College on Problems of Drug Dependence, 17 June, Acapulco, Mexico.

Reese Jones, John Mendleson, and Matthew Baggot at the Drug Dependence Research Center, University of California, San Francisco, have been studying MDMA and its pharmacological, pharmacokinetic, physiological, and subjective effects in humans. In one study, designed to evaluate several effects of MDMA, eight volunteers each received a low dose (0.5 mg/kg) or a moderate dose (1.5 mg/kg) of MDMA or placebo in a double-blind, ascending-dose cross-over study. When compared with the placebo condition, the moderate dose, but not the low dose, produced statistically significant increases in blood pressure, heart rate, and the cardiovascular indicator rate pressure, which is calculated by multiplying heart rate and blood pressure. The results were comparable in terms of cardiovascular response to those produced by stimulants. Peak physiologic values occurred 1 to $2\frac{1}{2}$ hours after administration. The moderate-dose MDMA caused a number of significant subjective effects with a peak at two hours after dosing, including some effects typically associated with stimulant drugs, hallucinogens, and the so-called entactogens. Rise in cortisol correlated with an increase in heart rate and drug liking. A rise in DHEA, a steroid hormone that is a precursor to both testosterone and progesterone, correlated with euphoria.

With the same study design as the latter study, this group of investigators also obtained plasma and urine samples at regular intervals for forty-eight hours after dosing. They found that the metabolism and breakdown of MDMA were selective based on the specific structure of MDMA, favoring one of the two possible mirror-image structures. Both maximum plasma concentration and the area under the curve (the plotting of concentration vs. time), two important indicators of the metabolism and disposition of MDMA, were higher for the R-enantiomer than the reportedly more active S-enantiomer. The selectivity of the breakdown of MDMA based on chemical structure is reflected in metabolite formation. Initially, greater plasma and urine concentrations of the S-(+)-MDA were recorded; R-(–)-MDA was the more prevalent enantiomer in later urine samples. [Recall from "The Chemistry of MDMA" that (–)-MDA has more hallucinogenic effects resembling LSD, but (+)-MDA has more of a stimulant effect and is shorter in duration of action. The (+)-isomers also are considered more toxic to the neuron's axon terminals.—Ed.]

In another study the Drug Dependence Research Center also reported that the metabolism and disposal of MDMA are dose-dependent. This means that the larger the dose of MDMA ingested, the longer it takes the body to metabolize the drug, and the faster the amount of MDMA will rise in the blood stream. For example, clearance decreased by approximately 65 percent when the dose of MDMA was increased by a factor of 3 (from 0.5 to 1.5 mg/kg). This finding suggests that small increases in dose may result in large increases in plasma concentrations of MDMA.

In another study, this research group examined the cardiovascular characteristics of MDMA by using quantitative two-dimensional echocardiography one hour after one of two oral doses of MDMA (0.5 mg/kg or 1.5 mg/kg) or placebo in eight volunteers. This was done to determine the status of the heart and the cardiovascular system in general. The acute effects were compared with those of dobutamine, a medication that predictably increases heart rate, blood pressure, and myocardial oxygen consumption, or the amount of oxygen that the heart utilizes while pumping blood. In a dose-dependent fashion, 1.5 mg/kg of MDMA increased blood pressure, heart rate, myocardial oxygen consumption, and the rate-pressure product, an indicator of cardiovascular status, peaking at 1 to $2^{1}/_{2}$ hours after dosing. These effects were comparable in magnitude to the effects of 20–40 mg/kg/mL IV dobutamine. In contrast to dobutamine, MDMA had no measurable inotropic effects (strengthening the contraction of the heart muscle), nor did it cause any heart wall motion abnormalities. MDMA did not produce any apparent toxicity to the heart.

More human studies are planned to elucidate the pharmacodynamic and pharmacokinetic properties of MDMA. One aim of future research is to better understand whether MDMA belongs in a unique pharmacological class, the entactogens, or whether its behavior more closely resembles that of other phenethylamines.

References

Everhart, E. T., P. Jacob III, P. Shwonek, M. Baggott, R. T. Jones, and J. Mendelson. 2000. Estimation of the metabolic disposition of MDMA and MDA enantiomers in humans. In Problems of drug dependence, edited by L. S. Harris. Washington D.C.: U.S. Government Printing Office.

Harris, D., M. Baggott, R. T. Jones, and J. Mendelson. 2000. MDMA pharmacokinetics and physiological and subjective effects in humans. In Problems of drug dependence, edited by L. S. Harris. Washington, D.C.: U.S. Government Printing Office.

Lester, S., M. Baggott, S. Welm, et al. 2000. The cardiovascular effects of Ecstasy, 3-4-methylenedioxymethamphetamine (MDMA). *Ann. Intern. Med.* 133(12):969–73.

Charles Grob and colleagues from the Harbor-UCLA Medical Center have conducted various studies designed to determine the psychological and biological effects of MDMA in humans. Eighteen subjects received MDMA at two different doses in a double-blind, placebo-controlled research design, in an attempt to examine psychological, physiological, and neuroendocrine responses to the drug. The subjects involved in the study were healthy adult volunteers with a history of Ecstasy use. The potential subjects underwent a psychiatric and physical examination and could not participate in the study if they had a history of any major psychiatric or chronic medical illness, heart disease, seizure disorder, or substance abuse. Also excluded were those who were taking any medication or who were pregnant. The eighteen subjects— five women and thirteen men—were asked to abstain from using Ecstasy or other illicit drugs for one month before the study began. Subjects enrolled in the study took part in three separate randomized, double-blind experimental sessions. During each session, each subject received one of three treatments: placebo or one of two different doses of MDMA, ranging from 0.25 mg/kg to 2.5 mg/kg. These higher doses were chosen to correspond to typical recreational doses of Ecstasy.

Each experimental session lasted for eight hours. During each session, blood was drawn from the subject at thirty-minute intervals, four times before receiving the drug and twelve times after. The subject's body temperature, heart rate, and blood pressure were measured at thirty-minute intervals. Research volunteers indicated their psychological state by periodically responding to several different test measures. Arousal and hedonic (that is, pleasant vs. unpleasant) states were assessed with the Altered States Graphic Profile, and anxiety was measured with the State-Trait Anxiety Inventory. Subjects also responded to the Profile of Mood States, a self-reported assessment of mood. All blood samples were assayed to determine the pharmacokinetics of MDMA (how its concentration varied in the blood over time) as well as concentration in the blood of cortisol, prolactin, and ACTH, which stimulates cortisol release. Subjects experienced various changes in physiological and psychological states after ingesting MDMA. Most of the changes were dose-dependent. There were a few nonlinear relationships between dose and response found in the study. Thus, there were some changes in the subject's state, which were greater or less than what might be predicted by the dose ingested.

When compared with placebo, MDMA produced a moderate increase in heart rate, which was most evident after doses of 1 mg/kg or more. Ingestion of MDMA produced a dose-dependent rise in body temperature. MDMA ingestion also significantly and dose-dependently increased both systolic and diastolic blood pressure when compared with placebo. Subjects who received MDMA did not show an enhancement of anxiety or negative mood when compared with the effects of placebo, but they reported increases in both pleasure and arousal, based on components of the Altered States Graphic Profile. Subjects also experienced dose-dependent increases in hedonic, pleasurable feelings, with higher doses producing more euphoria and positive mood. Oddly, the highest doses of MDMA, more than 2.0 mg/kg, produced a little less arousal than lower doses. Subjects receiving MDMA had significantly elevated levels of three hormones—ACTH, cortisol, and prolactin. The effects of MDMA on hormone levels occurred in a dose-dependent fashion, with higher doses of MDMA corresponding to greater increases in levels of the hormones in the blood. Increased hormone levels correlated with changes in the subjects' psychological state over time. Grob concluded from these data that while MDMA ingestion appears to pose certain risks to people through its effects on the cardiovascular system, the drug does not pose any grave health risks when it is administered in a controlled setting. This inves-

tigation also established that therapeutic doses of MDMA in a clinical setting lead to elevations in mood and arousal and seem to cause little or no
psychological distress, at least in experienced users.

In two separate investigations, Grob, along with collaborators, studied
the possibility that MDMA use damages human brains. The question arose
out of the data from animal studies that show damage to serotonin nerve
endings when large doses of MDMA are administered. In one study, highly
technical radiological tests, called SPECT (single positron emission computed tomography) scans, were done on the brains of Ecstasy users and age-
matched control subjects, and comparisons were made of the measures of
blood flow in the brain. In another study, differences in the quantity of several chemical markers for neuronal (brain cell) death were investigated using
another radiological method, called proton magnetic resonance imaging or
MR-Spectroscopy (MR SPECT). The subjects for these studies were healthy
adults, and exclusion criteria were similar to the ones used in the dose-response study. People who used low doses of Ecstasy were sought for these
studies, and recreational use was defined as occurring six or more times per
year. Subjects in the control group had never taken Ecstasy, according to self-
reports.

In the first of the two studies, blood flow within the brain was measured
in forty-two people (twenty-one in the study group and the control group,
respectively). Each group consisted of seventeen men and four women. Subjects enrolled in this study first underwent MRI and then SPECT scans.
Cerebral blood flow was examined with various models of analysis, taking
into account baseline, post-MDMA, and control findings. Several methods
were used to spot relationships between parameters of MDMA use and alterations in the brain. Key factors included blood flow in the brain, brain
volume, percentage of cerebrospinal fluid (the fluid that bathes the brain and
spinal cord), cumulative life exposure to Ecstasy, and last dose of MDMA.
Both Ecstasy users and controls had normal MRI evaluations.

Compared with baseline radiological scans, post-MDMA ingestion scans
in eight of ten Ecstasy users who had just received two doses of MDMA
showed a slight reduction in cerebral blood flow in most regions of the brain.
While Ecstasy users and matched controls did not differ in terms of baseline
regional blood flow throughout the brain, post-MDMA ingestion scans (two

to three weeks after MDMA was administered) showed mildly reduced regional blood flow to certain areas of the brain when compared with control scans and when compared to baseline scans of MDMA subjects. Reduction in blood flow in specific areas of the brain was more pronounced in subjects who had received higher doses of MDMA compared with those who had received lower doses. Two of the ten subjects who received MDMA were scanned nearly two months after drug administration (forty-three days and eighty days after MDMA was administered, respectively), and their post-MDMA ingestion scans indicated an increase in global blood flow in the brain compared with scans performed at baseline.

Because of the lack of difference in the baseline scans between Ecstasy users and controls, Grob concludes that recreational use of Ecstasy does not appear to alter cerebral blood flow. This suggests that Ecstasy use does not produce any lasting changes in the brain or the brain's metabolism, but experimental administration of MDMA does seem to produce transient changes in blood flow in certain regions of the brain two to three weeks after use. There is an apparent return to normal patterns of blood flow in the brain after MDMA use, perhaps with some signs of increased cerebral blood flow two months after using MDMA.

In the second of the two studies investigating the possibility of harmful effects of Ecstasy ingestion on the brain, evidence of neurochemical abnormalities in Ecstasy users was sought. This was accomplished by comparing the concentration in the brain of specific brain chemicals, or markers, in Ecstasy users compared with the concentrations found in non-Ecstasy users. Markers included N-acetylaspartate (NA), myoinositol (MI), and myoinositol/creatine ratios. NA is a chemical compound that is a known marker, or biological sign, of brain cell death. MI is a compound that is a marker for glial cell proliferation, or gliosis, a process that takes place after an insult to the brain, similar to a scar after an insult to the skin.

Healthy adult volunteers were enrolled in the study—twenty-one people with a history of Ecstasy use and thirty-seven without such a history. Both MRI and MR SPECT were performed in three distinct regions of the brain, and measures of the levels of chemicals important in elucidating brain activity and damage were taken. No differences were found between NA values in Ecstasy users and in control subjects in any of the three evaluated regions of the brain. Normal NA concentrations suggest lack of significant neuronal injury in these recreational Ecstasy users. Significant differences were discovered, however, between MI values in Ecstasy users and control subjects. Ecstasy users had higher MI levels and higher MI/creatine ratios than controls. Grob concluded that Ecstasy use seems to impose some stress on the brain, as evidenced by increases in MI. Greater lifetime exposure to Ecstasy produces greater amounts of MI in certain brain regions, suggesting cumulative effects. Ecstasy use does not seem to cause any neuronal or brain damage per se, since both users and control subjects possess comparable amounts of NA in all regions of the brain.

In another study, Grob attempted to describe the neuropsychological effects of Ecstasy use. Twenty-four people with an extensive history of Ecstasy use were recruited for the study. Sixteen men and eight women, screened to exclude a history of major psychiatric or medical illnesses, underwent MRI to ensure that their brains were free of any lesions or structural abnormalities. The subjects in this study completed a battery of neuropsychological tests designed to assess attention, memory, and cognitive performance. Intelligence was measured through the Wechsler Adult Intelligence Scale–Revised (WAIS-R), quantifying verbal and performance intelligence. The Digit-Span Memory Test, a subtest of the WAIS, measured attention and concentration and immediate recall. Information processing was measured with the Digit Symbol Test, also a subtest of the WAIS, and the Stroop Task. The Rey-Osterreith Complex Figure served as a measure of constructional ability. Verbal memory was measured with the Rey Auditory Verbal Learning Test, the Logical Memory subtest of the WAIS, and the Warrington Recognition Memory Test. Visual memory was assessed through the Rey-Osterrieth Complex Figure three-minute delayed-recall test, the Continuous Visual Memory Test, and the Visual Reproduction Test, a subtest of the Wechsler Memory Scale. Executive function (decision making and planning) was assessed through the Stroop Task, Auditory Consonant Trigrams and the Wisconsin Card Sorting Task, and the Controlled Oral Word Association test of verbal fluency.

Fourteen of the twenty-four subjects completed these tests twice, once at baseline and once after receiving their second experimental dose of MDMA, similar to a recreational-use dose. All other subjects completed the tests once.

After scoring the subjects' performance on each test, researchers compared test scores with published norms available for each test. Analysis did not find any significant differences on the neuropsychological tests between the Ecstasy users and the control group at baseline. There was also no appreciable difference before and after MDMA administration within the subjects. The subjects as a whole performed at levels that fell within or above the published norms for most of the tests, except for the Wisconsin Card Sorting Task, which correlates to decision making and planning ability. Subjects with greater frequency of Ecstasy use scored worse on measures of visual memory and verbal recognition memory and better on tests of mental speed and cognitive inhibition. Length of abstinence, in months, for the subjects was positively related to performance on tests of divided attention, working memory, and visual memory. The longer the time without Ecstasy use, the better the subjects performed on these tests.

Grob concluded that a single dose of MDMA does not produce any measurable deficit in attention, memory, intelligence, or executive function. People taking frequent doses of MDMA may perform less well on tests of attention and memory, but their performance is not necessarily below average. Only performances on tests of decision making and planning ability are diminished in Ecstasy users, though a single dose does not further affect this ability. According to Grob, this may reflect preexisting differences between Ecstasy users and the general public or show evidence that chronic Ecstasy use can reduce function in the frontal lobes.

Dr. Grob plans to continue his attempt to secure approval from the regulatory agencies to investigate the safety and efficacy of MDMA in the treatment of the psychological distress and refractory pain associated with end-stage cancer.

References

Chang, L., C. S. Grob, T. Ernst, et al. 2000. Effect of ecstasy (3,4-methylenedioxy-methamphetamine [MDMA]) on cerebral blood flow: A co-registered SPECT and MRI study. *Psychiatry Res.* 98:15–28.

Chang, L., T. Ernst, C. S. Grob, and R. E. Poland. 1999. Cerebral (1)H MRS alterations in recreational 3,4-methylenedioxymethamphetamine (MDMA, "ecstasy") users. *J. Magn. Reson. Imaging* 10:521–6.

Grob, C. S., R. E. Poland, L. Chang, and T. Ernst. 1996. Psychobiologic effects of 3,4-

methylenedioxymethamphetamine in humans: Methodological considerations and preliminary observations. *Behav. Brain Res.* 73:103–7.

Grob, C. S. 1998. MDMA research: preliminary investigations with human subjects. *Int. J. Drug Policy* 9:119–24.

Michael C. Mithoefer and Kathleen Brady at the Medical University of South Carolina in Charleston are planning to study the potential use of MDMA in patients with chronic PTSD. They submitted a protocol to the Food and Drug Administration in June 2001, and at the time of this book's publication approval is pending. This pilot study will gather preliminary information about the safety and efficacy of MDMA-assisted psychotherapy in stimulating therapeutic processing of traumatic experiences, with the goal of reducing or relieving symptoms of PTSD. The research subjects, between the ages of eighteen and sixty-five years, will meet criteria for chronic PTSD and will have undergone at least one unsuccessful attempt at treatment with medications and/or psychotherapy. These carefully selected volunteers will receive two oral doses of 125 mg of MDMA. The doses will be given four to six weeks apart in an open-label pilot study. The treatment team, composed of a male psychiatrist and a female nurse, will perform twelve ninety-minute preliminary and follow-up therapy sessions. The two MDMA-assisted psychotherapy sessions will occur approximately four to six weeks apart. The Clinician-Administered PTSD Symptom Scale and the Impact of Events Scale, administered at the outset of the study and again at four weeks and at four months after the last treatment session, will be used as outcome measurements.

Conclusion

Many of the cited studies have supported one another's findings. For instance, MDMA seems to increase certain cardiac parameters, such as blood pressure and heart rate, predictably, and there is an enantiomer-specific disposition in MDMA metabolism. Other findings by these researchers have not been corroborated, simply because there are too few clinical MDMA studies under way. For a drug being used by millions of people around the world, one would expect more data to be generated at this point in the history of MDMA.

One obstacle in the path to widespread research is MDMA's legal status as a Schedule I drug, which makes many projects difficult to initiate. Another problem is that because MDMA was patented in the last century, no pharmaceutical company has any interest in funding human studies. Unfortunately, the U. S. government is much more interested in funding risk as opposed to benefit-oriented research. To further the cause of benefit-oriented research, proceeds of this book's sales will be donated to the Holland Fund for Therapeutic MDMA Research. If you are interested in seeing more clinical studies looking at potential benefits of MDMA-assisted psychotherapy, please make a donation at drholland.com.

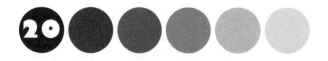

GIVING MDMA TO HUMAN VOLUNTEERS IN SWITZERLAND

Alex Gamma, Ph.D.,
Matthias E. Liechti, M.D.,
and Franz X. Vollenweider, M.D.

Introduction

Half a decade ago, public awareness of MDMA as a recreational drug called "Ecstasy" reached its first peak in Switzerland. From a researcher's point of view, MDMA mainly raised interest because of its purported unique psychological effects. Early scientific investigations reported that MDMA produces an "easily controlled altered state of consciousness with emotional and sensual overtones" and suggested that MDMA might be useful as an adjunct to insight-oriented psychotherapy (Nichols 1986; Shulgin 1986). MDMA was described as a relatively mild, short-acting drug capable of facilitating heightened states of introspection and intimacy along with temporary freedom from anxiety and depression. Moreover, it produced minimal distracting alterations in perception, body image, or sense of self (Greer 1985; Downing 1986; Greer and Tolbert 1986; Gasser 1996). It seemed to have few of the typical effects of hallucinogens and stimulants with which it shares a common chemical basis. Considering these unique psychotropic effects, it was suggested that MDMA and related drugs (for example, MDA, MDE, and MBDB) constitute a novel pharmacological class termed "entactogens" (from the Greek, meaning "touching within") (Nichols 1986; Hermle et al. 1993; Gouzoulis-Mayfrank et al. 1999).

In animal studies, MDMA has been shown to be a potent releaser of serotonin (5-HT) (Schmidt 1987) and, to a lesser extent, of dopamine (DA) (Yamamoto and Spanos 1988). It appeared to us that research into the neurochemical mechanism of action of MDMA in humans might further our understanding of the neurobiological basis of human mood and of the affective disorders in which these neurotransmitters had been implicated. Furthermore, in view of its extensive recreational use, information on the psychological, physiological, and behavioral effects of MDMA seemed important to assess possible risks to Ecstasy users.

Based on this rationale, we have conducted several studies in a total of seventy-four healthy volunteers (fifty-four men and twenty women), aimed at a broad characterization of the psychological and behavioral effects of MDMA and the concomitant neurochemical and neurophysiological changes underlying them. These studies were made legally possible on the basis of Swiss drug legislation that allows the use of MDMA for medical or research purposes, depending on case-by-case permission from the Swiss Federal Health Office. Our studies also were approved by the local ethics committee.

All studies were prospective and involved the oral administration of a single dose of MDMA (1.35–1.7 mg/kg of body weight) to healthy, mostly MDMA-naive subjects in double-blind, placebo-controlled experimental settings. Before admission to one of the studies, all subjects were screened by psychiatric interview and by medical examination to minimize any possible risks related to MDMA administration. After being informed of the procedures involved in the experiments and the possible risks and benefits of MDMA administration, all subjects gave their written consent. Participants were mostly university students, ages twenty to thirty, who had a personal or scientific interest in the study. This chapter summarizes the effects of MDMA on psychophysiological measures, sensory information processing, and brain activity. For more details the reader is referred to the original literature.

Psychological Effects of MDMA

When we started our research with MDMA, most reports available on its psychological effects were retrospective and anecdotal and lacked drug and dose identification. This situation was partly due to the fact that using MDMA for prospective clinical studies was illegal in most countries and that Ecstasy tablets sold for recreational use often contained other psychoactive compounds, so that their effects could not be ascribed reliably to MDMA alone. To avoid these limitations and to obtain robust data on the subjective effects of pure MDMA, we used prospective within-subject study designs with standardized psychometric ratings obtained during the peak effect of the drug.

The Altered States of Consciousness rating scale (OAV) is a visual-analog scale that measures alterations in mood, thought processes, and experiences of the self/ego and of the environment (Bodmer 1989; Dittrich 1998). The OAV consists of three dimensions. The first dimension, OB (Oceanic Boundlessness), measures derealization and depersonalization associated with a positive basic mood and alterations in the sense of time. The second dimension, VR (Visionary Restructuralization), refers to visual illusions, elementary and complex hallucinations, synesthesia, facilitated imagination, and the altered experience of meaning. The third dimension, AED (Anxious Ego Dissolution), measures thought disorder, ego disintegration, and loss of body and thought control associated with arousal and anxiety. The Adjective Mood rating scale (AM) (Janke and Debus 1978) consists of fourteen scales measuring efficiency/activation, self-confidence, heightened mood, apprehension/anxiety, depression, thoughtfulness/contemplativeness, extroversion, introversion, inactivation, dazed state, tiredness, sensitivity, aggression/anger, and emotional excitation.

The subjective effects of MDMA turned out to be highly robust, despite some differences in the experimental settings (Vollenweider et al. 1998; Gamma et al. 2000b; Liechti and Vollenweider 2000a,b; Liechti et al. 2000a,b). Analysis of the pooled data of all studies, including seventy-four subjects (Liechti et al. 2001a), showed that most subjects under MDMA experienced a state of profound well-being and happiness, increased extroversion and sociability, heightened emotional sensitivity, and slight derealization. In general, subjects felt carefree and relaxed. Physical sensations were described as more pleasurable than usual. The perception of space and time was altered, and subjects felt dreamy or lost in thought. MDMA induced few perceptual changes.

There was only a single report of scenic or complex visual hallucinations, but elementary hallucinations, such as distorted objects, flashes of light, and simple patterns, were common. Colors appeared more lively, and sounds seemed to move closer or farther away. The dose according to body weight of MDMA (mg/kg) positively correlated with the intensity of perceptual alterations, particularly in women. Thus, higher doses of MDMA, in the range of 1.35–1.7 mg/kg, produced more hallucinogen-like perceptual changes (Liechti et al. 2001a). MDMA also led to thought disturbances that included impaired decision making, accelerated thinking, and losing track of one's thoughts. The slight depersonalization and mild ego impairment during MDMA were not experienced as problematic or psychotic but as a pleasurable state of loosened ego boundaries. Transient dysphoric reactions associated with anxiety occurred in a few subjects at onset of the drug's action, but this mostly passed when subjects became acquainted with the drug effect and were reassured by the experimenter.

Women generally showed stronger responses to MDMA than men, though baseline psychometric ratings did not differ between the two genders (Liechti et al. 2001a). Women had significantly higher ratings for positive mood, depersonalization, and altered perception of time and space. Women also reported stronger perceptual changes, in particular a higher frequency of elementary hallucinations and optical illusions. Finally, women scored higher on anxiety-related measures. These increases were due to feelings of helplessness and defenselessness and an increased need for protection. Thought disturbances also were more pronounced in women, particularly greater fear of loss of body control. The women's increased sensitivity to MDMA even extended to its side effects: more women than men experienced jaw clenching, difficulty concentrating, dry mouth, thirst, impaired balance, and lack of appetite.

The psychological profile of MDMA that emerges from these studies is in agreement with anecdotal reports from recreational Ecstasy users, with possibly one exception. In our experimental setting, the stimulant, or activating effect of MDMA was much less pronounced than at raves or dance clubs. Perhaps this is a purely psychological effect of the recreational setting, in particular, the infectious effect of loud techno music and the many dancing people. It also may be that the activation Ecstasy users report comes from amphetamine, which often is contained in Ecstasy tablets or consumed separately at raves. Besides only moderate stimulant effects, MDMA's hallucinogen-like effects were also very mild in our studies and consisted mainly of intensified perception of color, touch, and sound as well as slight distortion of objects. The predominant, typical component of the MDMA experience was a feeling of emotional warmth associated with enhanced well-being, contentment, and openness toward other people, which is not adequately described as typical of either stimulants or hallucinogens. Our findings therefore confirm a unique psychological profile of MDMA and support its proposed classification as an entactogen.

The clear-cut gender differences in the behavioral responses to MDMA are striking with regard to the well-documented female preponderance for mood disorders, especially depression and anxiety. Our findings may signify an increased sensitivity of women to MDMA-induced serotonin depletion, which may reflect a sensitivity to serotonergic changes that arise from an internal cause as well. This heightened sensitivity may manifest as an increased susceptibility to mood disorders, since endogenously caused serotonergic alterations are implicated in mood disorders.

Cardiovascular Effects of MDMA

MDMA increased both diastolic and systolic blood pressure. This is the only effect that was more pronounced in men. The peak increase in blood pressure after MDMA was about 30 mm Hg for systolic blood pressure and 15 mm Hg for diastolic blood pressure. One-third of the subjects had systolic blood pressure values of more than 160 mm Hg, and 10 percent reached values above 180 mm Hg. One man had a hypertensive reaction (240/145 mm Hg) without other signs of hypertensive crisis. MDMA also increased heart rate by about 13 beats per minute.

Adverse Effects of MDMA

Acute adverse effects included jaw clenching, dry mouth, and loss of appetite. At the onset of the MDMA effect some subjects reported nausea, hot flashes, paresthesia (a tingling feeling), and dizziness. Tremor and increased restlessness were noted in about one-third of the subjects. Side effects were generally considered mild and were similar to those reported by Ecstasy users.

There were no complications requiring medical intervention. Some acute effects of MDMA lasted up to the next day, including lack of appetite, dry mouth, and increased jaw muscle tension. Newly occurring aftereffects were fatigue, muscle ache, and headache in about half of the subjects. Up to one-third of the subjects reported slightly depressed mood, including emotional irritability, lack of energy, brooding, and bad dreams. These side effects lasted up to three days in a few subjects. Women reported significantly more of these adverse aftereffects than men.

Neurobiological Processes Associated with MDMA Effects

Having elucidated several important phenomenological and physiological aspects of the MDMA experience, we used different strategies to investigate the neurobiological processes that could be responsible for the distinct psychological effects of MDMA in humans. The approaches to addressing this question were to examine the neurotransmitters involved in the neurochemical action of MDMA, to use functional brain imaging to identify brain regions involved in mediating its effects, and to investigate the effects of MDMA on information processing.

Effects of MDMA on Neurotransmitter Systems

In animals, MDMA mainly releases serotonin (5-HT) (Schmidt 1987) via interaction with the serotonin transporter, and, to a lesser extent, it releases dopamine (Yamamoto and Spanos 1988) and norepinephrine (Fitzgerald and Reid 1990). In addition, MDMA has been shown to have moderate affinity for the serotonergic 5-HT2 receptors (Battaglia et al. 1988a). [For a review of the pharmacological action of MDMA, see "How MDMA Works in the Brain."] Based on these findings, we hypothesized that the effects of MDMA in humans would be primarily due to its principal neurochemical action, 5-HT transporter-mediated 5-HT release. This view is supported by the finding that selective serotonin reuptake inhibitors (SSRIs) blocked MDMA-induced 5-HT release or the behavioral effects of MDMA in animals (Schmidt 1987; Hekmatpanah and Peroutka 1990; Gudelsky and Nash 1996). Second, given the fact that postsynaptic serotonergic 5-HT2 receptors have been implicated in the effects of classic hallucinogens (Sanders-Bush and Conn 1987; Vollenweider et al. 1998b), we speculated that 5-HT2 receptor stimulation might be responsible for the mild hallucinogen-like action of MDMA. Third, since dopamine is thought to play an important role in the mediation of euphoria produced by classic stimulants, such as d-amphetamine and cocaine (Lieberman et al. 1990; Laruelle et al. 1995; Schlaepfer et al. 1997; Volkow et al. 1997), increased dopamine activity also might contribute to the positive mood effects elicited by MDMA.

To test these hypotheses, we assessed the psychophysiological effects of MDMA (1.5 mg/kg taken by mouth [PO]) in humans after pretreatment with the SSRI citalopram (40 mg IV) in sixteen subjects, the serotonergic 5-HT2 antagonist ketanserin (50 mg PO) in fourteen subjects, and the dopaminergic D_2 antagonist haloperidol (1.4 mg/kg PO) in fourteen subjects. Each of the three studies used a double-blind, placebo-controlled, within-subject design. Thus, all subjects participated in four experimental sessions involving administration of placebo, pretreatment alone, MDMA alone, and pretreatment plus MDMA. As in our other studies (Vollenweider et al. 1998a, Gamma et al. 2000a), we used the OAV and the AM scale to assess subjective peak changes after drug intake.

The SSRI citalopram markedly reduced most psychoactive effects of MDMA, as evidenced by similar reductions in all scales of the OAV. MDMA-induced positive mood (OB), thought disturbances, and reduced control over thought and body (AED) as well as perceptual alterations (VR) were all attenuated after citalopram pretreatment (Liechti et al. 2000a). In addition, citalopram also lessened the acute cardiovascular response to and side effects of MDMA (Liechti and Vollenweider 2000b). It thus appears that the SSRI prevented the interaction of MDMA with the serotonin transporter and thereby "buffered" the overall MDMA experience. Of note, the subjective effects of MDMA were not only attenuated, but also at the same time markedly prolonged after citalopram pretreatment.

In contrast to citalopram, pretreatment with the 5-HT2 antagonist ketanserin resulted in only a moderate attenuation of the subjective MDMA experience (Liechti et al. 2000b). Similarly to studies with serotonergic hallucinogens such as psilocybin, however, ketanserin significantly decreased the perceptual effects of MDMA. These results suggest that stimulation of

5-HT2 receptors may mediate the hallucinogen-like action of MDMA in humans. Finally, pretreatment with the dopaminergic D2 antagonist haloperidol selectively reduced the euphoric (OB) effect of MDMA (Liechti et al. 2000a) but increased the negative effects of MDMA, such as anxious derealization. These findings are in agreement with the view that dopamine may contribute to the euphoric effects of MDMA. It is also notable that haloperidol did not lessen cardiovascular responses to MDMA (Liechti and Vollenweider 2000a). It appears, then, that other neurotransmitters, such as serotonin and/or norepinephrine, or receptor sites other than dopamine D_2 receptors may be involved in these effects of MDMA.

In sum, our pharmacological studies described here indicate that the psychological effects of MDMA in humans largely depend on serotonin release through interaction of MDMA with the 5-HT uptake carrier. Positive mood effects of MDMA may be related in part to dopaminergic D_2 receptor stimulation. The mild hallucinogen-like perceptual effects of MDMA appear to be due to 5-HT2 receptor stimulation. The role of other neurotransmitters such as norepinephrine, and of recognition sites such as the alpha-2, dopamine D_1, and 5-HT1 receptors, in the action of MDMA remains to be elucidated.

Effects of MDMA on Brain Activity

To identify brain regions modulated by MDMA, we conducted a positron emission tomography (PET) study in sixteen healthy, MDMA-naive subjects (Gamma et al. 2000b). A single oral dose of 1.7 mg/kg MDMA or placebo was administered in a double-blind, randomized, and counterbalanced fashion. Regional cerebral blood flow as an index of brain activity was measured by $[H_2O^{15}]$-PET seventy-five minutes after drug intake, when the plateau of MDMA effects typically is reached (Vollenweider et al. 1998a). Ratings of subjective experience during the PET measurement were obtained four hours after drug intake, using the OAV and the AM mood rating scales.

MDMA produced marked alterations of brain activity in limbic, paralimbic, and neocortical areas. Blood flow was increased bilaterally in the ventromedial prefrontal cortex, the ventral anterior cingulate, the inferior temporal lobe, the medial occipital lobe, and the entire cerebellum. MDMA decreased blood flow bilaterally in the pre- and paracentral cortex, the dorsal anterior and posterior cingulate, and the superior temporal gyrus, insula, and thalamus. Unilateral decreases were noted in the left amygdala and right parahippocampal formation and uncus. Furthermore, blood flow in the left amygdala tended to correlate with scores for anxious derealization (AED).

These results show that distributed changes in cerebral blood flow and brain activity underlie the subjective effects of MDMA. MDMA affects a variety of brain regions that have been shown to be involved in mood regulation and emotional processing—these are the limbic (amygdala) and paralimbic (cingulate, orbitofrontal cortex, temporal cortex) brain structures along with their associated neocortical areas in the frontal lobe. Modulation of these sites likely plays a substantial role in the mood-enhancing and prosocial properties of MDMA. Within this network of brain regions, the amygdala, in particular, has a well-established function in mediating the fear response and its conditioning (Mulan and Penfield 1959; Le Doux 1995). Our study and many previous functional imaging studies (Schneider et al. 1995; Ketter et al. 1996; Kalin et al. 1997) likewise found higher left amygdala activity to be correlated with higher scores in anxiety-related psychometric measures. Other brain imaging studies have found that the reverse also is true: lower activity in the left amygdala correlated with pleasurable mood states, including euphoria (Ketter et al. 1996). These results raise the possibility that reduced activity in the amygdala, as found in our subjects soon after taking MDMA, may correlate with MDMA-induced enhancement of mood and well-being.

Effects of MDMA on Information Processing

We investigated the effects of MDMA on pre-pulse inhibition (PPI) of the acoustic startle reflex in forty-four subjects (Vollenweider et al. 1999b; Liechti et al. 2001b). The startle reflex is a contraction of the skeletal and facial musculature in response to a sudden intense stimulus, such as a loud noise. In humans, the eye-blink component of the startle reflex is measured using electromyography of the orbicularis oculi muscle, which circles the eye. PPI is the unlearned suppression of startle when the startling stimulus is preceded by a weaker pre-stimulus by 30 to 500 milliseconds. For instance, if a softer noise precedes a louder noise, there is typically a blunted response to the louder noise. PPI is regarded as a measure of sensorimotor gating, or filtering of cognitive and sensory information, and it is a way of measuring pre-attentional deficits that are frequently seen in schizophrenia and other psychiatric disorders. The pharmacological effects of MDMA-like drugs on PPI have been studied extensively in rodents (Geyer and Callaway 1994). Entactogens, including MDMA, MDE, and AET (alpha-ethyltryptamine), as well as the serotonin releaser fenfluramine, impair PPI of the startle reflex in rodents, and this impairment is reduced by pretreatment with SSRIs.

Surprisingly, we found that MDMA (1.7 mg/kg PO) increased PPI in healthy volunteers, thus having an opposite effect on sensorimotor gating in humans versus animals (Vollenweider et al. 1999b). In addition, this effect of MDMA was attenuated by pretreatment with the SSRI citalopram but not by haloperidol or ketanserin (Liechti et al. 2001b). The observed difference in the effects of MDMA on PPI in humans and rats was unexpected. It appears that the effect of MDMA on PPI in humans is due to MDMA-induced release of serotonin, as it is in animals. It is also obvious, however, that some of the functional consequences of the released serotonin differ between rats and humans, since MDMA has opposite effects on PPI. It is unclear whether methodological differences or true differences within the serotonergic system between rodents and humans account for this discrepancy. These studies indicate that MDMA might have effects in humans that are different from those in animals, and they underscore the need for comparison studies in animals and humans.

Conclusion

Our neurochemical investigations indicate that the subjective effects of MDMA are based mainly on an enhancement of serotonergic neurotransmission through an interaction with the presynaptic 5-HT uptake site. This finding is in agreement with the marked limbic, paralimbic, and neocortical modulation of brain activity in our PET study. These areas are rich in serotonergic innervation and form an interconnected network that has been shown to be crucially involved in the regulation of mood and emotion. Thus, it appears likely that MDMA exerts its strong effects on mood and emotion by modulating serotonergic transmission, particularly in limbic and paralimbic and associated neocortical areas.

Women showed a markedly increased subjective responsiveness to MDMA compared with men. It is an intriguing possibility deserving further study that this gender difference may be related to the fact that women are also more susceptible to mood disorders, such as depression and anxiety, in which the 5-HT system has been implicated. The opposite effects of MDMA on PPI in rodents compared with human beings point to the limitations of animal models of human function and emphasize the importance of human studies.

These studies were supported in part by the Swiss Science Foundation (SNF grants 31–52989.97), the Swiss Federal Office of Health (BAG grant 316.98.0686), and the Heffter Research Institute, Santa Fe, New Mexico.

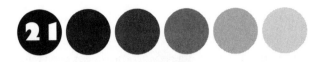

GIVING MDMA TO HUMAN VOLUNTEERS IN THE UNITED STATES

An Interview with Charles Grob, M.D.

JH: I think I would like to start by having you introduce yourself and explain what sort of work you do.

CG: I'm the director of the Division of Child and Adolescent Psychiatry at Harbor-UCLA Medical Center, and I'm a Professor of Psychiatry at the UCLA School of Medicine. I've been a psychiatrist for more than twenty years. I've had a long-standing interest in the history of research with hallucinogens within the field of psychiatry and, more recently, an interest in MDMA.

JH: Before you had heard about MDMA, you were interested perhaps in the use of LSD in psychiatry?

CG: Absolutely. I feel that these substances have extraordinary potential to help us learn about the mind—the mind/brain interface—to improve our understanding of mental illness, and to develop innovative and more effective treatments. I think they have great potential value to psychiatry, if they're used under optimal conditions. I always stipulate that as the limiting factor, they be used appropriately and not misused. It is essential to distinguish between the appropriate use within a controlled investigation or a controlled treatment setting versus uncontrolled recreational use by people who often are poorly prepared, do not understand the nature of the substance they're taking, and do not know how to establish proper safeguards and protective factors.

JH: When you performed your clinical research with MDMA and you obtained informed consent from your subjects and explained the potential risks and benefits of the procedure, what sort of risks did you outline?

CG: Our research subjects were all normal volunteers who had prior experience with MDMA, so they already understood the psychological state induced by MDMA. When we obtained their consent, we conducted an extensive discussion of what was known to date about the potential for adverse effects of the drug, both immediate and long-term, established and speculative. We really did not discuss benefits to any great degree, because we were not looking to explore the potential benefits of MDMA in this study. We were simply looking to establish a foundation for doing human research and getting a baseline set of physiological and psychological data from human subjects. It was not a treatment study. That's important to emphasize, because the media, on occasion, have stated incorrectly that we conducted a treatment study. We have not done so as yet, although we have submitted several protocols to do so, which have not been approved.

JH: What is your view of the risks of unsupervised MDMA use?

CG: There are many dangers with the recreational model, not the least of which is that there is more and more drug substitution with Ecstasy, so that young people often do not know what they are taking. Besides the drug substitution problem, there is often an appreciable degree of polydrug use going on. And there are the issues concerning the context in which this kind of drug use often occurs. The problem with using a drug like MDMA in a rave setting is that most people engage in prolonged and vigorous exercise in a place where the ambient environment is frequently hot and has poor ventilation. There is also the problem with fluid replacement, in that sometimes participants in these marathon dances forget to take breaks and replace body fluids. At times, the management of establishments where raves are taking place has not made adequate fluids available. Also, people who may have a great deal of premorbid psychopathology, specifically previous serious psychiatric disturbances, who get involved with MDMA as a simple extension of other drug use may be at risk for particular kinds of adverse side effects.

JH: Is it fair to say, in your view, that the risks associated with clinical research are minimal and controllable?

CG: I believe that it is possible to administer MDMA safely within the context of an approved research study and to learn a great deal from that. However, one needs to be wary of particular kinds of side effects. I'll explain that by describing a couple of clinical examples. In our research model, we had three experimental sessions. During two of them subjects received two different doses of MDMA, and on one occasion they were given an inactive placebo. These sessions were randomized and double-blind, so neither the subject nor my research staff and I knew what was being administered on any particular occasion. One person, a young man, came to us for his third experimental session. He had tolerated the other two with no problems. During the third session, after about an hour he sustained a rapid elevation of blood pressure, from a baseline of about 120/80 to around 220/100. I was quite alarmed, but I also realized that something had to be different from the other two occasions. I knew that on at least one of those other occasions he had been administered MDMA. So I asked him what was different this time.

He replied that he hadn't thought it important enough to let us know, but the day before the session he had spent the night at a friend's house who lived close to the hospital, so that he could get to the research center early in the morning. His friend had a cat, and apparently he's allergic to cats. He had had an allergic reaction and experienced some respiratory distress, so his friend had suggested that he take some asthma medication. The subject had not thought this was important enough to let us know earlier. What was induced by the interaction between this medicine and the MDMA was a fairly serious hypertensive reaction. Fortunately, his blood pressure came down rapidly, and there were no negative consequences. It did highlight, however, what I thought was a relevant concern in terms of the additional risks of taking the drug in a recreational setting—that people who are concurrently on particular medications most likely are not aware of the risks of interactions and the likelihood of increasing adverse consequences.

Another example of this is cited in a 1999 article in the *Archives of Internal Medicine*. This was a case of a man who was being treated with the HIV drug ritonavir, which is a protease inhibitor. He apparently took MDMA and had a dangerous cardiovascular reaction, which was attributed to the fact that ritonavir was inhibiting the metabolism of MDMA at the level of the hepatic cytochrome P450 2D6 enzyme system. This man had taken MDMA earlier in his life when he was not on any HIV medications and had tolerated it without any problems. The message here is that one has to be very cautious about potential medication interactions.

Going back to the questions of our study, we recruited a total of nineteen subjects, eighteen of whom went through the entire study. After about an hour, the one other subject complained of anxiety during his first and only session. He became very distressed and agitated and attributed it to the fact that when he is on a drug like MDMA, he becomes highly sensitized to his environment. He told us that the cause for his angst was that he was "picking up on all the negative vibes in the hospital." I told the subject that the rules of the study were such that he had to commit to spending the night at the hospital, for safety reasons, but that he could leave in the morning. He did not have to return for the two subsequent sessions. I made it clear to him that he had the option of dropping out of the study at that point, which is the course he decided to take. He informed me that he was not going to return to the hospital and that he wanted to withdraw from the study entirely. Later, since he had formally withdrawn from the study, we were able to break the blind to see how much MDMA he had taken. To our great surprise, we discovered that he had been administered an inactive placebo. The lesson there is never to underestimate the power of suggestion and the power of the placebo response.

JH: I remember that you told me this story back when it happened, and it really stayed with me. It's important, because people often ask me about anxiety reactions and panic reactions, and I think that a good part of those reactions is just people's expectations about what their experience is going to be.

CG: Speaking of panic reactions, do you remember that there was a brief article in the *American Journal of Psychiatry* about ten years ago? It was from New York City, and it described two young people who had panic attacks after taking MDMA. The authors speculated about the implication of a serotonergic mechanism for panic attacks and warned that panic episodes were potential adverse effects of taking MDMA. They did mention the context in which the panic attack occurred, but they didn't make much of it. The two young people were on a New York City subway train. It is important never to underestimate the importance of set and setting. I can tell you that I lived in New York for many years, and drawing upon that experience I would conjecture that you don't need to be on a mind-altering drug to have a panic attack on a New York subway.

JH: All this really underscores the tremendous difference between using MDMA in a supervised clinical setting versus . . .

CG: The supervised setting markedly diminishes risks. We identified a related issue—that the MDMA we were provided with, by David Nichols of Purdue University, was extremely pure, unlike the drug often sold on the illicit market. This MDMA was originally synthesized under a private contract to provide material suitable for preclinical toxicology studies [see "MDMA's Promise as a Prescription Medicine"], and his product was assayed as 99.98 percent pure. Our subjects, particularly those with a great deal of experience with recreational Ecstasy, told me that the quality of their experience during the experimental drug session was quite different from what they were accustomed to. They said that it was a much "cleaner and clearer" altered state, without many of the side effects they were used to with their black market Ecstasy.

JH: One of the things that I'm attentive to is when people talk about MDMA versus Ecstasy. It's always important to differentiate the two. When people talk about a rave setting, where anyone can buy anything, I always insist they refer to it as Ecstasy, which is a group of unknown drugs. I think that you and I are both irate about a lot of published scientific articles in which researchers are studying ravers and polydrug users who take Ecstasy and making assertions about MDMA causing certain abnormalities.

CG: There are very poorly controlled studies conducted by some investigators. One problem that has arisen repeatedly in the neuropsychiatric literature, and also in the media, is confusing the apparent effects of recreational Ecstasy with those of MDMA. These days, because of rampant drug substitution, there is no assurance that Ecstasy is MDMA. At some raves, less than 50 percent of Ecstasy is found on assay to be MDMA. Also, many hardcore ravers ingest a variety of other drugs, some of which have very powerful central nervous system effects. It concerns me that some investigators minimize the significance of the polysubstance use histories of their subjects, which is often extensive, and are inattentive to the strong likelihood that much of the Ecstasy they are taking is not MDMA. There is also a pattern in these studies of attributing the dysfunctional lifestyles and behavior of these high-risk-taking people solely to MDMA. They ignore the very strong contributing factor that there are many other drugs that these people are taking. They also tend to ignore the significance of the fact that these people often are strongly identified with the rave culture and engage in a lifestyle where every weekend they subject themselves to prolonged periods of sleep and nutritional deprivation and ingest a variety of different drugs.

I believe that it is important to acknowledge that many of these high-risk people had severe baseline psychopathological vulnerabilities that predicted they would engage in this kind of lifestyle. Some of the research reports purporting to establish dangerous consequences from MDMA use—as well as the peer review processes that has supported their generous government funding and their publication, at times in the most prestigious medical and psychiatric journals—are in need of serious reexamination. It is important ultimately not only to answer questions related to the true range of effects of MDMA but also to restore scientific credibility to the field.

JH: I agree that much research, especially the projects that have received a lot of media attention, is severely flawed. There also have been problems with serious statistical manipulations of data, leading to deceptive conclusions. Some of the memory studies coming out are a good example. Researchers are giving a large battery of tests and then playing with the numbers.

CG: One of the first human MDMA studies is a good example. The claim was that the MDMA users who had spinal taps to measure the serotonin metabolite 5-HIAA in their spinal fluid had abnormally low levels. It was not appropriately appreciated that the controls for the study were patients with chronic pain, and it is known that people with chronic pain syndromes often have elevated levels of 5-HIAA in their spinal fluid. I think that was somewhat deceptive, but even worse was a subsequent study in which researchers performed L-tryptophan challenge tests, an indirect measurement of serotonergic function. They did this test on subjects who had a history of taking MDMA; even though there were no statistically significant findings, the investigators had sufficient concern from their findings to conclude that MDMA damages the serotonin system. The report did not reveal—and this gets to the heart of the problem with the integrity of this research—that these MDMA-using subjects were not randomly recruited. Apparently, they had been studied previously in the cerebrospinal fluid 5-HIAA study, and these were the subjects who scored at the bottom, at the lower end of the spectrum. They were preselected! There was a preselection bias in choosing subjects. This is all right insofar as it might be interesting to know how two different markers of serotonergic function correlate. But it was not appropriate in this case that the published article did not reveal that these subjects had been recruited based on previous testing. This article was published in one of the most prestigious psychiatric journals and has never been retracted or even corrected.

JH: There is another problem with these studies. If you're taking a group of people who have used Ecstasy two hundred or four hundred times, it's pretty clear that you are preselecting for some sort of psychopathologic characteristics—impulse control disorders or compulsive behavior or perhaps depression. There is something "off" about these people. At the very least, you could surmise that these are people with some sort of serotonergic dysfunction. They are clearly self-medicating and finding that taking a serotonin agonist repeatedly is what they need to feel well.

CG: Absolutely.

JH: Isn't it true that one of the control groups in the memory studies was a group of graduate students?

CG: This is what the investigators told us in England, at the Novartis meetings. They were presenting their data on neuropsychological deficits in

Ecstasy users, and I asked who the controls were. The reply was that many of the controls were graduate students from the Baltimore and Washington D.C. areas who participated to make a little extra money. Now I suspect that even graduate students will indulge in substance use, but I strongly doubt that it will be to the same degree as the hard-living, heavy-drug-taking subjects who identify so strongly with the rave culture.

JH: Also, you have to think about who volunteers for studies of memory. For the most part, it is people who consider themselves to have good memories. Was education controlled for in these studies? Were the Ecstasy users graduate students also?

CG: Not likely. This was a very poor control group. The investigators also tended to minimize the degree to which their Ecstasy-using subjects also had used a lot of other drugs.

JH: This is a very important point. Certainly drugs like ketamine and dextromethorphan, which are known to interfere with memory processing and are likely to be used in a rave setting, should be mentioned specifically, and these users should be excluded from the studies.

CG: Ketamine and dextromethorphan have been substituted for MDMA in Ecstasy pills and also seem to be taken to an increasing degree for their own effect. Most of these drugs are going to have powerful effects on central nervous system function. Disregarding the potential impact of drugs like ketamine and dextromethorphan, which is what has been occurring, and attributing all identified and suspected pathologic effects to MDMA use, will only obfuscate the truth and further erode confidence in the veracity of these reports.

JH: I certainly agree with you. I would like to change gears for a minute. I want to have an understanding of what kind of research you have done with MDMA thus far and what your plans are for future work. Perhaps the way to lead into that subject is to talk about how you first learned about MDMA and became interested in performing clinical research with MDMA.

CG: I first heard about MDMA when I was working at the Johns Hopkins Hospital, in the Division of Child and Adolescent Psychiatry. I remember that one of the other child psychiatrists at Hopkins attended an Esalen ARUPA meeting [see "MDMA's Promise as a Prescription Medicine" for more information]. He later told me about the meeting and the MDMA experience he had had there. I was quite struck by how enthusiastic he was about what he considered to be the potential therapeutic application of MDMA. This particular doctor was fairly insightful and intelligent, so I was intrigued by what he was saying, and I started reading. He provided me with a few articles, and I did a literature search and found some other reports. What I read was very interesting.

JH: Was this before or after the media attention began in 1985?

CG: Yes, it was about then. At that time I was living in Baltimore and fairly cut off from anyone who had an interest in hallucinogens. I kept my interest to myself and did a lot of reading on the topic. My main focus at that time was completing my psychiatric training. I was primarily busy learning my craft, developing my skills as a psychiatrist and child psychiatrist. I finished my training at Johns Hopkins and stayed there for several years on the full-time faculty. Concerning MDMA and hallucinogens, I felt that this area of research could be potentially very important to look into, but I was in no position to do so until I moved to California in 1987. At the University of California I got to know Gary Bravo and Roger Walsh, who shared the vision that these drugs had an unrealized role in psychiatry. Together with Mitchel Liester, we developed a research study. We interviewed psychiatrists who had had personal experiences with MDMA in the early and mid-eighties (Liester et al. 1992). The study was basically to examine why they took it, what their experiences were, and what short- and long-term sequelae they might have sustained, both positive and negative. We felt that this would be a subject population with some expertise in identifying and describing intra-psychic states.

None of our subjects, by the way, had ever administered MDMA to a patient. Their knowledge was entirely from their first-hand experience. Quite a number of them told us that they believed that when used under optimal conditions, MDMA has profound implications as a treatment. I was also struck by the degree to which their views on MDMA were consistent with the old literature on hallucinogen-augmented therapy from the 1950s and 1960s. By the early seventies, political pressures had forced the closure of established hallucinogen research programs. This important area of investigation has remained virtually taboo since then, with very limited exceptions. I've always felt that literature to be very rich in descriptive material, which, at the very least, should encourage us to examine in a more systematic and controlled manner whether those substances could have therapeutic action, particularly in conditions that are refractory to conventional treatment.

JH: Which conditions interested you in terms of MDMA-assisted psychotherapy?

CG: The protocol I eventually submitted to the Food and Drug Administration (FDA) examined the safety and efficacy of a single dose of MDMA in end-stage cancer patients with severe psychological demoralization, existential depression, isolation, and physical pain. That would be a group for which modern medicine often can do very little. We were not looking to treat their medical condition; instead we were looking to alleviate some of their psychological and spiritual suffering, to help facilitate a *rapprochement* and enhancement of communication with important family and friends, from whom they were often quite isolated emotionally. When I was in medical school, one of the most inspiring articles I read was Stanislav Grof's article in 1972 in the journal *International Pharmacopsychiatry*, reporting on his work administering LSD and DPT (dipropyltryptamine) to terminal cancer patients. His findings were quite impressive and included improved mood, reduction of anxiety, diminished pain and need for narcotic pain control, and enhanced bonding and communication with family. I later read Grof's book *Human Encounters with Death*, which I found to be an excellent description of the potentials of this research model that has been too long neglected.

JH: I assume that you had similar goals when you handed in your protocol to the FDA.

CG: The goal of our MDMA protocol submitted to the FDA was to conduct a similar study, but we also felt that there were advantages to using MDMA over classic hallucinogens like LSD. It is shorter acting, it facilitates communication and articulation, it is more easily controlled, and there is far less likelihood of a frightening experience, dysphoria, or general ego fragmentation.

JH: What about the potential analgesic or pain-killing properties of MDMA?

CG: There is an important case reported by George Greer. In the early eighties, before the drug was scheduled, he was conducting psychotherapy with a man who had multiple myeloma. The man had numerous bone lesions that caused terrible pain; he was on high-dose narcotics to treat the pain. In the context of this ongoing therapy, Greer administered MDMA to the man, and he experienced a dramatic alleviation of pain, not only during the several hours when he was under the acute effects of MDMA but also for weeks and even months afterward. Greer ended up treating him three times over about eight months and found marked reduction in his need for narcotics to treat bone pain [see "Clinical Experience with MDMA-Assisted Psychotherapy" for more information].

JH: I am remembering that video of the 48 Hours program from the fall of 2000 of Sue and Shane, a couple who used MDMA late in Shane's illness with kidney cancer. In this video he says that he is pain free during the session and mentions to Sue how nice it is to "not have cancer" for a night. Are there any other anecdotal reports of MDMA-induced analgesia?

CG: Except for discussions in the MAPS bulletin, there aren't any other published clinical cases that I know of. There are some animal studies from the late seventies and early eighties, including one that Sasha Shulgin worked on. In that study, animals given MDMA were noted to have seemingly greater tolerance to painful stimuli. Also, MDMA appeared to augment the action of morphine in animals.

JH: I have read personal testimonials from family members of cancer patients in the MAPS bulletin. I have also received e-mail from people describing the analgesic effect of MDMA.

CG: I also have heard anecdotal accounts of people who describe their own experience or that of a family member. In these accounts, there was a severe medical condition with very pronounced pain. Following treatment with MDMA—often single-dose treatment—there was a fairly dramatic and sustained alleviation of pain and an apparent improvement in the psychological condition as well.

JH: I have read enough testimonials that suggest that if pain relief is not sustained after the experience, at least there is less pain for the three or four hours that the patient is under the influence of MDMA. There are two things that make MDMA a unique medicine. First, it is a non-sedating analgesic; morphine and many other potent pain medications cause drowsiness and a clouding of the consciousness, but MDMA keeps you clear. It is also a non-sedating anxiolytic (anxiety-reducing medication), and we have nothing like that in psychiatry. All the anti-anxiety medicines cause sedation as well. I think that as a result of this effect alone, MDMA deserves to be studied as a unique pharmacological tool.

CG: When you're talking about using MDMA in treatment, I think that it is important always to point out that you're not talking about ongoing medication administration as a treatment regimen. Rather you're talking very often of single-dose administration or perhaps two or three doses interspersed by months, or even years, over the life of the patient.

JH: What is ongoing, what is long-term, though, is the supportive psychotherapy, to prepare the patient and to process what arises out of the MDMA-assisted sessions.

CG: Greer's patient also was trying to use self-hypnosis exercises to treat his pain, and he found that after the MDMA session he had far greater success. His self-hypnosis techniques became more effective in alleviating his pain. Arthur Hastings wrote an article in which he described working with a few subjects who had a history of taking MDMA. He put them into a hypnotic trance that he felt was very similar to the MDMA state. Having had the MDMA experience, these people were more able to be hypnotized, specifically with regard to inducing features reminiscent of that earlier MDMA experience. This finding raises interesting potential research questions that I think are worth pursuing.

JH: That's one of the things I remember hearing about MDMA early on—that it is a type of altered state that one can reproduce later without the drug, as opposed to LSD.

CG: The early model with MDMA was that it was a drug that people would not need to take very often or for very long, maybe only one time. The common statement going around in the mid-eighties was "Once you get the message, you can hang up the phone." You don't need to take it repeatedly.

JH: I always liked that quote. I also wanted to cover what else you've studied, including the SPECT studies (single positron emission computed tomography).

CG: We ran eighteen subjects through the entire study. We examined effects of MDMA on vital signs—temperature, respiratory rate, heart rate, blood pressure. We examined psychological effects using questionnaires. We used indwelling intravenous catheters, and every thirty minutes we took blood for assays of pharmacokinetics (how MDMA is metabolized) and also for neuroendocrine assays (how MDMA affects hormone levels). On some, but not all, of the subjects, we conducted SPECT scans to look at blood flow in the brain—a baseline study before drug administration and a follow-up study several weeks after the last MDMA administration. We also did baseline MR SPECT (magnetic resonance spectroscopy) studies. We found no difference between the Ecstasy users, with an average Ecstasy exposure of 214 times, and the normal controls on their SPECT scan results before administration of MDMA.

JH: Did you notice any temperature changes with administration of MDMA in a clinical setting?

CG: There was a very modest elevation in temperature. I don't think that it exceeded a degree, even at the highest doses. But these were people lying comfortably in bed who were encouraged to drink fluids.

JH: What, if anything, did you see of significance on the SPECT scans?

CG: At two or three weeks after MDMA administration, we found modest decrements in blood flow in particular regions, but the baseline values were normal. Whatever process was occurring in the short term seemed to correct itself over time. Or it could parallel what you see with serotonin axonal degeneration followed by axonal regeneration. That's speculative, but it may correlate to that. [See "Does MDMA Cause Brain Damage?" for more information.]

JH: Didn't you also repeat the scans later on, to see if the hypoperfusion [low blood flow] corrected itself?

CG: Most of our subjects received only baseline SPECTs and then repeated SPECTs three weeks after the last drug dose. The changes were modest, but we did see some changes in blood flow. Two subjects were scanned again forty-three days and eighty days after MDMA was administered, and they showed signs of increased blood flow. It should be noted that with MR SPECT, you can identify some neurochemical factors. One of the markers for brain injury is a compound called N-acetylaspartate [NA], and there have been studies that have shown reductions of NA in a variety of clinical conditions, including methamphetamine use. We were very interested in looking at that, and we found that with the Ecstasy users, there was no difference in this marker from our control population. A normal NA concentration suggests lack of significant neuronal injury in these recreational Ecstasy users. We did find a slight increase in myoinositol, but we're not sure about the significance of that or whether it would hold up in future studies.

JH: What about the neuropsychological data? That data derived from these same eighteen patients?

CG: Yes. The neuropsychological data indicated no appreciable difference before and after MDMA administration within subjects or between the Ecstasy group and the control group at baseline.

JH: What are your future research plans?

CG: The main study we want to do is the clinical treatment study of patients with end-stage cancer.

JH: What has been your experience getting permission from the government to do this work?

CG: I've had some very pleasant conversations with people at the FDA, and they've had constructive input for the treatment protocol, but let me back up a bit. Initially, the FDA response was surprisingly positive. Those were the days when Curtis Wright was still there, and he was very pro-active about the need to open up hitherto taboo areas of study. Unfortunately, after Curtis Wright left the FDA, communication became more difficult. Although the FDA has approved two other MDMA administration studies of normal volunteers, so far they have not approved clinical treatment studies. Last year, because of the growing publicity of the MDMA neurotoxicity issue in the media and by NIDA [National Institute on Drug Abuse], I wrote an extensive review critiquing the MDMA neurotoxicity field [Grob 2000]. I plan to resubmit the end-stage cancer research study protocol to the FDA later this year [2001].

JH: I'm glad your article has been published. It's a great article and should encourage researchers in the fields of psychiatry and neuroscience to reexamine the MDMA neurotoxicity issue. Where do you see things going in the future? Do you see yourself giving MDMA to patients?

CG: I remain very determined to conduct an approved pilot study to examine the safety and efficacy of MDMA, as well as other hallucinogens, in selected groups of patients. Besides end-stage cancer patients, there are two other prospective groups that are often very difficult to treat using conventional treatment methods. These are patients with chronic post-traumatic stress disorder and patients with refractory substance abuse problems. Both MDMA and other hallucinogens have great potential in these areas, especially ayahuasca in the treatment of drug addiction and alcoholism.

JH: What do you think the pitfalls are in the future? What do we have to look out for in the field of clinical MDMA research?

CG: First, there is the question of the degree to which our culture has recovered from the turmoil of the late 1960s. Have we reached the point where we no longer have the model of Timothy Leary hanging over our heads, stopping any effective movement in the field? I think we have. We need to be able to learn from the mistakes of that time, however. In particular, we need to learn that polarizing political issues will hamper our capacity to progress in this field. We need to make inroads into the mainstream medical, psychiatric, and neuroscience research community and establish a dialogue with them. Once more influential investigators perceive that it is finally possible to conduct research safely with these compounds, we will see vigorous and pro-active efforts to explore the untapped potentials for MDMA and the hallucinogens as agents of healing. Keep in mind, however, that one of the more substantial obstacles blocking the field from moving forward, particularly with MDMA, has been the persistent high degree of recreational use and abuse.

JH: Do you think that the rave phenomenon is hindering the progress of the therapeutic research agenda?

CG: Absolutely. I think that is a major concern. With MDMA, the way the drug is used recreationally tends to exacerbate potential risks. I've gone so far as to say that if someone plans to take MDMA, a rave would be one of the most dangerous place to do so. That's an enormous issue that needs to be addressed. Ideally, one would almost want to propose a moratorium on the recreational use of the drug, so that the therapeutic value can be investigated. Of course, that will never happen. The bottom line is that millions of teenagers and young adults taking the drug under hazardous circumstances—and taking a variety of drugs—are putting themselves at significant risk. This widespread recreational use makes it much more difficult to move the field of therapeutic investigations forward. These are powerful tools, and, in the hands of people who fully understand the safety parameters and how to optimally utilize them, they can work wonders. In the hands of irresponsible people with limited knowledge who are prone to risk taking, however, they can be very hazardous. I hope that in the future we will see an evolution toward more honest and effective drug education leading to minimized levels of risk. Concurrently, the acceptance and elaboration of the MDMA- and hallucinogen-augmented treatment models in psychiatry should allow for the development of safer and more effective treatment models.

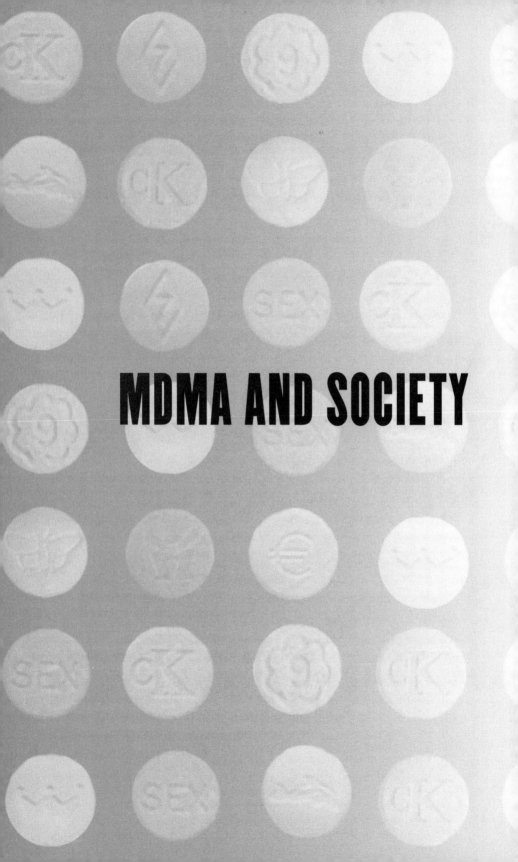

MDMA AND SOCIETY

Introduction

As humans, one of our most basic defining characteristics is that we are so-cial beings. We are expected to commune with others. It is in our nature to crave and create a community, a network, and a culture to surround us. The newly formed culture provides structure, with rules informing its members about expected behavior and about which actions will lead to expulsion from the group. These guidelines help define the group and create boundaries and parameters to enhance the feelings of connection among members. At our healthiest, we gravitate toward connection with others; at our most ill, we isolate ourselves from the group.

When an individual member of a group is in need, the community may substitute for the family in caring for that person, helping him or her feel protected and nurtured. Present-day examples include church communities, labor unions, neighborhood watches, and even crack houses. Anywhere that one finds shared interests, there will be a community creating guidelines for accepted behavior and benefits from membership. The Internet is a prime example, with its multitude of chat rooms, and e-mail forums. Cell phones are another recent testament to our universal desire to be constantly con-nected to others. Many would argue that the club scene, the rave commu-nity, in particular, provides just such a cohesive unit and culture. Like people affected with group hysteria or a flock of birds moving as one to the dictates of a "group mind," the community of ravers loses its sense of self in favor of a larger, stronger, and perhaps healthier entity. The tenets of peace, love, unity, and respect are advertised and adhered to.

Being a productive member of a community, conforming to its mores and tenets, and helping maintain the structure of the group can lead to a more meaningful and happier life. A sense of belonging and giving to the group, as opposed to being "on the dole" and taking from the community, can help enhance a person's self-esteem and sense of purpose. We not only crave, but we indeed thrive on these connections. When mental illness or drug use cuts us off from the rest of society and when the shame and guilt drive us to hide from others, the subsequent isolation compounds the effects of the illness. One of the many unique effects of MDMA is a feeling of connection to others—the sense that we are not isolated, that we belong to a clan larger than ourselves. This has therapeutic implications not only for the individual but for our society as well.

The Tribal Dance

Reminiscent of the ancient Dionysian rituals, the rave brings its participants together through the loss of self into a redefined whole. Dancing to music with a beat not coincidentally approximating the rhythm of an exercising heart or a resting fetus, ravers are as bonded to one another as members of a single tribe dancing around the fire. They celebrate life, the intensity and purity of being, and the present. How can the ravers not be transformed by this experience? The euphoric sense of release, of mass transcendence, leaves its indelible mark on all those who join the rave.

The symbol of a lost childhood, of a desire to play or frolic, is evident in the pacifier worn around the necks of the dancing ravers. Truly they are getting in touch with their "inner child" as they lose themselves in the dance. And although many will make a distinction between therapeutic use and recreational use of the drug, it is fair to say that at its best, the rave is a wonderful kind of group therapy. Some adolescents involved in this movement have never felt so comfortable with themselves and their place in society as when they are at a rave.

The Politics of Ecstasy

Our society makes few distinctions concerning illegal drugs. Lines are seldom drawn between what may be useful to some and harmful to others. The media, the government, parents, and teachers simply advise against drug use in toto. Fear of the unknown is a potent dissuader. At heart, our society is afraid of all drugs, and this fear is turned into aggression; to calm society's collective anxiety, people go on the attack. The bottom line is that drugs scare people, and fear makes great copy. The media is frequently hysterical about drugs, especially a new drug. Most television coverage of MDMA takes full advantage of this fear, citing claims that just one pill can cause death or brain damage.

Often, use of a particular drug will be linked to sex. The U.S. media, for example, tags most new street drugs, such as GHB, rohypnol, or MDMA, as "date rape drugs" or "truth serums." Some people believe that when we are blissful, we are vulnerable. What will happen if we let down our guard, if we tell the dirty little secrets that we are all so ashamed to harbor? The media insists that the public must be protected from this exposure.

The experience of Ecstasy must be a sin. In line with the puritanical tradition of "guilty pleasures," it must be bad for you if it feels so good. Current drug policy logic dictates that if a drug causes euphoria or pleasure or bliss it needs to be outlawed, for surely it is dangerous, of no use to anyone, and subject to abuse. The popular sixties philosopher Alan Watts spoke of the "taboo against knowing who you are," which may somehow threaten our politics of complacency. Our society is much more apt to condone a mind- or body-numbing drug like alcohol than a mind-manifesting and -enhancing drug. A drug that stimulates discovery or creativity is more threatening to our government than a form of opium for the masses. MDMA is like the forbidden fruit from the Tree of Knowledge. Surely free access to self-knowledge is damaging.

The hesitance to be happy and relaxed, full of self-knowledge and self-love, comes from our comfort with our own self-hatred. On a very deep subconscious level we are sure that we do not deserve love and happiness. We believe that we have done bad things in our lives and deserve to be punished. And more than that: it is bad to shine, to be proud, to take the time to learn to be comfortable in our own skin and to love ourselves. The politics of Ecstasy rests on the bedrock of this fear—the fear of self-love, of enlightenment, and of our own greatness, purity, and strength. In our culture we have been taught that we must have guilt with pleasure, because we do not deserve pure pleasure. The ecstatic experience is proscribed and its adherents prosecuted and punished, because Ecstasy—and enlightenment—are subversive.

But what of the group ecstatic experience? It remains to be seen what the impact on society will be from weekly bacchanals with tens of thousands of euphoric revelers loving themselves and those around them. There are those who feel there has been a cultural response already, helping solidify the global village through tribal dance and communion. MDMA has catalyzed the worldwide rave movement, with its tenets of Peace, Love, Unity, and Respect, touching and perhaps in some way revolutionizing numerous cultures throughout the world.

It is possible that MDMA could be of substantial use to us, possibly helping us evolve as a society and become more caring and attentive toward others. Within a therapeutic framework, MDMA may help us become more nurturing toward ourselves and more relaxed, empathic, and connected to others. It is possible it could make us more hopeful—about ourselves and our potential, individually and as a culture.

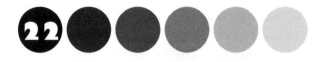

ECSTASY: PRESCRIPTION FOR CULTURAL RENAISSANCE

Douglas Rushkoff

Every culture and subculture gets the drugs that it deserves. In fact, almost every major cultural movement in history can be traced back to the chemicals they did or did not have. While ancient nomadic tribes experienced regular psychedelic excursions by eating the mushrooms that grew on the dung of the cattle herds they followed, early agrarian cultures were denied the privilege (and spared the hazards) of such a drug-inspired social system. Historians tracing the shift in value systems toward property ownership, and in psychology toward the development and maintenance of ego, too often ignore the impact that these natural psychedelics must have had on these early cultures. Similarly, the coffee beans imported from Morocco to Europe in the fourteenth and fifteenth centuries gave rise to the late-night discussions and midnight oil–burning artistic reverie that launched what we now call the Renaissance. Young coffee drinkers, empowered by the stimulant beverage to stay awake after normal working hours, embarked on a reconsideration of the foundations of their reality. They developed everything from calculus to perspective painting as their apprehension of our world's dimensionality took a leap forward.

That's what a renaissance is—a rebirth of old ideas in a new context. We gain the ability to reframe many facets of our existence with a greater sense of dimensionality. Whether it's understanding that the globe itself is a sphere instead of a plane or that paintings can have depth and vanishing points, renaissance insight marks an increase in an understanding of dimension. It is a moment when we go "meta." Just such a renaissance moment has been under way in the popular culture of the West since the 1960s. Foreshadowed by breakthroughs in relativity and quantum physics, this leap in dimensionality finally hit public consciousness with the escape of the so-called CIA brainwashing drug LSD into academic and subcultural circles.

The psychedelic revolution, though limited to an underground phenomenon, led to a rebirth of ancient ideas in a new, scientific context. Psychologists such as Timothy Leary, eager to comprehend the nature of the LSD trance, turned to spiritual systems from the East, such as those outlined in *The Tibetan Book of the Dead.* This book chronicled the process by which the insights acquired on a transdimensional vision quest could be incorporated into a person's daily existence through a "conscious rebirth" at trip's end.

Just as participants in the earlier Renaissance had come to grips with the three-dimensional reality of the sphere on which they walked, psychedelic pioneers began to perceive the planet as a living system, interconnected and interdependent. Biologists and philosophers alike strove to develop new theories to explain this phenomenon. James Lovelock, for example, came up with a "Gaia hypothesis" that credits the planet with the properties of a self-regulating form of life. Meanwhile, mathematicians emerged from their psychedelic experiences with a new appreciation for the dimensionality of the numbers with which they worked. Systems theory posited a new set of dynamic mathematical relationships between the members of natural systems and large populations. People began working with long-detested nonlinear equations, discovering "fractional dimensionality," or fractals, which allowed for the mathematical comprehension of formerly unfathomable systems. By granting a cloud its fractional dimensionality, rather than reducing it to a simple sphere, mathematicians were finally able to reckon with its previously untenable surface area.

Just as the sixteenth century brought with it a new technique for depicting our newfound perspective, the 1970s saw the emergence of holographic technologies, which went even further, to add dimensionality to our representations. In addition to depicting depth, the hologram can represent the passage of time. As the viewer moves across the holographic image, the image itself can move—a woman can blink her eyes, and a bird can flap its wings. More remarkably, the holographic plate itself stores information in a way that forces us to reevaluate the nature of matter. If a holographic plate depicting a flying bird is smashed into hundreds of pieces, each piece will contain an image of the entire bird, albeit blurry. Through each separate piece of the hologram, the viewer sees the bird from a distinct angle—as if the viewer had rubbed away frost from different parts of a window. When the image is left intact, the separate images are resolved into a single image with all the necessary information. The implication, which is currently under scrutiny in fields as diverse as brain anatomy and cultural anthropology, is that each part of a system somehow contains a faint representation of the whole. When properly networked, the total picture of reality is resolved.

The original Renaissance also was inspired, in part, by a new communications technology: the printing press. Thanks to Gutenberg, the masses became literate. The Bible and other texts were no longer to be read only by the upper classes and the religious elite. This led to an increasingly level playing field in terms of the dissemination of information and eventually provoked a religious reformation known as Protestantism.

By the 1980s, our current renaissance found its technological equivalent to the printing press: the personal computer. People were empowered not merely with access to information but also with the ability to self-publish across global networks. This marked a clear dimensional upscaling of the relationship of the individual to society at large. Each human being with a computer linked to the Internet became a node in a dynamic system, capable of feedback and iteration. We are still only beginning to reckon with the social impact of this new human interactivity.

Our computer networks give us the best clue to the nature of our latest increase in dimensional thinking as well as to the reason why MDMA, in particular, became the drug of choice among the newly "networked." Much of early cyberculture was founded by people with psychedelic experience. It seemed that those who had experience navigating the hallucinatory realm of the LSD trip were most comfortable learning the languages and confronting the yet uninvented worlds of cyberspace. As fledgling Silicon Alley firms became dependent on Grateful Deadheads and other psychedelics users as programmers, cyberculture became known as a "cyberdelic" movement. The values of 1960s psychedelia found new life as they trickled up from a subculture to what was soon to become America's leading industry.

As if in an effort to actualize physically and experientially the networked culture they were building in cyberspace, young, hi-tech San Franciscans developed their own version of the electronic music parties they heard about from friends who had traveled to Britain and Ibiza. In Europe, the huge parties called raves were already commonplace. Thousands of revelers would gather in abandoned warehouses or on remote fields to dance until dawn to the throbbing beat of "acid house" music recorded originally by Detroit-based African Americans. When the first imported raves were held in the San Francisco Bay area, however, they took on a more self-consciously evolutionary agenda. San Francisco raves were designed to be like the famous acid tests thrown by Ken Kesey and the Merry Pranksters. Just like the 1960s "happenings" on which they were based, a rave's music, lighting, and ambience are all fine-tuned to elicit and augment altered states of consciousness. The rhythm of the music was precisely 120 beats per minute, the frequency of the fetal heart rate and the same beat used by South American shamans to bring their tribes into a trance state. Through dancing together, without prescribed movements or even partners, rave dancers sought to reach group consciousness on a level they had never experienced before. The object of a rave was to experience a reality that went beyond the self. Ravers aspired to an awareness of the group organism. Inspired by the holograms and fractals on their computers, they sought to create a dynamic system in which each member could experience the essence of the whole. The drug they chose to assist them in this quest was MDMA.

Most of them already had experienced LSD. But the LSD trip was a personal, introspective experience. Although most people report a sensation of connectedness with the universe at the peak of an LSD experience, this realization of the oneness of reality is a largely intellectual revelation, on the order of an intense spiritual insight. For the LSD trip is epic in structure, like the Homeric arc of a heroic journey. A rising euphoria climaxes in an ego-shattering epiphany of self-realization. Ego is destroyed, at least temporarily, and the foundations of ego and self are revealed as artificial constructs of mind. But the trip itself is spent challenging and destroying these constructs. Eventually, the tripper takes the long journey back to waking state consciousness, clutching to the insights he or she has garnered in the rebirth back into an ego-defined existence.

MDMA, which gained notoriety as an empathogen through its use by psychotherapists before its reclassification as an illegal substance in the 1980s, offered a trip more appropriate to the purposes of the rave. Unlike LSD, Ecstasy—which most ravers simply called E—provided a more even plateau of duration than the highly arced LSD trip. Users took the drug and experienced its full effects in less time. Instead of rising to a crescendo and then releasing users into free fall, Ecstasy came on more subtly, gently coaxing its users into a mild and communicative euphoria. Instead of journeying inward, E users found themselves venturing outward. Ecstasy's flatter and correspondingly more predictable onset and duration made it a much more practical enhancement to an eight-hour party. Its amphetamine-like side effects helped users dance longer and with greater energy than they might otherwise, guaranteeing that they would be out on the floor with their newfound friends during the group's peak moments. No one wanted to be left out.

The climax of a group E experience is not individual but collective. Where LSD subjected its users to the harsh crucible of self-analysis, E immediately proved itself a carefree, social drug. Rather than burning through an individual's obstacles to self-awareness, it melted away a group's obstacles to intimacy. Although MDMA became notorious for fostering "inappropriate bonding" in a romantic setting, it also was just as celebrated for developing group cohesion at a larger gathering. Like alcohol, E served as a social lubricant, dissolving inhibitions and catalyzing an almost tribal sensibility. Instead of doing this by amplifying an individual's sense of power and invincibility, E's effect was to generate a sense of identification between people. It was as if a group of people taking E together became empowered collectively. The sense of individualism and personal gain one strove for in the workaday reality suddenly seemed a hollow illusion, promoted by economics, marketing, and one's own fear of exposure. Competition between people, and even the notion of individuated personhood, seemed a farce. On MDMA, users came to regard such personal strivings and associated anguish as laughable distractions from the real business at hand: forging intimate relationships on a level previously unimaginable.

Nothing could have been more aligned with the rave's stated purpose. Although it was not mandatory, dosing with E was deemed extremely beneficial to a group of several thousand strangers hoping to shift itself into the head space and heart space of collective awareness. The rave gathering offered experiential evidence of the dimensional leap that had been calculated and depicted by holograms and fractals. It made physical the sorts of social networking that had been practiced only on a virtual level through the Internet. Stripped of personal ambition and provoked to form emotional bonds, the revelers at a rave gathering were enabled to push their experiments in group dynamics beyond what their egos and inhibitions would have permitted otherwise. Ecstasy seemed to serve as a fuel. While some users believed that the MDMA molecule had an almost conscious agenda of its own, more users tended to identify their new sensibility as coming directly from the heart, uncovered and activated at last by the drug's catalytic power.

It was a three-part process. First, Ecstasy stripped away the user's inhibitions to self-expression. On E, lies are inefficient, and the peculiarities or weaknesses they are meant to obscure no longer seem like offenses against nature. Young men who had long repressed their feminine sides felt an irrepressible urge to express their anima, their female spirit. While a few experimented with homosexuality, it usually had less to do with defining sexual identity than with eradicating overly determined and intimacy-restricting social roles. In this first stage of the Ecstasy trip, users experience themselves in full spectrum and without reservation. Old or young, gay or straight, muscular or nerd—everyone is okay and beautiful just exactly as he or she is.

This first stage is also the time when psychological discomfort generally will occur, if it occurs at all. Although it is extremely minor compared with the harrowing, hallucinatory nightmare of a bad LSD trip, a difficult E experience typically results from the user's resistance to the emotional needs or personality traits he or she has been repressing all along. The reason that negative experiences are so rare is that MDMA does not parade people's hidden traits before them, demanding that they give voice to them. Instead, E makes people feel so open and accepting that these orphaned personality constructs finally rise to the surface, where they can manifest without shame. The user is so open-minded and emotionally giving that he or she welcomes the formerly rejected sentiments with open arms. Instead of feeling overwhelmed, the user generally feels consolidated and whole for the first time.

Once this process of self-acceptance is completed, the user still feels a burning need to accept more. This is when the second stage begins in earnest, and one seeks to recognize and embrace the emotional needs and personality traits of others. With the same openness and judgment-free enthusiasm with which they embraced themselves, users strive to accept the hearts, minds, and bodies of those around them. They understand that their friends are also experiencing and expressing new parts of themselves and seeing the world through the same non-prejudicial eyes. The overwhelming need to empathize with one another outweighs every other consideration. This is why almost no one on Ecstasy looks to score sexual conquests or increase his or her social status. People are too busy accepting and embracing each other to care about themselves.

This is when the third stage, the action of E most important to the group as a whole, finally takes effect. The majority of the crowd soon realizes that speech and one-to-one contact is no longer a sufficient means of reaching out and accepting the thousands of other people present. That's why they turn to the dance. As part of the collective, ten-thousand-armed dancing mass, everyone gains the ability to accept and embrace the totality of the group simultaneously. Everyone has liberated themselves personally, accepted one another individually, and must now accept the totality of the group itself in their hearts. In a sense, they go "meta." Like quantum physicists who realize they cannot make an observation without finding themselves under the magnifying glass, ravers realize that they are part of the very thing they are trying to accept.

This is the magic moment of the rave that so many people talk about for months or even years afterward. Unlike a rock concert, which unites its audience in mutual adoration for the sexy singers on stage, the rave unites its audience in mutual adoration of one another. The disc jockey providing the rhythm is more of an anonymous shaman than a performer, mixing records from a remote corner of the room. The stage is the dance floor, and the stars are the ravers themselves. The group celebrates itself.

The peak of the E experience is when the drug and dance ritual brings the revelers into a state of collective consciousness. Descriptions of these extended moments of group awareness often fall into cliché, but they are profound, life-changing events for those who have experienced them. The dancers achieve what can only be called "group organism." That is, the individuals form a dynamic system like a coral reef, where each person experiences himself or herself more as a member of the collective entity than as an individuated being. But in lower-order hive minds, the individual members, whether bees or plankton, have little or no awareness of their own participation in the collective. Their service is instinctual. The collective to which they belong has no purpose other than mutual survival. The collective formed purposefully by E-charged ravers is the result of a ritual self-consciously performed for no purpose other than the sensibility of group mind itself. The mass spectacle results in a fleeting but undeniable rush of collective awareness. The dancing mass becomes a single being with thousands of pairs of eyes. To catch a fellow raver's glance is akin to seeing oneself in the mirror. It is as if each person is an extension of the same being, encountering itself.

The collective awareness achieved through mass MDMA use perfectly matched the social agenda of the subculture it came to serve. In their quest to find a drug capable of forging new social bonds, the rave underground happened upon a chemical that exceeded their original expectations. Ecstasy broke social inhibitions while engendering an empathic imperative that fostered new levels of emotional bonding. But the intensity of these bonds, augmented by the self-consciously inclusive and egalitarian environment that the users had engineered for themselves, led to an entirely new and unexpected way of understanding the relationship of individuals to the larger groups they form.

Like a hologram, the human project itself is understood as a collective enterprise. Each person contains the entire process—albeit a fuzzy, unresolved picture of that process—within himself or herself. The only way to resolve the picture is to bring those individuals together into a single coordinated and multidimensional being. For those keen on enacting a renaissance of this magnitude—and hoping to do so before human beings had the ability to accept themselves, much less one another—MDMA served as a crucial social medicine.

Ironically, perhaps, just as the hi-tech Internet tended to encourage what the media theorist Marshall McLuhan predicted would be "tribal" affiliations and a sense of electronic Global Village, the laboratory-born MDMA molecule spawned a similar network of tribal communities. Like primitive tribal people who, after ingesting various combinations of rain-forest psychotropic drugs, would dance in a group trance around the shaman's fire, young, techno-savvy ravers find their newfound tribal imperative actualized on the dance floor and catalyzed by a chemical. Although it is ingested by individuals, this powerful molecule's greatest action might be on the group.

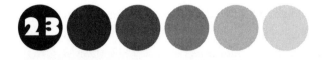

MDMA AND SPIRITUALITY:
An Interview with Rabbi Zalman Schachter

JH: How did you first hear about MDMA?

ZS: In 1956 I read Aldous Huxley's *Doors of Perception*, and in 1962 Timothy Leary took me on my first acid trip. I got to MDMA via the other psychedelics. I really can't remember from whom I first heard about it. It was in the air, not before the late seventies or perhaps the early eighties. I can't remember the circumstances surrounding the first opportunity I had to take it, but I felt the great delight of loving the universe and feeling loved by the universe. I don't recall whether there were any difficult aftereffects. I think the transition was very smooth. Since that time, I've taken it a few times with my wife. Certainly it enhanced a sense of deep sharing. The first question that comes from that is the issue of public policy. MDMA isn't something that should be given over the counter. I remember that Ram Dass [a.k.a. Richard Alpert, Ph.D.] once said to me that to smoke grass you should have to have a driver's license the same as for driving a car, and for acid you should have to have a pilot's license the same as for flying a jet.

Wine originally was turned into a sacramental drink, and people wanted to turn sexuality into a sacramental act as well. This is why in Judaism sex is called kiddushin and in Catholicism it is the sacrament of marriage. So the question is, why haven't the psychedelic substances, the mood lifters, been made sacramental? I've had the opportunity to be with Native Americans at peyote rituals, and there I have seen the great value of making such substances sacramental. Ayahuasca circles also are performed in sacramental settings. When people go to raves and bring in MDMA, I have the sense that it might be a good way to create a sacramental feeling. From the Jewish perspective, the proviso is that you would first make a *brakhah*. You know that word?

JH: You say a blessing. You bless the act, and the fact that it is blessed makes it special and sacramental.

ZS: That's right. Under those circumstances someone would not take it and decide to go downtown. I remember hearing about people dropping acid and then going to see *Yellow Submarine.*

JH: Probably not the best use of their time with that tool.

ZS: When it comes to breakthroughs, the "responsible people" didn't want to take responsibility, so the irresponsible people took risks. And that, of course, is always a problem.

JH: I'm curious about your own history. When was your rabbinical training?

ZS: I was ordained in 1947.

JH: When you first took MDMA you were already a rabbi?

ZS: Yes.

JH: And did you have a congregation at that time?

ZS: By that time I was past the congregation phase, and I had served as campus clergy and as a professor. During the time that I took MDMA, I was teaching religion at Temple University.

JH: Can you take me through the process from when you first had your personal experience with MDMA to the point when you decided that you wanted to share it with other people?

ZS: I haven't yet done that . . . the sharing with other people. There's always the circumspection of the problems that it can raise, so I'm careful about that.

JH: Before it was made illegal, there was no time that you shared it with a congregation?

ZS: I would tell my students about it. I was not hesitant to talk about it, because anything that is kept under the table or under wraps assumes different proportions than if it is really seen and understood. I found that many of the people with whom I spoke nodded, as if they had experienced it. It's a self-selected group that hangs out with me, so often these were people who had had some drug experiences. I recall one man who told me that he got a stash of MDMA to give out to couples for their honeymoon. Of course, he did this only with friends.

JH: I think I misunderstood your history. I thought that there was a time in Philadelphia where you were sharing MDMA with others or leading them on some kind of "vision quest."

ZS: It's wonderful that I have such a reputation! I would do that vision quest and all the other things but not necessarily with substances.

JH: Some of this book is about using MDMA in psychotherapy—with individuals, for instance, those who have been traumatized in the past or who are depressed; or with couples; or in palliative care, working with the dying population, where I really think it could be useful.

ZS: Let me talk about that. Years ago, I met Abe Maslow ["hierarchy of needs" theorist] on a plane, and we had a good conversation about certain forms of psychology. I said something about the ability of psychedelics to demonstrate his description of peak experiences. At first he viewed this idea with disdain. It would be like taking a cable car up to Mont Blanc. It's not fair. We disagreed about that. I felt that it's important to domesticate peak experiences. If somebody has a wonderful experience in some area, it is good to be able to replicate it, and drugs are great facilitators. He didn't like the idea. Later on he had a heart attack and retired from Brandeis University and went to Palo Alto. He hung out with Ram Dass, and eventually did experience LSD. I don't remember whether he wrote about it, but it had great bearing on his move from humanistic psychology to transpersonal psychology.

Do you remember when Aldous Huxley was about do die? He wanted to get some LSD and he asked his doctor to give it to him. His doctor said, "I wouldn't advise it." He called another doctor, who came over and administered it to him so that he could pass the last two hours of life under its influence. He had written a book called *Island*. At the end of *Island* a woman named Sushilla is dying of cancer of the throat, and he describes her deathbed scene. As he was dying, he had his wife, Laura, read him the deathbed scene that he had written. That's a beautiful thing. If you can imagine that the fear people have of death can be overcome—those who are in hospices and AIDS centers and so on—that's an important thing, because it reconciles people to their ends. They aren't dragged kicking and screaming.

JH: How did you feel when the Drug Enforcement Administration placed MDMA in Schedule I on an emergency basis? Did the scheduling surprise you, or did it upset you? Did it change the course of your actions in any way?

ZS: No, I wasn't surprised. Yes, it upset me, but I wasn't surprised. I thought that if anyone comes up with anything that gives you euphoria, which the establishment doesn't control or make money from, that the establishment will create an interdiction. I think it was Gerald Heard [author of *What Is Love? The Power of Wonder*] who once told me that the warriors, the Kshatriya, in India are into alcohol. The Brahmins are into grass. He was pointing out that for some people, it's a cultural thing. The guys who are couch potatoes who drink beer are certainly not going to like the consciousness that comes with MDMA. So the fear in people is that to have experiences that ask for greater sharing rather than for more tightness will undermine the common collusion. Politics is involved.

JH: It does seem as if fear plays a large role, particularly fear of the unknown.

ZS: It is also fear of having to give up, though the noetic quality of MDMA is not as upsetting. It doesn't "take" you. I don't know of anyone who has had a bad trip on it.

JH: I imagine that it's pretty tricky to have a bad experience, but I have heard that some people have had a rough time. They're few and far between, as I understand it.

ZS: It may be partly that the oceanic feeling that occurs is something that may seem as though it could drown a person. It may be threatening in that way.

JH: What you were talking about before, with the couch potatoes, I just thought of the phrase "ignorance is bliss." MDMA does not offer ignorance. That's not what it's about.

ZS: It offers a bliss that isn't ignorance. That's right. People who wear a lot of body armor feel threatened by it. The armor comes loose on MDMA.

JH: Yes, it does. The defenses seem to subside, to surrender, and the walls come down. I think the masks come off, which possibly can be frightening. Maybe not while the person is experiencing MDMA, since there is that sense of strength and calm and security. But it might be frightening to someone hearing about it, like the fear of the "truth serum" aspect.

ZS: The question is always, what is the psychoprophylaxis? There should be something to prepare people.

JH: Yes, I definitely believe that people should be prepared. I don't know exactly how to phrase this—and it's a large question—but most of my thinking about MDMA has been about psychology and psychiatry and therapy. I haven't thought too much about where religion and spirituality really fit in with MDMA.

ZS: Someone once asked me if I had a spiritual take on the chemical substances, and I said this: "When God saw that people, instead of turning to God, were turning to the medicine cabinet, God made himself available in the medicine cabinet. So Satan came and said, 'If that's how easy it's going to be, I'm out of a job.' God said, 'I did what I had to do; you do what you have to do.' And Satan became a pusher." You get the idea that the issue is the application and the safeguards and so on. More than that, most of the time the mind does not expand to wrap itself around what the soul knows. What the soul knows at one moment becomes a fleeting experience. People can't recall it, because they haven't taken the time to digest it with their minds and with their affect and their actions. So they haven't assimilated the insights that they've taken from one of those experiences. It's important to integrate these insights afterward. Are you acquainted with Kohlberg's moral development theories?

JH: Yes.

ZS: Most of the time psychology and psychiatry talk about climbing out of the pathological realms. Once a person has adjusted to outer society, unless you go to transpersonal psychology or humanistic psychology, there isn't a scale. You're off the scale for pathology.

Much of medicine begins with going to the pathology lab and working on dead people. In the gross anatomy lab, that's what you do. You work with pathological conditions most of the time. The notion of health and wellness only recently has been introduced into this kind of thinking, right? Itzhak Bentov wrote a book called *Stalking the Wild Pendulum,* in which he talked about how earth, in order to heal herself, is "hothousing" certain levels of awareness in people.

JH: Is this where religion and spirituality come in? Once you get past pathology and into issues of personal growth and a higher awareness?

ZS: That's right. I want to say spirituality and not necessarily religion. Many times, religion deals with getting brownie points, social brownie points from people in your environment. Most of the religious systems have said that they will not allow for transformation. They're there to sugarcoat the status quo with an aura of holiness. It's not quite the same thing as spirituality. Dr. Roberto Assagioli [the founder of psychosynthesis] wrote a remarkable book about psychological disturbances as a result of spiritual growth [*Psychosynthesis: A Collection of Basic Writings*].

JH: I sometimes come across a patient who is experiencing a manic or psychotic episode, and it seems very much like a religious "peak experience" or a mystical epiphany. It's the kind of debate that gets stirred up every once in a while in the emergency room along the lines of "who's to say this person isn't a seer or a mystic or a saint?" I also have heard the term "kundalini explosion" to describe a manic episode.

ZS: Most doctors don't know how to handle that. They get anxious themselves when somebody. . . . How should I put this? Have you heard of a man called John Rosen? He was doing what he called "direct analysis." He would go into a ward with schizophrenic or manic-depressive patients, and he would enter into conversation with people on the level at which they were experiencing things. Frieda Fromm Reichman, who wrote *I Never Promised You a*

Rose Garden, did something similar. It's difficult to help people, but, on the other hand, if you don't go into those places, you can't help them. Very often, people get into high speed, like a mind fever, in which they know a convergence of everything. It feels and sounds like the kind of peak experience you'd like to share with them, but not with the same wind velocity. I think a big mistake is being made by people who will not release such patients from mental institutions until they have sworn off the insights that they had while they were in that psychotic moment. That's why I feel that it's very important for psychiatrists to have spiritual and psychedelic experiences. That's why they used to call them psychotomimetics. They meant to say that if you're going to work with psychotics without having visited your own inner world, you aren't going to be worth much. Empathy is what's called for at that moment—feeling that you still belong within the circle of human beings.

JH: It's important to commune with them. I think one of the most important characteristics of MDMA is that there is a sense of connectedness to other people and to the culture. One of the most pitiful problems of psychiatric patients is that they are isolated. Being disconnected from the rest of humanity, from their families, without friends, is utterly debilitating. One of the ways I can envision MDMA helping psychiatric patients is by allowing them to feel reconnected.

ZS: There is a certain amount of solipsism in the effect of regular psychedelics. Nobody can follow you into the deep recesses of your experience. With MDMA it's a different story. You're out there; you're not in the recesses of your mind as much. You're looking at people, and you see them looking at you, and there is a loving feeling. There are also some noetic issues that come up. It's not only the warm visceral stuff. I think that can lead to certain kinds of trust rebuilding and insight.

JH: Trust on what level?

ZS: Trusting other people, seeing that people are people. Everybody has a longing, and everybody wants to be loved.

JH: Yes, and also that everyone is basically insecure on some level and needs that connection with others.

ZS: You see the eyes shifting a little bit when a person gets to the question of whether it is okay to stay open, and then the reassurance comes. The other person says, "I'm open to you, and you can be open to me. Both of us have our issues, but so what?"

JH: I suppose you could think of a rave as the ultimate Havurah, or group sharing.

ZS: That's right.

JH: MDMA seems to be on a smaller, more manageable level than some of the stronger psychedelics, in terms of that opening.

ZS: The experience is also a little bit shorter lived. But can you imagine on a shabbas [sabbath] afternoon of a nice summer day, a group sitting outdoors and experiencing MDMA, singing songs and sharing food?

JH: I was imagining that, and I thought that's what we were going to talk about today!

ZS: We are right back to what we talked about. I think that there could be wonderful ways in which one could utilize MDMA in a group setting. I'll give you an example. Take a man who called me a couple of weeks ago. He is seventy-five years old; he wants to bring together his children and grand-children and have a party with them. There are some children who are more observant and some who are less observant. For the crowning moments of his relationship with his family, he would like to have them become united and have a feast together. I could imagine—though I couldn't tell him such a thing—the whole family taking MDMA together. Once a woman brought her husband to see me. He was of a very brittle kind of theological turn of mind. His mind was locked into a way of thinking that didn't allow him to be as nonverbally communicative with his wife. I dared to say at that moment, "Why don't you smoke some grass?" He snapped back—recoiled—and they left immediately. How did I dare make such a suggestion?

JH: That brings up a question. In your role as a rabbi, I think that you must find that there are some people who probably are taken aback that you have any kind of openness to these sorts of mind-altering substances. I wonder how you broach the subject with them? How would you introduce the idea? How do you allay their fear of the unknown?

ZS: I wouldn't do it next time! I tell you, there is something very funny. You go into a group of people, and you don't know who is Jewish and who isn't. Pretty soon, you have conversations with the people, and they drop a few words.

JH: It's as if they want you to know.

ZS: They want you to know. And it's the same thing with altering consciousness. The people who want you to know find ways to let you know.

JH: It's very true.

ZS: They talk about a mind move, a "flip," an insight. Then you know, "Aha, that's a buddy. That's a water brother."

JH: I, too, have noticed that when I meet someone, I may make a casual mention of marijuana just to gauge the person's reaction.

ZS: To ask, "Is it safe?"

JH: Right! Can we talk about this?

ZS: Right!

JH: Let's say that if it were not illegal to do so, and if you wanted to, you could introduce MDMA to a group of people or to a congregation. Would you want to do that?

ZS: The answer is yes. A definite yes.

JH: What do you think would be your goals in having a group session?

ZS: It would create a collusion of ethics. Right now the ethics are dog eat dog. There is a Greek word that speaks about the love that you have for the people in your group—*agape*. To create an agape community and then to work with the people in the group about what will be the ethics that will work in the community and the kind of ethics to try to bring into the world—

I think that would be a very beautiful thing to do. I can imagine that the seder that would happen among people who have had MDMA would be such a wonderful, deep experience.

JH: I keep coming back to the word love. That is the bottom line—the likely outcome of a group experience and what people would want to take away from the experience and share with others.

ZS: Right. The question is how to digest that. I think the preparation of people before the experience and the processing afterward are going to be important.

JH: There's no question that the set and the setting, as with any drug experience, are crucial. I also agree that what is learned, what is communicated between the participants, and then what is communicated with others all are important.

ZS: Yes. Then there is the issue of guilt. There are some people who carry heavy burdens of guilt. To be able to enter a place of forgiveness, assisted by MDMA, would make a great deal of difference.

JH: I think about acceptance a lot, but I don't usually think of it in terms of forgiveness or its application to guilt.

ZS: When you begin with acceptance first, you include yourself and the other one in the circle of humanity. And then there is a way of saying "I forgive" from that place, which you couldn't say before acceptance.

JH: It does seem very healing, the ideas of acceptance and forgiveness.

ZS: I think the intergenerational use of MDMA would be a remarkable thing.

JH: One of the optimal goals of most people's therapies is to forgive their parents.

ZS: Have you ever heard of the Hoffman Quadrinity Process? There's a group of people who are doing things in one week in California that really open the field for reconciliation with parents. I did it when I was sixty years old, and it goes from the somatic way of getting rid of the anger by thrashing it out—killing the parents, as it were—to a point where you defend your parents. You get to a place where you are angry with God and then become reconciled. It's a remarkable process. A couple of weeks after I was finished with that, I went to see my mother. For the first time in years, I was able to see her in the present, not as an ogre who would eat me up alive. That was very helpful.

JH: There is so much anger and hurt and confusion buried between family members. I imagine an MDMA-assisted family therapy session could go a long way toward resolving these sentiments and bringing about a sense of forgiveness. This reconciliation, with the family, and perhaps even with God, seems like a beautiful and serene sabbath.

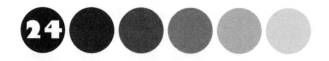

MDMA'S PROMISE AS A PRESCRIPTION MEDICINE
An Interview with
Rick Doblin, Ph.D.

JH: Dr. Doblin, how did you first hear about MDMA?

RD: I first heard about MDMA in 1982. I was going back to college as a freshman to study psychedelics, after having dropped out ten years before to devote myself to integrating difficult psychedelic experiences of my own. Just as I was supposed to start the school year, I learned of a month-long workshop at Esalen given by Stan Grof. Stan was teaching a breathing technique that was a legal alternative to the use of psychedelics. I managed to arrange for off-campus learning and went to the workshop. While I was there, I heard about MDMA. My first impression was "Why bother?" I was told that it helps you feel deeper emotions and get close to people, but it just seemed like a mild "feel-good" drug. It didn't seem as if you could dredge up the depths of your soul and wrestle with your demons, and it didn't seem possible that you could have any powerful transformations, such as the ones catalyzed by LSD. It seemed somehow superficial and not profound.

JH: Did it sound too easy?

RD: Yes, too easy. I wasn't interested in it. I don't drink alcohol, and I don't smoke cigarettes. I generally don't use drugs to feel good.

JH: You use them to get work done?

RD: I'm more results-oriented. It just seemed as if it would be soft and sweet, like taking a tranquilizer. I just didn't quite see the point of it. On the other hand, several people who had tried it told me that they had found it to be of substantial value.

JH: Of value for what?

RD: It was of value for understanding their emotional struggles and in communicating with their significant others. My inquisitive nature triumphed, and I decided that I would go ahead and get some MDMA, bring it home, and take it with my girlfriend. There was a degree of excitement and anticipation, but no real great expectation on the day we set aside to try MDMA. It was in October 1982. To our great surprise, the experience was quite valuable in helping us blend with each other and talk at a deep level. It was marvelous. We had a sense of astonishment at how little difference there was between the MDMA experience and our normal way of being together. The MDMA experience was so subtle, so clear. It didn't really affect our processes of thinking or our perceptions. It wasn't in any way like LSD. This was completely different—a much more gentle change—and yet it was profound. I was amazed at how easy it had been for me to dismiss it earlier and yet how utterly useful and important I saw it could be. The central point of it was that we both felt that it wasn't the drug talking; it was us, expressing our love to each other. It was a drug that helped us reach levels of ourselves that were genuine, that represented our deeper feelings. We weren't always able to speak from that depth; this was a glimpse of our potential and what we were able to accomplish in special moments, but it didn't seem in any way artificial. It felt very true.

JH: I think that it takes away a lot of the fear that we have in expressing ourselves and our love for one another.

RD: There's a certain responsibility that comes from having that experience and then trying to act at that depth at other times of your life, when you're not under the influence of the drug. It takes a lot of learning and a lot of work to be that honest, clear, and open about potentially critical information. One way to deal with it is to recognize these difficulties and to work hard to bring that depth into your daily life. The other way, psychologically speaking—which is what a lot of people do—is to say, "Well, that was a false experience, and I don't have to try to live up to that because that wasn't real. That was a drug experience." Then you accept an easier, lower level of daily functioning. I would rather live with the knowledge that there is a depth that I'm not reaching as the result of limitations that I have to work on, rather than to deny the reality of those moments that MDMA shows are within our potential.

JH: I'm very glad you said that. I think there are many people who discount the MDMA experience, as if it is a completely artificial state as opposed to a more highly developed one. What you glimpse in the midst of an MDMA experience is like seeing the peak of a mountain, and you can see the path that will take you to the top. It gives you the vision and the motivation to keep on hiking. You get a taste of what your ultimate self could be, and maybe you even see what steps you have to take to actualize that vision. Another way it is described is like seeing the picture on the jigsaw puzzle box. You get to see the way the picture should come together, the finished product, and it motivates and helps you try to construct that.

It is somewhat enigmatic. This is a powerful tool, but the shift in consciousness is very subtle. You've described it, and so have I, as akin to the feeling after a deep, cleansing breath. And I have had people tell me that the experience can't be that gentle. I think that in a therapeutic setting, when you're relaxed and it's quiet and you're not dancing at a club, the shift really is that mild.

RD: One of the tragedies of the war on drugs is that MDMA research could help us understand the processes of love and acceptance. You would think that with something that affects those basic emotions, that reduces fear to help one express love and to accept and integrate deeply painful but necessary emotions, we would have hundreds of psychologists doing their dissertations on MDMA. MDMA helps strengthen the ego so that you can hear—you really want to hear—what people think of you and feel about you in an honest way. You can accept the information without having it shatter your ego. There's a whole empowering of your self, an acceptance of yourself. Those are such crucial aspects of being alive and human. You would think that there would be a tremendous amount of research, not so much on MDMA's therapeutic potential or on MDMA's neurotoxicity but into the basic psychological processes of how we experience love and how we build ego strength and self-acceptance. None of that research is happening.

It's just so sad to see MDMA being portrayed inaccurately in the media, and by the government, particularly, as a drug whose main effect is death and destruction and producing holes in a person's brain. It's been more than twenty years of lost opportunities. Fundamental areas of human functioning could have been looked at through the lens of MDMA, and substantial amounts of productive therapeutic work could have been conducted, but this has not happened. It's impossible to quantify these lost benefits, but I feel confident that they drastically outweigh any harms that the prohibition of MDMA has reduced.

JH: Let's talk about those twenty years. What were the steps you took after your initial MDMA experience to approach the government?

RD: When I first learned about MDMA in 1982, it was still legal. In contrast, I had learned about and started appreciating LSD in 1971, after it had been made illegal and the government crackdown on research was almost complete. I was in the tail end of the sixties generation, and I unfortunately missed the golden era, when it was possible to investigate psychedelics scientifically. When I learned about MDMA, I realized that this was an extraordinary situation in which there was a semisecret underground river that was nourishing the psychedelic community. I realized that there were people in respected social, academic, and even government positions who might be willing to try the drug while it was legal but would not do so after it was made illegal. If they had valuable experiences, these people could help defend the use of MDMA when the inevitable government effort to criminalize it eventually would begin. So I began contacting these sorts of people.

JH: Who?

RD: In particular, I got in touch with Robert Muller, the Assistant Secretary-General of the United Nations. He had written a book called *New Genesis: Shaping a Global Spirituality*. The thesis of the book was that at the core of each religion there is a certain mystical understanding of our shared humanity that is relatively similar and leads to tolerance, understanding, and respect. Yet there are still many wars that are products of religious hatred and intolerance that are as deadly and as common as the wars based on nationalism. Robert Muller proposed that the United Nations be supplemented by an organization that represented the world's religions, to provide a context for them to find common ground. I was very impressed with what he had to say. Here was a person in a politically powerful position who was talking about the importance of spirituality. I thought perhaps he might be interested in helping promote research into the spiritual potential of psychedelics. I wrote a letter to him saying that I was inspired by his arguments but wanted to request that he extend his analysis a bit to include the idea that psychedelics were tools to understand and explore spirituality. I mentioned that every new method of killing gets virtually unlimited research money from the militaries around the world, yet psychedelic research into spirituality was politically blocked. I asked him, "Would you help out in trying to support psychedelic research?" I felt as though I was somebody who was stranded on a deserted island and was throwing out a message in a bottle to see if anyone would respond.

Here I was an undergraduate at college, with no credentials, and an Assistant Secretary-General of the United Nations wrote me back! He sent a handwritten letter saying that he agreed with what I was proposing and that he would help. He sent a list of several people, Christian and Zen monks, scholars of religion, whom he wanted me to contact and have them evaluate what I had to say. I had discussed MDMA in the letter and read into his letter a little subtext, which was to send them MDMA. I contacted a few of these people, and some of them were willing to have me send them MDMA and then report back to him, which they did.

My sister worked for a congressman and has never chosen to take any drugs, but she was willing to help me build a case for psychedelic research. She helped me contact Dr. Carleton Turner, the Reagan-era equivalent of "drug czar." I made an appeal to him about the importance of studying psychedelics, discussed the political suppression of research, and asked if he would help. He responded, which surprised me, and referred me to a colleague for further discussions, though not involving actual use of MDMA. Those were my two main political contacts, one with the United Nations and one with the U.S. government. I also contacted various people in academic institutions.

JH: Tell me about the ARUPA conference you helped coordinate.

RD: Every few years or so, the psychedelic community used to have small invitation-only conferences at Esalen. Dick Price, the co-founder of Esalen, came up with the name ARUPA, which stands for the Association for the Responsible Use of Psychedelic Agents. It's also a Sanskrit word meaning "formless," since the group organizing the conferences was never formally incorporated and involved a shifting cast of characters. A copy of the letter that I had written to Robert Muller found its way to Laura Huxley, the wife of Aldous Huxley. She spoke to Alise Agar about it, and Alise invited me to one of these Esalen conferences. Alise is a remarkable woman who knit together the psychedelic community. After attending one conference, I worked to help organize another one in 1984, which focused in part on MDMA. Dr. Carleton Turner even sent a representative. At about this time, Debby Harlow, Alise Agar, and I established a nonprofit organization to support psychedelic research. The organization was called Earth Metabolic Design Laboratories.

JH: Who attended that ARUPA conference?

RD: Dick Price, Leo Zeff, Sasha Shulgin, Stan Grof, and Terence McKenna, among others. Terence and I had an important interaction that led to the first biomedical study of the physical effects of MDMA in humans. Terence, as you know, was very sympathetic with the potential of plant medicines.

JH: I know. He and I had several conversations about why he could never really get behind MDMA—it was a synthetic molecule and didn't come directly out of the earth.

RD: Terence was talking about MDMA's riskiness due to its being a synthetic drug. I asked for proof and said, "Terence, we should arrange for a study of MDMA, and we should do it now, while it's still legal. I'll put up a thousand dollars for a study of MDMA." And then Dick Price said, "I'll put up a thousand dollars, too." And that was the genesis for Dr. Jack Downing's study of the effects of a single dose of MDMA on about twenty volunteers, which later took place under the auspices of Leo Zeff and was published in the *Journal of Psychoactive Drugs* [Downing 1986].

JH: Were you one of the subjects in that study?

RD: I was one of the helpers, not one of the subjects; I was there as one of the funders and coordinators. It was just a beautiful experience. It took place at a house on Stinson Beach, in northern California, on the ocean. This was in 1984. I had been trying since 1983 to get studies started on the basic safety of MDMA, but ones that could be kept quiet at first. I was worried that if they were made public, the government would act precipitously against MDMA.

JH: Next in the timeline came the Drug Enforcement Administration trials.

RD: In July 1984, Sasha [Shulgin] learned of the DEA's intention of placing MDMA in Schedule I. The DEA had published in the *Federal Register* its intent to criminalize MDMA and announced a legally required thirty-day comment period. I wanted to put my energy into fighting the DEA's efforts, as did Debby and Alise. We had been doing a lot of proselytizing during 1983–84, not just through Robert Muller but through all sorts of connections—previous psychedelic researchers, academic experts, Lester Grinspoon at Harvard, all sorts of people with whom we had communicated about the potential of MDMA. We decided to organize a formal protest to the DEA's proposed scheduling of MDMA. Sasha suggested that I contact a lawyer in Washington, Richard Cotton, who might be willing to work with us. We had to pay for some expenses, but his firm took the case pro bono. We outlined a strategy that involved gathering a respected group of people willing to sign a request for a hearing. I gathered those petitions and then walked into DEA headquarters to hand-deliver the request for a hearing. That was a sweet moment. I later learned that the DEA had absolutely no knowledge of the underground therapeutic use of MDMA and were taken totally by surprise by our petition. The DEA administrative law judge saw that we had sufficiently credible people requesting a hearing and decided to grant our request.

Once we got the DEA hearing, it became clear that the DEA was trying to criminalize MDMA not only in the United States but also internationally through the World Heath Organization [WHO]. This was when I asked Robert Muller for help. He helped me arrange to meet with the crucial people at UNESCO [United Nations Educational Scientific and Cultural Organization] and the WHO in Geneva, where I went in February 1985, bringing information about the therapeutic use of MDMA. Through unbelievable coincidence and synchronicity, Stan Grof's brother was the head of the Expert Committee at WHO that was going to help decide the fate of MDMA internationally.

JH: Oh, God!

RD: Stan Grof's brother is a respected psychiatrist in Canada who has conducted more traditional psychiatric research. He was appointed the chair of this Expert Committee. He was the only member who objected to the scheduling of MDMA, fearing that it would impede research. In any case, while I was in Geneva, I met Bob Schuster, who was the scientific consultant to the Expert Committee. I discussed MDMA's therapeutic potential, and he told me about George Ricaurte's neurotoxicity findings.

JH: With MDA, not MDMA.

RD: Right. Bob Schuster wasn't alarmist; he simply noted that there were some small effects of MDA on serotonin levels. He thought MDMA should be on Schedule III, which made any nonmedical use criminal but still allowed physicians to administer the drug legally to patients. When I came back from Geneva in February, there was starting to be some publicity about MDMA and about the upcoming DEA hearings. For several years starting in the early 1980s, Sasha and others had been able to dissuade the media from reporting on MDMA, but once the DEA moved against MDMA and we had demanded a hearing, media interest started to develop. The *Phil Donahue Show* contacted me and asked me to help organize a panel to appear. I agreed and suggested Dr. Rick Ingrasci, a psychiatrist who had given MDMA to many patients. I also recommended that Bob Schuster be invited to participate.

This took place at a time when I was being contacted quite a lot by the media. The crucial difficulty for me was that reporters asked, "Your organization is fighting for therapeutic use, but what do you think about criminalizing recreational use?" I felt compelled to say that the drug war was counterproductive and that I didn't feel that making the recreational use of MDMA criminal was wise. That caused a lot of tension within Earth Metabolic Design Laboratories (EMD). Some of the doctors and other people with established reputations and credentials were willing to be identified in public as supporting medical use but not recreational use. Right before the Donahue show was to be taped, I decided to resign from EMD rather than split the organization; I appeared in the audience and not on the program. I spoke a little bit about the need for MDMA research, but from the floor and not as a member of the panel. Unexpectedly, the Donahue show was the key event that led to the DEA's emergency scheduling of MDMA.

JH: Because of Schuster?

RD: Gene Haslip of the DEA was on the show, and that's the first time that anybody from the DEA had heard about potential MDMA neurotoxicity.

JH: Wasn't it your fault that Schuster was on that show? Do you feel bad about that at all?

RD: You can't always predict what's going to happen. Schuster's point of view was that MDMA should be put in Schedule III, which was the same position we were requesting in the DEA hearings. I thought that here we had an influential scientist who was working with the World Health Organization and felt that MDMA should be made available to doctors, so why not put him on the show? About a year later, the DEA's emergency scheduling was voided, since the DEA had not been delegated the authority by the Attorney General to schedule drugs on an emergency basis. Moreover, Schuster subsequently was appointed as the head of the National Institute on Drug Abuse (NIDA).

JH: Isn't he now working in conjunction with Manny Tancer to do clinical research with MDMA?

RD: Yes! You can read about it on the MAPS website (www.maps.org/newsletters/v07n3/07305tan.html).

JH: Did Schuster speak at the DEA trials?

RD: No. Lewis Seiden, a research associate of Bob Schuster's at the University of Chicago, spoke on the neurotoxicity of MDA.

JH: Did you go to all the DEA trials?

RD: Yes, we coordinated that process. I thought it likely that we would not be able to keep MDMA legally available to physicians and concluded that the only avenue that was going to be left was working through the Food and Drug Administration to develop MDMA as a prescription medicine. Shortly before I left EMD, I initiated twenty-eight-day toxicity studies of MDMA in dogs and rats, to put us in position to do human studies sanctioned by the FDA. I contacted Dave Nichols, a medicinal chemist at Purdue University, to make a kilogram of MDMA for research purposes. We paid him four thousand dollars—four dollars a gram! This is the MDMA that has been used for all the FDA-approved human research in the United States. Raising money for the animal studies was difficult, as you can imagine, because a lot of people in the psychedelic community don't believe in animal testing.

JH: And the animals have to be killed.

RD: Yes, definitely.

JH: How did you feel at the end of the DEA hearings?

RD: I felt proud. We had educated a lot of people through the media about the therapeutic benefits of MDMA and created a public record of support for MDMA's therapeutic potential. We delayed the criminalization of MDMA by about seven months, so I felt satisfaction in thinking of all those people who had legal MDMA experiences in that time who would not have done so otherwise. I had never thought that we would win anyway.

JH: But initially you won. The DEA administrative law judge who presided over all the trials, after nearly two years of testimony and three separate court dates, ruled in favor of Schedule III.

RD: Right, but then the head of the DEA overruled him.

JH: When Judge Francis Young ruled in favor of Schedule III, you were surprised?

RD: Yes.

JH: And you weren't surprised when John Lawn overturned it?

RD: Not at all. It always seemed to me as if we were going to lose. We were in the Reagan era; the drug war was escalating. But the victory was communicating to the public the potential benefits of MDMA.

JH: You got through to me. I hope that's something.

RD: Exactly. I felt great about it. Then, when we finally lost, it was clear that in the long run the only way MDMA was going to be saved was through the FDA. After I left EMD, I started a new organization, the Multidisciplinary Association for Psychedelic Studies [MAPS]. It took me a while to get a new nonprofit group organized and approved, and it took a while for the animal studies to get done, but what I asked for in exchange for leaving EMD was that the animal data become the property of MAPS. I used that data to open the Drug Master File for MDMA at the FDA.

Through an ironic twist of fate, I needed to use the data in the Drug Master File on behalf of my own grandmother. She had had a recurrence of severe unipolar depression. This time she was treatment-resistant and failed to obtain relief after several courses of electroconvulsive therapy, lithium, and numerous other medications. Underlying her depression was debilitating fear and anxiety, which I thought might be alleviated to some degree, if only for a short period of time, by MDMA. After consulting with her psychiatrist, my mother and my father, a physician, agreed to go forward, but only if I could obtain legal permission for the experiment. Although a psychiatrist experienced in psychedelic research and I both negotiated with the FDA, we met with irrational resistance. The FDA claimed that my grandmother needed to be protected from the risk of neurotoxic effects, despite an appeal from her and her family stating her willingness to accept that risk. She stopped eating and had to be force-fed, but still the FDA prevented us from giving her MDMA. I even appealed to the Assistant Secretary for Health, to no avail. After she died, with her depression still in full flower, I coped by committing myself even more to opening the door to the full exploration of MDMA's therapeutic potential.

JH: What would you say is the mission of MAPS?

RD: MAPS is supposed to ensure that what happened to my grandmother does not happen to anyone else. It is designed to support scientific research into the risks and benefits of psychedelics and marijuana. We recruit researchers who may be interested in these topics, and we offer them assistance in protocol design, working through the regulatory system, funding, and contacting other scientists to establish collaborative networks. We move as efficiently as we can in a strategic manner toward an opening of the regulatory system to permit legal access to these substances, initially in the treatment of disease but also eventually for broader purposes, meaning personal growth, creativity, spirituality. The point of greatest leverage for MAPS is FDA-approved research into medical applications. We are not a lobbying organization to change laws, since we work within the current regulatory system.

JH: When did you enter the doctoral program at Harvard?

RD: I started at the Kennedy School of Government in 1988 in a two-year program, for a master's in public policy. That led me into the Ph.D. program, which I have just completed. When I started at New College in 1982, I was studying psychology and psychedelic research. Since I first took LSD in 1971, I had been training to become a psychedelic therapist, underground if necessary. But when I graduated from New College in 1987, I was rejected at all the clinical psychology Ph.D. programs to which I applied. I got very close several times, but when I mentioned my desire to conduct MDMA psychotherapy research for my dissertation, I encountered resistance among a few faculty members, enough to remove me from the A-list. After my last rejection, I realized that since politics was in the way of what I really wanted to study, I might as well study politics. During the DEA hearings, I had created a tutorial in drug policy, which fascinated me. Suing the DEA led me to the Kennedy School!

JH: Did you ever perform any underground MDMA-assisted psychotherapy?

RD: Yes. In fact, it has proved to be the thread that is now becoming my major focus with MAPS, to conduct MDMA post-traumatic stress disorder research. In early 1984, before MDMA was scheduled, I attended another month-long workshop at Esalen with Stan Grof, this one on spiritual emergencies. The day after I returned home, I received a phone call from a friend of mine, who asked me to consider working with his ex-girlfriend. They had taken MDMA together, during which time past episodes of sexual abuse flooded her awareness unexpectedly. This had disturbed her so much that she subsequently checked herself into a hospital so that she wouldn't commit suicide. She had been suicidal and in and out of hospitals before he met her. She had been brutally raped in an earlier period of her life and also had had other horrible things happen to her. The psychiatrists in her past and during her most recent hospitalization had given her all the typical antidepressant medications that cover the symptoms but don't deal with the problem.

JH: I'm glad you mentioned that.

RD: He said that after she was released from the hospital, she still felt suicidal and hopeless about finding the help she needed. He asked me if I would try to help her, as a last resort. I agreed to try, with a substantial amount of trepidation. I spoke to her and said, "If you promise not to commit suicide while you're with me, I'll try my best to be helpful." She came down, and we structured a three-week process. She was under round-the-clock supervision by me or her friends at school. She agreed to stop taking her antidepressants. We conducted an MDMA session for PTSD. We also did a subsequent combination LSD and MDMA session.

These sessions helped her substantially. They didn't solve all her problems, but they helped her start to find a process to work through things. Because of that experience sixteen years ago, she has changed her career goals. She is studying to become a licensed therapist, is in a master's program in transpersonal psychology at Naropa Institute, and is working as a co-therapist in Spain on the MAPS-funded MDMA/PTSD project. It's that sort of depth of time and experience that gives me a lot of courage. She tells me that in her life those experiences have proved to be valuable not just at that time, in the short run, but over the long term. She looks back on her life and identifies that as a turning point. [For her personal account, see www.maps.org/research/mdma/marcela.html.]

JH: You were obviously impressed with the clinical utility of using MDMA in psychotherapy.

RD: Completely. In 1984, I also worked with a friend of mine, a musician in his mid-thirties who had cancer of the esophagus. He and his girlfriend had moved into his parent's home so that he could die near his family, and he and his girlfriend asked me to conduct an MDMA session with them. At the time we did the session, he couldn't eat and was being fed through a tube. He was on massive amounts of morphine, but the pain was still there. The morphine was so strong that he really wasn't present; he was nodding out most of the time. We worked with MDMA, and they had a beautiful, life-affirming experience. It was so scary for me, because I was thinking, "My God, what if he dies while we are doing this?" He was so near death anyway. First of all, he ended up being pain free and completely lucid for an extended period of time. Second, they went through a beautiful review of their relationship; they were clearly saying good-bye. He died six days later. He slept peacefully every night until then. I remember leaving that night in elation. I was so glad that I had taken the risk to try to help him. The last thing he said to me as I walked out the door was "Rick, you under-dosed me."

JH: I'm glad that you mention not only PTSD but also palliative care and treatment of the dying patient. This is a group of patients with minimal treatment options. Doctors talk about keeping people comfortable, but they don't always do a very good job. There is so much fear surrounding death that I think it exacerbates the pain. And the families and loved ones are in pain too.

RD: I have one more story about a friend's father, who was in his fifties and dying of cancer. My friend was very close to her dad, and she decided to share some MDMA with him. I talked to him about it ahead of time and then afterward. He said, "You know, I used to deny the fact that I was dying, but now with the help of MDMA, I've accepted it. That has brought me a lot of peace, but I'm wondering if this acceptance of death is actually going to make me die sooner." We talked about that, and together we came up with the idea that by accepting death, he was no longer using his energy to fight against the truth of his disease. Instead he had liberated his attention to appreciate each remaining moment of his life, which would prolong the experience. He increased his ability to really enjoy the time that he had left.

JH: MDMA can help improve the quality of life you have left, not just for the patient but for the family as well.

RD: Exactly. And he felt that by virtue of enjoying every day . . .

JH: He could make it last that much longer.

RD: Yes. And he did survive longer than people thought he would. He hung on, fighting but not denying. I have had several experiences performing MDMA-assisted psychotherapy with people who had PTSD, people who were dying, people in relationships. I know a married couple who couldn't conceive a child. They had not been using birth control for about a year and a half. Under the influence of MDMA one night, they spoke with each other about their struggles trying to get pregnant and their fears and anxieties about becoming parents. The wife felt something shift somehow inside her body, and she had an intuition that she could now get pregnant. They had sex right then and conceived. Their daughter is now fourteen years old.

JH: That brings us to another potential therapeutic use, which is mind/body medicine. MDMA could be a useful tool not just for psychiatry but also for medicine.

RD: I once sat with a doctor who took MDMA. During the experience, his whole right arm became paralyzed. I had learned from Stan and others, from breath work, and from LSD-catalyzed psychotherapy that there is a mind/body connection and that psychological issues can be expressed symbolically in the body. Instead of panicking and saying, "Oh, my God, let's get him to the emergency room; he's paralyzed," I said, "Okay, what does this mean?" And he told me a story about how he had a very conflicted relationship with his father and, in fact, that he had hated his father. But when his father drew near the end of his life and was dying, the family came to him and said, "Your dad is not really conscious. He's just on life support, and we need somebody in the family to pull the plug." And he physically pulled the plug.

JH: With that hand.

RD: With that hand. Once we talked it all out at the end of the session, he could move his hand again. It's amazing the kind of mind/body connections that MDMA really opens up.

JH: What do you see as the future for MDMA as a prescription medicine?

RD: My dissertation was about just that. First, I believe that there is a way to regulate the use of MDMA as a prescription medicine so that society will obtain substantially more benefits than risks. I think we can control it in any number of ways through training requirements for psychiatrists, regulations for the facilities in which it's used, reporting systems, and patient registries. I believe that MDMA has tremendous potential as a prescription medicine to aid psychiatrists and psychotherapists. I think it would be about a five-million-dollar, five-year research project. If we had no political obstacles and just were able to work with the FDA the way any other pharmaceutical company could, I believe that in that time frame and with those finances, we could make MDMA into a prescription medicine for PTSD. That's what MAPS is working toward.

JH: Is your dissertation online? Is there somewhere people can go to learn more about the details of your proposal?

RD: Yes, they can check it out on the MAPS Web site at www.maps.org/docs/doblindissertation.pdf. I'll just very briefly outline how I think it could be done. First, I think the same standards that the FDA uses to evaluate other drugs in terms of safety and efficacy are appropriate for evaluating MDMA. Even though it's a psychedelic drug and it has abuse potential, the same basic standards of safety and efficacy that the FDA uses to evaluate other drugs would apply.

JH: Other controlled drugs?

RD: Yes, like marijuana.

JH: Or Percocet [oxycodone], which also has an abuse liability but some medical utility.

RD: Yes. The next question is this: Can the drug be used safely as a prescription medicine in the way that most other drugs are approved? My answer to that is no. MDMA should not be simply a prescription drug that any doctor can prescribe. MDMA is never going to be like Prozac—it will never be a take-home drug. It should be taken under the supervision of a therapist. I think there needs to be a medical doctor on the treatment team who is medically responsible for the patient, but non-physicians also can be excellent therapists. However, the doctors or therapists who administer MDMA should be required to have special training. The MDMA experience can be therapeutic, not inherently but because it is part of a therapeutic relationship between the doctor and the patient that requires sophistication and special training to manage.

Another issue is preventing sexual abuse of patients. There is a certain willingness on the part of patients under the influence of MDMA toward self-disclosure and trust. There's a long-established awareness in psychotherapy that the intimacy of the relationship sometimes shades into sexual relationships between patient and therapist that are not to the advantage of the patient. That particular problem is relevant to the regulation of MDMA psychotherapy, because MDMA helps people open up in very intimate ways. I think that safeguards need to be established, so that MDMA is not used in that way. There is also the issue of what kinds of facilities are most appropriate for this sort of treatment. If you restrict the use to certain facilities, it gives the regulators an easier way to control use than if doctors can conduct therapy anywhere.

JH: That method also allows for tighter control to prevent diversion, which I know that the government is always worried about.

RD: It's also easier to track, easier to monitor. I think that we need to look at the models that the FDA has increasingly come to rely upon, where they try to limit the use of certain prescription drugs to people with particular training. With certain drugs there has to be written informed consent, even once you are past the experimental phase; there are documents outlining the risks, which patients have to sign. One of the new innovations that has developed in the scheduling of the medical use of drugs of abuse is bifurcated scheduling. Congress created a law that criminalizes GHB [gamma-hydroxybutyrate] and places it in Schedule I for the purposes of nonmedical use, and heavy penalties apply. But when it is used as a medical drug, it's in Schedule III, which means that it's easier for doctors to gain access to it; it's easier to ship and store . . .

JH: And perform research.

RD: Right. It's possible that MDMA could be another candidate for that kind of bifurcated scheduling. Enforcement against the nonmedical use of

MDMA, as long as that is considered a priority by our country, is not compromised by the approval of MDMA for medical use. Every concern that the DEA and the FDA can articulate regarding public safety associated with the therapeutic use of MDMA can be met in regulatory schemes that are legal, practical, and not too expensive. We can approve the medical use of MDMA-assisted psychotherapy within our current regulatory scheme, within the current range of powers that the FDA has. We also can pretty much guarantee that in this kind of tightly regulated system, we will be able to obtain substantial medical, therapeutic benefits with minimal health costs. That is the challenge that MAPS is working to address.

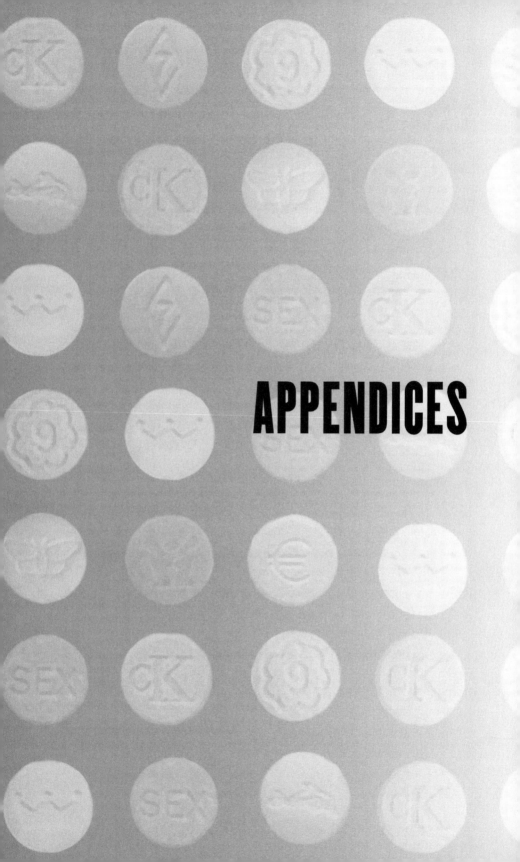

APPENDICES

HISTORY TIMELINE

1912   MDMA patent is filed by E. Merck in Darmstadt, Germany, on December 24.

1914   Patent is issued as number 274350 on May 16.

1924   Paper is published mentioning MDMA as intermediate in chemical synthesis.

1953   U.S. Army Chemical Center (contract no. DA-18-108-CML-5663) gives MDMA (code EA 1475) to laboratory animals at the University of Michigan.

1953   New York State Psychiatric Institute clinical research subject inadvertently killed with lethal dose of MDA (450 mg intravenous).

1960   Paper is published mentioning MDMA as intermediate in chemical synthesis.

1960s   Late in the decade MDA becomes popular and is nicknamed the "love drug."

1972   Gaston publishes street sample identified as MDMA, found in Chicago in 1970.

1973   Publication of Army Chemical Center's findings, declassified in 1969.

1976   Dr. Sasha Shulgin takes MDMA, 16 mg, for the first time on September 8, with no effect.

1976   Dr. Sasha Shulgin takes 81 mg of MDMA on September 27 and notes an effect.

1977   Shulgin introduces "Jacob," a therapist, to MDMA.

1977   MDMA is made illegal in the United Kingdom, added to the 1971 Misuse of Drugs Act.

1978   Sasha Shulgin and David Nichols publish first paper on human use of MDMA.

1970s–1980s   The mid-1970s to the mid-1980s sees the legal therapeutic use of MDMA in psychotherapy.

1980s   Popular use of MDMA begins in the United States in the early part of the decade.

1983   MPTP causes a Parkinson's-like syndrome in several Californian IV heroin abusers.

1983/4   Proto-raves with Balearic music begin on the Spanish island of Ibiza.

1984   On June 10, the *San Francisco Register* publishes first big story about MDMA.

1984   On July 27, DEA publishes plans in the *Federal Register* to put MDMA in Schedule I.

On September 10, Thomas Roberts, Ph.D.; George Greer, M.D.; Lester Grinspoon, M.D.; James Bakalar, Ph.D.; and their attorney, Richard Cotton, send a letter to the DEA administrator requesting hearings on the scheduling of MDMA.

1984–   Ecstasy use grows in popularity in Spain.
1986

mid-   MDMA appears on the street in Australia.
1980s

1985   On February 1, DEA holds first hearing in Washington, D.C. (attorneys only, no witnesses).

1985   On March 10–15, Earth Metabolic Design sponsors conference on MDMA at Esalen.

1985   Emerging recreational use in Texas captures attention of Senator Lloyd Bentsen.

1985   On May 31, DEA announces plan of emergency ban to place MDMA in Schedule I for one year.

1985   On June 10 and 11, DEA holds second hearing, in Los Angeles.

1985   On July 1, emergency scheduling of MDMA as Schedule I drug takes effect.

1985   Underground therapeutic use of MDMA continues in psychotherapy.

1985   On July 10 and 11, DEA holds third hearing, in Kansas City, Missouri.

1985   On October 8–11, DEA holds fourth hearing, in Washington, D.C.

1986   On February 11, MDMA is placed in Schedule I internationally by the United Nations' Commission on Narcotic Drug Laws.

1986   Greer and Tolbert publish their results from MDMA-assisted psychotherapy sessions.

1986   MAPS president Rick Doblin opens Drug Master File for MDMA at FDA (no. 6293).

1986   On May 18–19, Haight-Ashbury Free Clinic sponsors MDMA conference.

1986   On May 22, DEA administrative law judge Francis Young recommends Schedule III placement of MDMA.

1986   On May 30, MDMA is made illegal in Spain.

1986   On October 14, DEA publishes ruling in *Federal Register*, overruling Judge Young.

1986   On November 13, Schedule I status for MDMA takes effect.

1987   Dowling reports on five fatalities associated with Ecstasy use.

1987   Peroutka compares cerebrospinal fluid of Ecstasy users and controls and sees no difference in the level of the serotonin metabolite 5-HIAA.

1987   In the summer, Ecstasy use at discos increases in frequency on the Spanish island of Ibiza. That fall, the parties are exported back to Manchester, England.

1987   On September 18, the case of *Lester Grinspoon, M.D., v. DEA* begins in the First Circuit Court of Appeals in Boston, with Richard Cotton as attorney.

1987   December 22, 1987, to March 22, 1988, marks the "Grinspoon window": MDMA is briefly unscheduled owing to appeal process.

1988   On January 27, the DEA removes MDMA from Schedule I after court mandate 12/22/87.

1988   In February, the DEA publishes in *Federal Register* the intent to place MDMA in Schedule I, starting March 23, 1988.

1988   On March 23, MDMA is placed in Schedule I, with no subsequent appeals.

1988   In June the United Kingdom reports its first Ecstasy death, 21-year-old Ian Larcombe, who was alleged to have taken eighteen tablets at once.

1988   Britain's "Summer of Love" is marked by increased MDMA consumption.

1988   Psycholytic psychotherapy with MDMA begins in Switzerland.

1989   In the summer, large outdoor dance parties gain in popularity in the United Kingdom.

1990   Harlow and Beck present their findings from surveying psychiatrists who used MDMA in their practices.

1990   Ricaurte demonstrates a lower level of cerebrospinal fluid 5-HIAA levels in Ecstasy users versus chronic back pain patients.

1990s   Raves continue to grow in popularity among members of a large youth movement in Britain.

1991   One of the first large U.S. raves is held in San Francisco: "Toon Town" debuts.

1992–   Widespread MDMA use is noted in Spain.
1996

1992   Henry reports on cases of hyperthermia and hepatitis associated with Ecstasy use.

1992   On July 15, FDA meeting allows Dr. Charles Grob to perform clinical MDMA research.

1993   In January, the United Kingdom adopts Safer Dancing Campaign to diminish rave-associated injuries.

1993   Psycholytic psychotherapy ends in Switzerland.

1994   On May 18, Dr. Charles Grob gives first dose of MDMA to human subjects at UCLA.

1995   In February, Sasha Shulgin turns in his DEA license.

1995   Anna Woods, schoolgirl in Sidney, Australia, dies as the result of Ecstasy use.

1995   On November 16, England's Leah Betts dies. Her life support is removed five days after her eighteenth birthday, when she took one tablet of Ecstasy and drank copious amounts of water.

1999   In March, Sammy "the Bull" Gravano is arrested for running an Ecstasy ring in Arizona that distributed 25,000 pills per week.

1999   From August 30 to September 1, MAPS sponsors Israel MDMA conference.

1999   On December 2, NIDA launches multimedia campaign to educate the public about "club drugs," including website www.clubdrugs.org, and announces a $54 million budget.

2000   On May 25, the Club Drug Anti-Proliferation Act is introduced in Congress (HR 4553).

2000   On July 31, DEA sponsors the conference Ecstasy and Club Drugs: Dancing with Darkness.

2000   On September 27, modified Club Drug Act is signed by President Clinton.

2000   On November 9, Spain's José Carlos Bouso gives first dose of MDMA in PTSD study.

STATISTICS TIMELINE

1976   Ronald Siegel estimates that 10,000 doses of Ecstasy were consumed in America in that year (Siegel 1985).

1977–
1981   8 deaths are attributed to MDMA.

1980   Rick Doblin estimates that by 1980, more than 11 million doses of MDMA had been consumed worldwide (Rosenbaum and Doblin 1991).

1982   Harris opinion poll for the BBC in the United Kingdom reports that 31 percent of the people between the ages of 16 and 25 years admitted to taking Ecstasy, and 67 percent reported that their friends had tried the drug (Harris Research Center 1982).

1985   Ronald Siegel estimates that 30,000 doses are consumed per month in America (Siegel 1985).

1985   28 emergency room visits for MDMA use are reported in the United States.

1986   39 emergency room visits for MDMA use are reported in the United States.

1986   8 percent of the college students at Stanford report MDMA use (Calvert 1987).

1987   39 emergency room visits for MDMA use are reported in the United States.

1987   39 percent of Stanford students report having used Ecstasy (369 surveyed) (Peroutka 1987).

1987   20 percent of undergraduates at the University of Colorado report having used Ecstasy (Accola 1988).

1988   15.5 percent of Tulane University students (742 surveyed) report having used Ecstasy (Patterson et al. 1988).

1989   First significant seizures of Ecstasy are reported in the United Kingdom; 32,000 tablets are confiscated.

1991   Less than 200 emergency room visits for Ecstasy use are reported in the U.S. by DAWN.

1992   236 emergency room visits for Ecstasy use are reported in the United States.

1993   68 emergency room visits for Ecstasy use are reported in the United States.

1993   8 deaths are attributed to Ecstasy in England and Wales.

1993   NIDA survey: 2 percent of all college students report Ecstasy use in the past year.

1994   250 emergency room visits for Ecstasy use are reported in United States.

1994   24.3 percent of Tulane University students report having used Ecstasy (1,264 surveyed) (Cuomo et al. 1994).

1994   27 deaths are attributed to Ecstasy in England and Wales.

1994   1 death is attributed to Ecstasy in the United States.

1995   421 emergency room visits for Ecstasy use are reported in the United States.

1995   10 deaths are attributed to Ecstasy in England and Wales.

1995   6 deaths are attributed to Ecstasy in the United States.

1995   Nicholas Saunders estimates that 6 percent of 15-year-olds are using Ecstasy.

1996   English newspaper *Guardian* estimates 500,000 to 1 million people use Ecstasy each weekend and calls it the "largest youth phenomenon in British history."

1996   16 deaths are attributed to Ecstasy in England and Wales.

1996   8 deaths are attributed to Ecstasy in the United States.

1996   319 emergency room visits for Ecstasy use are cited in the United States.

1996   U.S. Department of Health and Human Services household survey reports that 1.1 percent of those 12 to 17, 4.2 percent of those 18 to 25, 2.5 percent of those 26 to 34, and 0.7 percent of those over 35 admitted to using Ecstasy at least once in their lives, totaling 1.5 percent of the U.S. population.

1996   Monitoring the Future Study reports 3.4 percent of eighth-graders, 5.6 percent of tenth-graders, and 6.1 percent of twelfth-graders admitted to using Ecstasy at least once in their lives.

1997   637 emergency room visits for Ecstasy use are reported in the United States.

1997   11 deaths are attributed to Ecstasy in England and Wales.

1997   3 deaths are attributed to Ecstasy in the United States.

1997   Household survey reports 1.3 percent of those 12 to 17, 4.6 percent of those 18 to 25, 3.1 percent of those 26 to 34, and 0.5 percent of those over 35 admitted to using Ecstasy at least once in their lives, totaling 1.5 percent of the U.S. population.

1997   Monitoring the Future Study reports that 3.2 percent of eighth-graders, 5.7 percent of tenth-graders, and 6.9 percent twelfth-graders admitted to using Ecstasy at least once in their lives.

1997   U.S. Customs reports seizures of 400,000 hits of Ecstasy.

1997   Drugs and dance survey indicates that 84 percent of people attending dance events in London reported use of Ecstasy.

1998   Household survey reports that 1.6 percent of those 12 to 17, 5.0 percent of those 18 to 25, 2.6 percent of those 26 to 34, and 0.5 percent of those over 35 admitted to using Ecstasy at least once in their lives, totaling 1.5 percent of the U.S. population.

1998   Monitoring the Future Study reports 2.7 percent of eighth-graders, 5.1 percent of tenth-graders, and 5.8 percent of twelfth-graders admitted to using Ecstasy at least once in their lives.

1998   1,143 emergency room visits for Ecstasy use are cited in the United States.

1998   9 deaths are attributed to Ecstasy in the United States.

1998   Household survey reports at least 3.4 million Americans 12 years and older have tried Ecstasy at least once in their lifetimes.

1998   DEA reports seizures of 750,000 hits of Ecstasy—tablets and powder combined (Cloud 2000).

1998   British Crime Survey reports that 10 percent of the people in the United Kingdom aged 16 to 29 years old have ever tried Ecstasy, and 4 percent had taken it in the last year (Ramsey et al. 1999).

1998   Federal Drug Identification Network Seizures reports that 1.2 million tablets were confiscated.

1999   2,850 emergency room visits for Ecstasy use are cited in the United States.

1999   Monitoring the Future Study reports 2.7 percent of eighth-graders, 6.0 percent of tenth-graders, and 8.0 percent of twelfth-graders admitted to using Ecstasy at least once in their lifetimes.

1999   DEA reports seizures of 5.4 million hits of Ecstasy—tablets and powder combined (Cloud 2000).

1999   Federal Drug Identification Network Seizures reports that 12.1 million tablets were confiscated.

2000   David Gauvin estimates at DEA club drug conference in July 2000 that 750,000 hits of Ecstasy are being used in New York and the New Jersey shore corridor every weekend, with 2 million tablets coming into the United States every week.

2000   Monitoring the Future Study reports 4.3 percent of eight-graders, 7.3 percent of tenth-graders, 11 percent of twelfth-graders admitted to using Ecstasy at least once in their lifetimes.

2000   U.S. Customs reports 9.3 million hits Ecstasy were seized.

Drug Abuse Warning Network (DAWN) data are found on the Web site www.samhsa.gov. England and Wales death statistics are from the Office of National Statistics drug-related deaths database. First results for England and Wales, 1993–97, are in *Health Statistics Quarterly*, vol. 5, Spring 2000. DAWN data before 1990 are found in Dowling (1990).

TABLE 1: Studies of Long-term Behavioral or Functional Changes after MDMA Exposure in Animals
by Matthew Baggot and John Mendelson, M.D.

Species and Strain	Neurotoxic MDMA Regimen	Significant Effects of MDMA Exposure	Measures not Significantly Different	Reference
Rhesus Monkeys	10 mg/kg IM, twice a day, for 4 days	Right shift in MDMA and d-fenfluramine dose-response curve for time estimation, learning task, and motivation tasks at post 1 mo.	Drug-free performance on all tasks at post 1 mo.	Frederick et al. 1998
Rhesus Monkeys	Escalating doses of 0.1, 0.3, 1.0, 1.75, 3.0, 5.6, 7.5, 10.0, 15.0, and 20 mg/kg, IM, twice daily for 14 consecutive days at each dose. (2 of 3 animals "skipped" the 1.75, 7.5, and 15 mg/kg dose levels). Preceded by one period of dose response testing using doses up to 1.75 mg/kg IM and followed by three two month periods of dose-response testing using doses up to 5.7 mg/kg IM.	Right shift in MDMA dose-response curve for time estimation, short-term memory, color and position discrimination, and motivation tasks post 5, 12, or 19 mo from chronic regimen (post 12 and 19 mo measures were post 5 mo from a dose-response determination).	Drug-free performance on all tasks at all time points.	Frederick et al. 1995
Sprague-Dawley Rats	20 mg/kg SC, twice a day for 4 days	None, although researchers note that 2 of 8 MDMA-exposed rats failed to acquire lever pressing with 20 sec reinforcement delays during the 8 hr session at post 14 days.	Acquisition of and behavior on a lever-press responding task at post 14 days.	Byrne et al. 2000
Sprague-Dawley Rats	10 mg/kg SC, twice a day for 4 days	Significant pretreatment × treatment × crossing times interaction, suggesting altered S(+)-MDMA-induced behavioral activation at post 21 days.	Drug-free locomotion at 21 days; RU24969-induced behavioral activation at 21 days.	Callaway and Geyer 1992
Wistar Rats	10 mg/kg SC, once a day for 4 days	Increased core temperature when placed in either 22°C or 28°C ambient temperature at post 4 or 14 wks.	None.	Dafters and Lynch 1998
Long-Evans Rats	40 mg/kg SC, twice a day for 4 days	None	Sexual behaviors at post 10 days; spontaneous motor activity.	Dornan et al. 1991

Strain	Dose	Finding	Other Measures	Reference
Sprague-Dawley Rats	20 mg/kg SC, twice a day for 4 days	Decreased cortical 5-HT release in response to electrical stimulation in DRN at post 10–12 days.	Electrical-stimulated 5-HT release in MRN or hippocampus at post 2 wks; number and firing pattern of classical 5-HT neurons and burst-firing neurons in DRN.	Gartside et al. 1996
Sprague-Dawley Rats	20 mg/kg SC, twice a day for 4 days	None.	DOI-induced head twitch responses, locomotion, and rearing activity at post 1 mo.	Granoff and Ashby 1998
Sprague-Dawley Rats	20 mg/kg SC, twice a day for 4 days	Increased conditioned place preference response to cocaine in MDMA group at 2 post wks.	None.	Horan et al. 2000
Sprague-Dawley Rats	5 mg/kg SC, once a day for 4 days, or 20 mg/kg SC, twice a day for 4 days, followed by 5 mg/kg MDMA 2 days later	Increased motor stimulant effects of 5.0 mg/kg SC MDMA in both MDMA-treated groups at post 11 days; increased motor stimulant effects of 15.0 mg/kg IP cocaine in both MDMA-treated groups at post 11 days; increased MDMA-stimulated DA release in the nucleus accumbens at post 2 wks.	Basal DA in nucleus accumbens at post 2 wks.	Kalivas et al. 1998
Sprague-Dawley Rats	15 mg/kg IP	Loss of rate-dependence of response of nigrostriatal cells to either quinpirole or apomorphine at post 1 wk.	Basal activity of nigrostriatal DA neurons; quinpirole-induced inhibition of nigrostriatal DA cell firing for all cells at post 1 wk.	Kelland et al. 1989
Sprague-Dawley Rats	6 mg/kg SC, twice a day for 4 days	Left shift in MDMA dose-response curve on DRL task in MDMA group at post 4 wks.	None.	Li et al. 1989
Lister Hooded Rats	Ascending regimen of 10, 15, and 20 mg/kg IP, each dose given twice daily for one day	Decreased performance in operant delayed match to nonsample task beginning at post 12 days.	Spontaneous behavior, body temperature, and skilled paw reach ("staircase task") up to post 16 days.	Marston et al. 1999
Sprague-Dawley Rats	20 mg/kg SC, twice a day for 4 days	Increased cocaine-induced dopamine release in nucleus accumbens in MDMA group at post 2 wks.	None.	Morgan et al. 1997

Species and Strain	Neurotoxic MDMA Regimen	Significant Effects of MDMA Exposure	Measures not Significantly Different	Reference
Sprague-Dawley Rats	20 mg/kg SC, twice a day for 4 days	Increased morphine-induced antinociception (assessed by tail flick test) at post 2 wks.	Drug-free behavior in tail flick test at post 2 wks.	Nencini et al. 1988
Sprague-Dawley Rats	20 mg/kg SC, twice a day for 4 days	Decreased inhibitory effects of DA and SKF38393 on glutamate-evoked firing in nucleus accumbens cells at post 9–15 days.	Inhibitory effects of GABA on glutamate-evoked firing in nucleus accumbens cells at post 9–15 days.	Obradovic et al. 1998
Sprague-Dawley Rats	20 mg/kg SC	Increased 8-OH-DPAT-induced prolactin release at post 2 wks. Decreased 8-OH-DPAT-stimulated ACTH release at post 2 wks.	Basal ACTH and prolactin concentrations and ACTH and prolactin response to saline injection at post 2 wks.	Poland 1990
Sprague-Dawley Rats	20 mg/kg SC	Increased d,l-fenfluramine-stimulated prolactin release at post 2 wks and 4 mo. Decreased d,l-fenfluramine-stimulated ACTH release at post 2 wks, 4 mo, and 8 mo.	d,l-fenfluramine-stimulated ACTH at post 12 mo; d,l-fenfluramine-stimulated prolactin at post 8 and 12 mo.	Poland et al. 1997
Sprague-Dawley Rats	20 mg/kg SC, twice a day for 4 days	Increased d,l-fenfluramine-stimulated prolactin release at post 4 and 8 mo. Decreased d,l-fenfluramine-stimulated ACTH release at post 4, 8, and 12 mo.	Saline-stimulated ACTH and prolactin release at post 2 weeks; d,l-fenfluramine-stimulated prolactin release at post 12 mo.	Poland et al. 1997
Long-Evans Rats	20 mg/kg SC, twice a day for 4 days with entire regimen repeated 1 wk later	None.	Performance in a spatial memory task using a T-maze (at post 7–10 wks) and scopolamine-induced changes in performance on this task (at post 15–16 wks).	Ricaurte et al. 1993
Sprague-Dawley Rats	10 mg/kg IP, twice a day for 4 days	None (increased time to find hidden platform in first trial of spatial navigation task at post 2 days).	Spatial navigation and learning set task at post 7–9 days, skilled reaching task at post 17–19 days, foraging task at post 26–29 days, with or without atropine pretreatment.	Robinson et al. 1993
Sprague-Dawley Rats	20 mg/kg SC, twice a day for 4 days	Decreased discrimination of 1.0 mg/kg MDMA from saline at post 13–15 days.	Discrimination of 0.5 or 1.5 mg/kg; conditioned place preference from MDMA at post 13–15 days.	Schechter 1991

Sprague-Dawley Rats	10, 20, and 40 mg/kg SC, twice a day for 4 days	None.	Food and water intake, schedule-controlled behavior, open field behavior, acquisition of one- and two-way avoidance, swimming ability, acquisition and extinction in 8-arm radial maze test, and morphine-induced antinociception at post 14–28 days.	Seiden, et al. 1996
Sprague-Dawley Rats	20 or 40 mg/kg IP, twice a day for 4 days	Decreased d-fenfluramine-stimulated 5-HT release in frontal cortex at post 2 wks.	None.	Series et al. 1994
Sprague-Dawley Rats	10 mg/kg IP, every 2 h for 4 injections	Decreased behavioral, hyperthermic, and 5-HT-releasing effects of MDMA at 1 wk after neurotoxic regimen.	None.	Shankaran and Gudelsky 1999
Sprague-Dawley Rats	20 mg/kg SC, twice a day for 4 days	Increased cerebral glucose utilization in molecular layer of dentate gyrus and in CA2 and CA3 fields of Ammon's horn in hippocampus at post 14 days.	Cerebral glucose utilization in neocortex, raphe nuclei, and some hippocampal areas at post 14 days.	Sharkey et al. 1991
Sprague-Dawley Rats	5 or 10 mg/kg PO, daily for 4 days	None.	Auditory startle, emergence from darkened chamber, complex maze navigation, response to hot plate, FI 90 operant behavioral task at post 2 to 4 weeks.	Slikker et al. 1989
Sprague-Dawley Rats	20 mg/kg, SC, twice a day for 4 days	Decreased S(+)-MDMA-appropriate responding after S(+)-MDMA and increased S(+)-MDMA-appropriate responding after saline at post 10 days.	None.	Virden and Baker 1999
Young Sprague-Dawley Rat Pups	10 mg/kg SC, every 12 hrs for 4 or 7 injections	Decreased rate of ultrasonic vocalization measured up to post 11 days.	Behavioral responses to the 5-HT$_A$ agonist 8-OH-DPAT, the 5-HT$_B$ agonist TFMPP, and the 5-HT2 agonist DOI at post 8 days.	Winslow and Insel 1990

Time from MDMA treatment is expressed as time from last exposure.

Abbreviations: DA - dopamine; DRN - dorsal raphe nucleus; DRL - differential reinforcement of low rate (behavioral task); FI - fixed interval of reinforcement (behavioral task); IM - intramuscular injection.

TABLE II: Reported Neurofunctional Differences Between Ecstasy Users and Nonusers
by Matthew Baggot and John Mendelson, M.D.

Putative Serotonergic Measures

Measure	Selective for Serotonergic Differences?	Relevant Animal Literature?	Correlated with MDMA Exposure?	Evidence for Recovery?	References
Decreased CSF 5-HIAA in 3 of 4 studies	Yes	**Decreased** up to 2 weeks after MDMA in squirrel monkeys (Ricaurte et al. 1988b) and 14 weeks after MDMA in rhesus monkeys (Insel et al. 1989)	No	No	**Decreased** in McCann et al. 1999b, 1994; Ricaurte et al. 1990. **Unchanged** in Peroutka et al. 1987
Decreased then **Increased** 5-HT2$_A$ receptor density in 1 of 1 studies	Yes	**Decreased** at 24 hr, **normal** at 21 d after MDMA in rats (Scheffel et al. 1992)	Yes	Not reported	**Increased** in Reneman et al. 2000a; **Decreased** then **increased** in Reneman et al. 2000b
Decreased neuroendocrine response to serotonergic drugs, in 4 of 6 studies	Yes	**Increased** at 2 mo. **normal** at 12 mo. in rats (Poland et al. 1997)	Yes in Gerra et al. 2000	No	**Decreased** in Gerra et al. 2000, 1998; Verkes et al. 2000; McCann et al. 1999a. **Unchanged** in Price et al. 1989; McCann et al. 1994
Decreased SERT density, estimated with PET, in 2 of 2 studies	Disputed—ligand kinetics may be altered by other changes (Kuikka & Ahonen 1998)	PET measures apparently decreased in one baboon up to 14 wks after MDMA (Scheffel et al. 1998)	Yes, though McCann included controls	Mixed (Yes in Semple; No in McCann)	Semple et al. 1999; McCann et al. 1998
Increased stimulus dependence for ERP EEG N1/P2 amplitudes in 1 of 1 studies	Disputed—5HT depletion did not change measure in one study (Dierks et al. 1999)	Unknown	No	Not reported	Tuchtenhagen et al. 2000

Nonspecific Neurofunctional Measures

Measure	Relevant Animal Literature	Correlated with MDMA Exposure	Evidence for Recovery	References
Increased brain myoinositol measured as by IH MRS in 1 of 1 studies	Unknown	Yes	Not reported	Chang et al. 1999
Decreased total sleep time (non-REM and stage 2 sleep) in 1 of 1 study	Unknown	No	Not reported	Allen et al. 1993
Altered cerebral blood flow or volume in 2 of 4 studies	**Increased** blood flow 6–9 wks after MDA in rats (McBean et al. 1990)	Yes	Yes	**Altered** in Reneman et al. 2000a,b and in Chang et al. 2000 **Unchanged** in Chang et al. 2000 (user-nonuser study) and Gamma et al. 2000b
Decreased cerebral glucose utilization in 1 of 1 studies	**Increased** in some hipppocampal areas 2 wks (Sharkey et al. 1991) after MDMA and 6–9 wks after MDA (McBean et al. 1990) in rats	No	No	Obrocki et al. 1999
Increased alpha and beta EEG power in 2 of 2 studies	Unknown	Yes	Not reported	Dafters et al. 1999; Gamma et al. 2000a

TABLE III: Memory Studies of Ecstasy Users vs. Nonusers
by Harry Sumnall

Memory feature	Studies finding significant effects of Ecstasy exposure	Studies finding no significant effects of Ecstasy exposure	Notes
Immediate Verbal	1 2 3 5 12 13 14	4 8 15 18	
Delayed Verbal	1 2 3 5 13 14 15	4 5	
Verbal learning		5 16	
Immediate Visual	1	8 14 18	
Delayed Visual	1 2 14		
Visuospatial		16	
Visuospatial span		10	
Working memory	2 3 5 17 18	9	[9] McCann et al. (1999) administered more than one type of working memory assessment
Working memory span		4 5	
Logical memory (delayed immediate)	11		
Prospective memory	6	6	
Remembering techniques		5	
Everyday memory		5	
Other	5 7 2	1 5 7 9	[1] found no difference using the Wechsler Memory Scale—Revised which contains measures of immediate verbal control, logical memory, learning and visual memory
			[7]Test information in this letter was incomplete but see Croft et al. (2000)

Reference	Correlation with past exposure? [a]	Self-reported total Ecstasy exposure [b]	Self-reported abstinence period [b]	Polydrug users? (Urinalysis?) [c]
1. Bolla et al. (1998)	Yes, although no differences based on Ecstasy exposure per se	Median 60 (25–300) doses over 4.75 (1–17) years at 2 (0–20) uses/month	Median 4 (2–36) weeks	Yes (Yes)
2. Croft et al. (2001)	Not assessed	41.9 (SD49.3) tablets over lifetime (25.7 ± 4.7 years)	>1 week	Yes (No)
3. Curran and Travill (1997)[†]	Not assessed	Not specified	Not specified	Yes (No)
4. Daffers et al. (1999)	No	14.04 (1–60) doses in previous 12 months	7 days	Yes (No)
5. Gouzoulis-Mayfrank et al. (2000)	Yes	934.4 (119.9) doses over 27 (18) months at 2.4 (1.6) uses/month	41 (71.1) days	Yes, only cannabis (Yes)
6. Heffernan et al. (submitted)	Not assessed	10 or more times within a month	Not reported	Yes (No)
7. Klugman et al. (1999)[‡]	Not assessed	235 (12–2600) doses over 4.3 (2.6) years	79 (2–400) days	Yes (No)
8. Krystal et al. (1992)	Not assessed	1.9 (1.7) doses over 5.1 (2.3) years	66 (50) days	Yes (No)
9. McCann et al. (1999b)	Yes	215 (30–725) doses over 4.52 (1–14) years	13.91 (3–147) weeks	Yes (Yes)
10. Morgan (1998)	Not assessed	35.6 doses over 2.12 (1.36) years at 2.94 (0.93) uses/month	20.4 (33.6) days	Yes (No)
11. Morgan (1999)	Not assessed	50 (20–160) doses	65 days	Yes (No)
12. Parrott and Lasky (1998)[†]	Not assessed	Not specified[‡]	Not specified	Yes (No)
13. Parrott et al. (1998)	Not assessed	>10 occasions; <10 occasions	Not specified	Not specified

Reference	Correlation with past exposure?[a]	Ecstasy exposure[b]	Abstinence period[b]	Polydrug users? (Urinalyis?)[c]
Rodgers et al. (2000)	Not assessed	20 uses over 5 years	2 months	Yes (No)
Reneman et al. (2000a)	Not assessed	218 (50–500) doses	4.6 (2–11) months	Yes (Yes)
Semple et al. (1999)	Yes	672 (50–1800) doses	18 (6–28) days	Yes (Yes)
Verkes et al. (2000)	Not assessed	169 (SD 252) tablets over 4.4 (2.4) years at 2.0 (1.1) tablets per occasion	15.7 (9.5) days	Yes (Yes)
Wareing et al. (2000)	Not assessed	Not specified. From drug use data provided, calculated to be 1280.91 for "previous" users and 1348.49 for "current" users	323.25 (130.05) days for "previous" users and 8.2 (5.75) days for "current" users	Yes (No)

[a] While correlation analysis may tell us about the interaction between lifetime drug exposure and cognitive deficits, basing this on self-reported drug use or the mean content of Ecstasy tablets is problematic. First, individuals may not accurately remember their lifetime consumption. This may lead to overestimation. Second, numerous forensic studies suggest that the actual MDMA content of Ecstasy tablets varies and many tablets contain other drugs or no active component.

[b] Mean (± SE) number of doses unless specified.

[c] Without performing qualitative urinalysis of samples obtained from volunteers on the day of testing it is not possible to reliably conclude that they are drug free, despite requests from the investigators or assurances from volunteers to the contrary.

† Subjects were tested during and after a Saturday night rave (in the case of Parrott and Lasky also before) and so these results reflect acute and residual drug effects rather than long term effects of Ecstasy per se.

* Space constraints precluded the publication of full test details. However, Croft et al. (2000) replicated the tests used in their later study

‡ "Regular" subjects reported using 1.8 Ecstasy tablets on the test night compared to 1.45 tablets in the novice group.

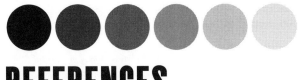

REFERENCES

Abramovsky, A. 2000. Ecstasy prosecution: State or federal law better for enforcement? *New York Law Journal*, 29 November.

Accola, J. 1988. MDMA: Studies of popular illicit drug raise questions about effects. *Rocky Mountain News*, 4 March, 72.

Adamson, S. ed. 1985. *Through the gateway of the heart: Accounts of experiences with MDMA and other empathogenic substances*. San Francisco: Four Trees.

Adamson, S., and R. Metzner. 1988. The nature of the MDMA experience and its role in healing, psychotherapy, and spiritual practice. *ReVision* 10(4):59–72.

Adler, J. 1985. Getting high on Ecstasy. *Newsweek*, 15 April.

Aguirre, N., S. Ballaz, B. Lasheras, and J. Del Rio. 1998. MDMA ("Ecstasy") enhances 5-HT1A receptor density and 8-OH-DPAT-induced hypothermia: Blockade by drugs preventing 5-hydroxytryptamine depletion. *Eur. J. Pharmacol.* 346:181–8.

Aguirre, N., M. Barrionuevo, M. J. Ramirez, J. Del Rio, and B. Lasheras. 1999. Alpha-lipoic acid prevents 3,4-methylenedioxymethamphetamine (MDMA)–induced neurotoxicity. *Neuroreport* 10:367–80.

Ajaelo, I., K. Koenig, and E. Snoey. 1998. Severe hyponatremia and inappropriate antidiuretic hormone secretion following ecstasy use. *Acad. Emerg. Med.* 5:839–40.

Albuquerque, A. 1992. Tratamiento del estrés postraumático en ex-combatientes. In *Avances en el tratamiento psicológico de los trastornos de ansiedad*, edited by E. Echeburúa. Madrid: Pirámide.

Alexander, G. E., M. L. Furey, C. L. Grady, et al. 1997. Association of premorbid intellectual function with cerebral metabolism in Alzheimer's disease: Implications for the cognitive reserve hypothesis. *Am. J. Psychiatry* 154:165–72.

Alexander, L., and L. Luborsky. 1986. Research on the Helping Alliance. In *The psychotherapeutic process: A research handbook*, edited by L. Greenberg and W. Pinsof. New York: Gilford Press.

Ali, S. F., G. D. Newport, A. C. Scallet, et al. 1993. Oral administration of 3,4-methylenedioxymethamphetamine (MDMA) produces selective serotonergic depletion in the nonhuman primate. *Neurotoxicol. Teratol.* 15:91–6.

Ali, S. F., G. D. Newport, R. R. Holson, W. Slikker Jr., and J. F. Bowyer. 1994. Low environmental temperatures or pharmacologic agents that produce hypothermia decrease methamphetamine neurotoxicity in mice. *Brain Res.* 658:33–8.

Allen, R. P., U. D. McCann, and G. A. Ricaurte. 1993. Persistent effects of (±)3,4-methylenedioxymethamphetamine (MDMA, "ecstasy") on human sleep. *Sleep* 16:560–4.

American Psychiatric Association. 1994. *Diagnostic and Statistical Manual of Mental Disorders*, 4th ed. Washington D.C.: American Psychiatric Association.

Ames, D., and W. C.Wirshing. 1993. Ecstasy, the serotonin syndrome, and neuroleptic malignant syndrome: A possible link? *JAMA* 269:869.

Anden, N. E., H. Corrodi, K. Fuxe, and J. L. Meek. 1974. Hallucinogenic phenylethylamines: Interactions with serotonin turnover and receptors. *Eur. J. Pharmacol.* 25:176–84.

Andreu, V., A. Mas, M. Bruguera. 1998. Ecstasy: A common cause of severe acute hepatotoxicity. *J. Hepatol.* 29(3):394–7.

Angrist, B. 1994. Amphetamine psychosis: Clinical variations of the syndrome. In *Amphetamine and its analogs: Psychopharmacology, toxicology, and abuse*, edited by A. K. Cho and D. S. Segal. New York: Academic Press. pp. 387–414.

Angrist, B., J. Rotrosen, and S. Gershon. 1980. Differential effects of amphetamine and neuroleptics on negative vs. positive symptoms in schizophrenia. *Psychopharmacology* 72:17–9.

Angrist, B., E. Peselow, M. Rubinstein, J. Corwin, and J. Rotrosen. 1982. Partial improvement in negative schizophrenic symptoms after amphetamine. *Psychopharmacology* 78:128–30.

Axt, K. J., L. A. Mamounas, and M. E. Molliver. 1994. Structural features of amphetamine neurotoxicity in the brain. In *Amphetamine and its analogs: Psychopharmacology, toxicology, and abuse*, edited by A. K. Cho and D. S. Segal. New York: Academic Press. pp. 315–67.

Ayd, F. J. 1995. *Lexicon of psychiatry, neurology, and the neurosciences*. Baltimore: Williams and Wilkins. p. 245.

Azmitia, E. C. 1999. Serotonin neurons, neuroplasticity, and homeostasis of neural tissue. *Neuropsychopharmacology* 21:33S–45S.

Baggott, M., B. Heifets, R. T. Jones, et al. 2000. *Chemical Analysis of Ecstasy Pills*. JAMA 1:2190

Ballard, P. A., J. W. Tetrud, and J. W. Langston. 1985. Permanent human parkinsonism due to 1-methyl-4-phenyl-1,2,3,6-tetrahydropyridine (MPTP): Seven cases. *Neurology* 35:949–56.

Bartels, S. J., and R. E. Drake. 1989. Depression in schizophrenia: Current guidelines to treatment. *Psychiatr. Q.* 60:337–57.

Bartzokis, G., M. Beckson, D. B. Hance, et al. 1999. Magnetic resonance imaging evidence of "silent" cerebrovascular toxicity in cocaine dependence. *Biol. Psychiatry* 45:1203–11.

Battaglia, G., B. P. Brooks, C. Kulsakdinum, and E. B. De Souza. 1988a. Pharmacologic profile of MDMA (3,4-methyldenedioxymethamphetamine) at various brain recognition sites. *Eur. J. Pharmacol.* 149:159–63.

Battaglia, G., S. Y. Yeh, and E. B. De Souza. 1988b. MDMA-induced neurotoxicity: Parameters of degeneration and recovery of brain serotonin neurons. *Pharmacol. Biochem. Behav.* 29:269–74.

Beatty, W. W., V. M. Katzung, V. J. Moreland, and S. J. Nixon. 1995. Neuropsychological performance of recently abstinent alcoholics and cocaine abusers. *Drug Alcohol Depend.* 37:247–53.

Beck, C. "MDMA—Die frühen Jahre." Paper presented at a meeting of the European College for the Study of Consciousness, Bad Boll, Germany, November 1997.

Beck, J., and M. Rosenbaum. 1994. *Pursuit of Ecstasy.* Albany: State University of New York Press.

Beck, A. T., R. A. Steer, M. Kovacs, and B. Garrison. 1985. Hopelessness and eventual suicide: A 10-year prospective study of patients hospitalized with suicidal ideation. *Am. J. Psychiatry* 142:599–63.

Beck, A. T., G. Brown, and R. A. Steer. 1989. Prediction of eventual suicide in psychiatric inpatients by clinical ratings of hopelessness. *J. Consult. Clin. Psychol.* 57(2)309–10.

Bell, D. S. 1965. Comparison of amphetamine psychosis and schizophrenia. *Br. J. Psychiatry* 111:701–7.

Benazzi, I., and M. Mazzoli. 1991. Psychiatric illness associated with ecstasy. *Lancet* 338:1520.

Bengel, D., D. L. Murphy, A. M. Andrews, C. H. Wichems, D. Feltner, A. Heils, R. Mossner, H. Westphal, and K. P. Lesch, 1998. Altered brain serotonin homeostasis and locomotor insensitivity to 3,4-methylenedioxymethamphetamine ("Ecstasy") in serotonin transporter-deficient mice. *Mol Pharmacol.* 53: 649–55.

Bendotti, C., S. Baldessari, M. Pende, et al. 1994. Does GFAP mRNA and mitochondrial benzodiazepine receptor binding detect serotonergic neuronal degeneration in rat? *Brain Res. Bull.* 34:389–94.

Berman, I., A. Kalinowski, S. M. Berman, J. Lengua, and A. I. Green. 1995. Obsessive and compulsive symptoms in chronic schizophrenia. *Compr. Psychiatry* 36:6–10.

Berman, S. B., and T. G. Hastings. 1999. Dopamine oxidation alters mitochondrial respiration and induces permeability transition in brain mitochondria: Implications for Parkinson's disease. *J. Neurochem.* 73:1127–37.

Bishop, M. G. 1963. *The discovery of love: A psychedelic experience with LSD-25.* New York: Dodd, Mead.

Blanchard, J., T. N. Tozer, and M. Rowland. 1997. Pharmacokinetic perspectives on megadoses of ascorbic acid [see Comments]. *Am. J. Clin. Nutr.* 66:1165–71.

Bodmer, I. 1989. Konstruktion des Fragebogens OAV zur quantitativen Erfassung aussergewoehnlicher Bewusstseinszustaende. Thesis, Institute of Psychology, University of Zurich, Zurich.

Bolla, K. I., U. D. McCann, and G. A. Ricaurte. 1998. Memory impairment in abstinent MDMA ("Ecstasy") users [see Comments]. *Neurology* 51:1532–7.

Bolla, K. I., R. Rothman, and J. L. Cadet. 1999. Dose-related neurobehavioral effects of chronic cocaine use. *J. Neuropsychiatry Clin. Neurosci.* 11:361–9.

Bonson, K. R., J. W. Buckholtz, and D. L. Murphy. 1996a. Chronic administration of serotonergic antidepressants attenuate the subjective effects of LSD in humans. *Neuropsychopharmacology* 14:425–36.

Bonson, K. R., Murphy, D.L. 1996b. Alterations in responses to LSD in humans associated with chronic administration of tricyclic antidepressants, monoamine oxidase inhibitors or lithium. *Behav. Brain Res.* 73:229–33.

Boot, B. P., I. S. McGregor, and W. Hall. 2000. MDMA (Ecstasy) neurotoxicity: Assessing and communicating the risks. *Lancet* 355:1818–21.

Boszormenyi, Z., and S. I. Szara. 1958. Dimethyltryptamine experiments with psychotics. *J. Ment. Sci.* 104:445–53.

Bowyer, J. F., B. Gough, W. Slikker Jr., G. W. Lipe, G. D. Newport, and R. R. Holson. 1993. Effects of a cold environment or age on methamphetamine-induced dopamine release in the caudate putamen of female rats. *Pharmacol. Biochem. Behav.* 44:87–98.

Brady, J. F., E. W. Di Stefano, and A. K. Cho. 1986. Spectral and inhibitory interactions of (±)-3,4-methylenedioxyamphetamine (MDA) and (±)-3,4 methylenedioxymethamphetamine (MDMA) with rat hepatic microsomes. *Life Sci.* 39:1457–64.

Broening, H. W., J. F. Bowyer, and W. Slikker Jr. 1995. Age-dependent sensitivity of rats to the long-term effects of the serotonergic neurotoxicant (±)-3,4-methylenedioxymethamphetamine (MDMA) correlates with the magnitude of the MDMA-induced thermal response. *J. Pharmacol. Exp. Ther.* 275:325–33.

Brothers L. 1996. Brain mechanisms of social cognition. *J. Psychopharmacol.* 10:2–8.

Brown, C., and J. Osterloh. 1987. Multiple severe complications from recreational ingestion of MDMA ("Ecstasy"). *JAMA* 258:780–1.

Brownell, A. L., B. G. Jenkins, and O. Isacson. 1999. Dopamine imaging markers and predictive mathematical models for progressive degeneration in Parkinson's disease. *Biomed. Pharmacother.* 53:131–40.

Bryden, A. A., P. J. Rothwell, and P. H. O'Reilly. 1995. Urinary retention with misuse of "ecstasy." *Br. Med. J.* 310:504.

Buchanan, J. 1985. *Ecstasy in the emergency department. Clinical toxicology update* 7. San Francisco Bay Area Regional Poison Center.

Burgess, C., A. O'Donohoe, and M. Gill. 2000. Agony and ecstasy: A review of MDMA effects and toxicity. *Eur. Psychiatry* 15: 287–94.

Burrows, K. B., and C. K. Meshul. 1999. High-dose methamphetamine treatment alters presynaptic GABA and glutamate immunoreactivity. *Neuroscience* 90:833–50.

Burrows, K. B., G. Gudelsky, and B. K. Yamamoto. 2000. Rapid and transient inhibition of mitochondrial function following methamphetamine or 3,4-methylenedioxymethamphetamine administration. *Eur. J. Pharmacol.* 398:11–8.

Buydens-Branchey, L., M. Branchey, P. Fergeson, J. Hudson, and C. McKernin. 1997. The meta-chlorophenylpiperazine challenge test in cocaine addicts: Hormonal and psychological responses. *Biol. Psychiatry* 41:1071–86.

Buydens-Branchey, L., M. Branchey, J. Hudson, M. Rothman, P. Fergeson, and C. McKernin. 1999. Serotonergic function in cocaine addicts: Prolactin responses to sequential D,L-fenfluramine challenges. *Biol. Psychiatry* 45:1300–6.

Byrne, T., L. E. Baker, and A. Poling. 2000. MDMA and learning: Effects of acute and neurotoxic exposure in the rat. *Pharmacol. Biochem. Behav.* 66:501–8.

Caccia, S., A. Bergami, C. Fracasso, S. Garattini, and B. Campbell. 1995. Oral kinetics of dexfenfluramine and dexnorfenfluramine in non-human primates. *Xenobiotica* 25:1143–50.

Cadet, J. L., and C. Brannock. 1998. Free radicals and the pathobiology of brain dopamine systems. *Neurochem. Int.* 32:117–31.

Cadet, J. L., B. Ladenheim, I. Baum, E. Carlson, and C. Epstein. 1994. CuZn-superoxide dismutase (CuZnSOD) transgenic mice show resistance to the lethal effects of methylenedioxyamphetamine (MDA) and of methylenedioxymethamphetamine (MDMA). *Brain Res.* 655:259–62.

Cadet, J. L., B. Ladenheim, H. Hirata, et al. 1995. Superoxide radicals mediate the biochemical effects of methylenedioxymethamphetamine (MDMA): Evidence from using CuZn-superoxide dismutase transgenic mice. *Synapse* 21:169–76.

Caldwell, C. B., and I. I. Gottesman. 1990. Schizophrenics kill themselves too: A review of the risk factors for suicide. *Schizophr. Bull.* 16:571–89.

Callaway, C. W., and M. A. Geyer. 1992. Tolerance and cross-tolerance to the activating effects of 3,4-methylenedioxymethamphetamine and a 5-hydroxytryptamine1B agonist. *J. Pharmacol. Exp. Ther.* 263:318–26.

Calne, D. B., J. W. Langston, W. R. Martin, et al. 1985. Positron emission tomography after MPTP: Observations relating to the cause of Parkinson's disease. *Nature* 317:246–8.

Calvert, C. 1987. Psychedelic drug use up on the farm. *Stanford Daily*, 3 March.

Camí, J., M. Farré, M. Mas, et al. 2000. Human pharmacology of 3,4-methylenedioxymethamphetamine ("Ecstasy"): Psychomotor performance and subjective effects. *J. Clin. Psychopharmacol.* 20:455–66.

Campbell, D. B. 1995. The use of toxicokinetics for the safety assessment of drugs acting in the brain. *Mol. Neurobiol.* 11:193–216.

———. 1996. Extrapolation from animals to man: The integration of pharmacokinetics and pharmacodynamics. *Ann. N. Y. Acad. Sci.* 801:116–35.

Campkin, N. T., and U. M. Davies. 1992. Another death from ecstasy. *J. R. Soc. Med.* 85:61.

Canton, G., L. Verriele, and F. C. Colpaert. 1990. Binding of typical and atypical antipsychotics to 5HT1c and 5HT2 sites: Clozapine potently interacts with 5HT1c sites. *Eur. J. Pharmacol.* 191:93–6.

Capdevilla, M. 1995. *MDMA o el exstasis quimico*. Barcelona: Los Libros De La Liebre De Marzo.

Carpenter, W. T. Jr., R. R. Conley, R. W. Buchanon, A. Breier, and C. A.Tamminga.

1995. Patient response and resource management: Another view of clozapine treatment of schizophrenia. *Am. J. Psychiatry* 152:827–32.

Castner, S. A., and P. S. Goldman-Rakic. 1999. Long-lasting psychotomimetic consequences of repeated low-dose amphetamine exposure in rhesus monkeys. *Neuropsychopharmacology* 20:10–28.

Cesarec, Z., and A. K. Nyman. 1985. Differential response to amphetamine in schizophrenia. *Acta Psychiatr. Scand.* 71:523–38.

Chadwick, I. S., A. Linsley, A. J. Freemont, B. Doran, and P. D. Curry. 1991. Ecstasy, 3,4-methylenedioxymethamphetamine (MDMA): A fatality associated with coagulopathy and hyperthermia. *J. R. Soc. Med.* 84:371.

Chang, L., T. Ernst, C. S. Grob, and R. E. Poland. 1999. Cerebral (1)H MRS alterations in recreational 3,4-methylenedioxymethamphetamine (MDMA, "ecstasy") users. *J. Magn. Reson. Imaging* 10:521–6.

Chang, L., C. S. Grob, T. Ernst, et al. 2000. Effect of ecstasy (3,4-methylenedioxymethamphetamine [MDMA]) on cerebral blood flow: A co-registered SPECT and MRI study. *Psychiatry Res.* 98:15–28.

Che, S., M. Johnson, G. R. Hanson, and J. W. Gibb. 1995. Body temperature effect on methylenedioxymethamphetamine-induced acute decrease in tryptophan hydroxylase activity. *Eur. J. Pharmacol.* 293:447–53.

Cho, A. K., M. Hiramatsu, E. W. Distefano, A. S. Chang, and D. J. Jenden. 1990. Stereochemical differences in the metabolism of 3,4-methylenedioxymethamphetamine in vivo and in vitro: A pharmacokinetic analysis. *Drug Metab. Dispos. Biol. Fate Chem.* 18:686–91.

Cho, K., A. Ennaceur, J. C. Cole, and C. K Suh. 2000. Chronic jet lag produces cognitive deficits. *J. Neurosci.* 20:RC66.

Cleare, A. J., and A. J. Bond. 1995. The effect of tryptophan depletion and enhancement on subjective and behavioural aggression in normal male subjects. *Psychopharmacology* 118:72–81.

Clineschmidt, B. V., A. G. Zacchei, J. A. Totaro, A. B. Pflueger, J. C. McGuffin, and T. I. Wishousky. 1978. Fenfluramine and brain serotonin. *Ann. N. Y. Acad. Sci.* 305:222–41.

Cloud, J. 2000. The lure of Ecstasy. *Time,* 5 June.

Coccaro, E. F., R. J. Kavoussi, T. B. Cooper, and R. L. Hauger. 1997. Central serotonin activity and aggression: Inverse relationship with prolactin response to *d*-fenfluramine, but not CSF 5-HIAA concentration, in human subjects. *Am. J. Psychiatry* 154:1430–5.

Coffey, C. E., J. A. Saxton, G. Ratcliff, R. N. Bryan, and J. F. Lucke. 1999. Relation of education to brain size in normal aging: Implications for the reserve hypothesis. *Neurology* 53:189–96.

Coffey, S. F., B. S. Dansky, M. H. Carrigan, and K. T. Brady. 2000. Acute and protracted cocaine abstinence in an outpatient population: A prospective study of mood, sleep and withdrawal symptoms. *Drug Alcohol Depend.* 59:277–86.

Cohen, R. S. 1995. Subjective reports on the effects of the MDMA (Ecstasy) experience in humans. *Prog. Psychopharmacol. Biol. Psychiatry* 19:1137–45.

Colado, M. I., and A. R. Green. 1995. The spin trap reagent alpha-phenyl-*N*-tert-butyl nitrone prevents "ecstasy"-induced neurodegeneration of 5-hydroxytryptamine neurons. *Eur. J. Pharmacol.* 280:343–6.

Colado, M. I., T. K. Murray, and A. R. Green. 1993. 5-HT loss in rat brain following 3,4-methylenedioxymethamphetamine (MDMA), *p*-chloroamphetamine and fenfluramine administration and effects of chlormethiazole and dizocilpine. *Br. J. Pharmacol.* 108:583–9.

Colado, M. I., J. L. Williams, and A. R. Green. 1995. The hyperthermic and neuro-toxic effects of "Ecstasy" (MDMA) and 3,4-methylenedioxy-amphetamine (MDA) in the Dark Agouti (DA) rat, a model of the CYP2D6 poor metabolizer phenotype. *Br. J. Pharmacol.* 115:1281–9.

Colado, M. I., E. O'Shea, R. Granados, A. Misra, T. K. Murray, and A. R. Green. 1997a. A study of the neurotoxic effect of MDMA ("ecstasy") on 5-HT neurones in the brains of mothers and neonates following administration of the drug during pregnancy. *Br. J. Pharmacol.* 121:827–33.

Colado, M. I., E. O'Shea, R. Granados, T. K. Murray, and A. R. Green. 1997b. In vivo evidence for free radical involvement in the degeneration of rat brain 5-HT following administration of MDMA ("ecstasy") and *p*-chloroamphetamine but not the degeneration following fenfluramine. *Br. J. Pharmacol.* 121:889–900.

Colado, M. I., R. Granados, E. O'Shea, B. Esteban, and A. R. Green. 1998. Role of hyperthermia in the protective action of clomethiazole against MDMA ("ecstasy")-induced neurodegeneration: Comparison with the novel NMDA channel blocker AR-R15896AR. *Br. J. Pharmacol.* 124:479–84.

Colado, M. I., B. Esteban, E. O'Shea, R. Granados, and A. R. Green. 1999a. Studies on the neuroprotective effect of pentobarbitone on MDMA-induced neurodegeneration. *Psychopharmacology (Berlin)* 142:421–5.

Colado, M. I., E. O'Shea, B. Esteban, R. Granados, and A. R. Green. 1999b. In vivo evidence against clomethiazole being neuroprotective against MDMA ("ecstasy")-induced degeneration of rat brain 5-HT nerve terminals by a free radical scaveng-ing mechanism. *Neuropharmacology* 38:307–14.

Collin, M., and J. Godfrey. 1997. *Altered state: The story of Ecstasy culture and acid house.* London: Serpent's Tail.

Commins, D. L., G. Vosmer, R. M. Virus, W. L. Woolverton, C. R. Schuster, and L. S. Seiden. 1987. Biochemical and histological evidence that methylenedioxymethamphetamine (MDMA) is toxic to neurons in the rat brain. *J. Pharmacol. Exp. Ther.* 241:338–45.

Connell, P. H. 1958. *Amphetamine psychosis.* Institute of Psychiatry Maudsley Mono-graphs no. 5. Oxford: Oxford University Press.

Cooper, S. J., C. B. Kelly, and D. J. King. 1992. 5-Hydroxyindoleacetic acid in cerebrospinal fluid and prediction of suicidal behavior in schizophrenia. *Lancet* 340:940–1.

Coppen, A. 1967. Biochemistry of affective disorders. *Br. J. Psychiatry* 113:1237–64.

Corral, P., E. Echeburúa, B. Sarasúa, and I. Zubizarreta 1992. Estrés postraumático en ex combatientes y en víctimas de agresiones sexuales: Nuevas perspectivas terapéuticas. *Bol. Psicol.* 35:7–24.

Corral, P., E. Echeburúa, B. Sarasúa, and I. Zubizarreta. 1995a. Tratamiento cognitivo-conductual del trastorno por estrés postraumático agudo en víctimas de agresiones sexuales: Un estudio piloto. *Psicol. Conduct.* 3(2):195–210.

Corral, P., E. Echeburúa, I. Zubizarreta, and B. Sarasua. 1995b. Tratamiento psicológico del trastorno de estrés postraumático crónico en víctimas de agresiones sexuales: un estudio experimental. *Análisis y Modificación de Conducta* 21(78):455–82.

Cousins, N. 1983. *The healing heart.* New York: W. W. Norton.

Creese, I., D. R. Burt, and S. H. Snyder. 1976. Dopamine receptor binding predicts clinical and pharmacological potencies of antischizophrenic drugs. *Science* 192:481–3.

Creighton, F. J., D. L. Black, and C. E. Hyde. 1991. "Ecstasy" psychosis and flashbacks [see Comments]. *Br. J. Psychiatry* 159:713–5.

Croft, R. C., A. J. Macay, A. T. D. Mills, and J. G. H. Gruzelier. 2001. The relative contributions of ecstasy and cannabis to cognitive impairment. *Psychopharmacology (Berlin)* 15 Jan. 153:373–79.

Crompton, M., S. Virji, V. Doyle, N. Johnson, and J. M. Ward. 1999. The mitochondrial permeability transition pore. *Biochem. Soc. Symp.* 66:167–79.

Crow, T. J. 1980. Molecular pathology of schizophrenia: More than one disease process? *Br. Med. J.* 280:66–8.

Cubells, J. F., S. Rayport, G. Rajendran, and D. Sulzer. 1994. Methamphetamine neurotoxicity involves vacuolization of endocytic organelles and dopamine-dependent intracellular oxidative stress. *J. Neurosci.* 14:2260–71.

Cuomo, M. J., P. G. Dyment, and V. M. Gammino. 1994. Increasing use of "Ecstasy" (MDMA) and other hallucinogens on a college campus. *J. Am. College Health* 42:271–4.

Curran, H. V., and R. A. Travill. 1997. Mood and cognitive effects of 3,4- methylene-dioxymethamphetamine (MDMA, "Ecstasy"): Weekend "high" followed by mid-week low. *Addiction* 92:821–31.

Dafters, R. I. 1994. Effect of ambient temperature on hyperthermia and hyperkinesis induced by 3,4-methylenedioxymethamphetamine (MDMA or "ecstasy") in rats. *Psychopharmacology (Berlin)* 114:505–8.

———. 1995. Hyperthermia following MDMA administration in rats: Effects of ambient temperature, water consumption, and chronic dosing. *Physiol. Behav.* 58:877–82.

Dafters, R. I., and E. Lynch. 1998. Persistent loss of thermoregulation in the rat induced by 3,4-methylenedioxymethamphetamine (MDMA or "Ecstasy") but not by fenfluramine. *Psychopharmacology (Berlin)* 138:207–12.

Dafters, R. I., F. Duffy, P. J. O'Donnell, and C. Bouquet. 1999. Level of use of 3,4-methylenedioxymethamphetamine (MDMA or Ecstasy) in humans correlates with EEG power and coherence. *Psychopharmacology (Berlin)* 145:82–90.

Davis, G. C., A. C. Williams, S. P. Markey, et al. 1979. Chronic parkinsonism secondary to intravenous injection of meperidine analogues. *Psychiatry Res.* 1:249–54.

Davison, D., and A. C. Parrott. 1997. Ecstasy (MDMA) in recreational users: Self-reported psychological and physiological effects. *Hum. Psychopharmacol. Clin. Exp.* 12:221–6.

Deakin, J. F. W. 1996. 5-HT, antidepressant drugs and the psychosocial origins of depression. *J. Psychopharmacol.* 10:31–8.

de la Torre, R., M. Farré, J. Ortuño, et al. 2000a. Non-linear pharmacokinetics of MDMA ("ecstasy") in humans. *Br. J. Clin. Pharmacol.* 49:104–9.

de la Torre, R., M. Farré, P. N. Roset, et al. 2000b. Pharmacology of MDMA in humans. *Ann. N. Y. Acad. Sci.* 914:225–37.

Delentre, P., J. Henrion, J. M. Jacques, M. Schapira, J. M. Ghilain, and J. M. Maisin. 1994. Toxic hepatitis due to ecstasy administration: Report of a possible case and literature review. *Acta Gastroenterol. Belg.* 57:341–5.

de Paul, J. 1995. Trastorno por Estrés Postraumático. In *Manual de psicopatología y trastornos psiquiátricos*, edited by V. E. Caballo, G. Buela-Casal and J. A. Carrobles. Madrid: Siglo XXI.

De Souza, E. B., G. Battaglia, and T. R. Insel. 1990. Neurotoxic effect of MDMA on brain serotonin neurons: Evidence from neurochemical and radioligand binding studies. *Ann. N. Y. Acad. Sci.* 600:682–97; discussion 697–8.

Deutch, A. Y. 1992. The regulation of subcortical dopamine systems by the prefrontal cortex: Interactions of central dopamine systems and the pathogenesis of schizophrenia. *J. Neural Transm. Suppl.* 36:61–89.

Dierks, T., S. Barta, L. Demisch et al. 1999. Intensity dependence of auditory evoked potentials (AEPs) as biological marker for cerebral serotonin levels: effects of tryptophan depletion in healthy subjects. *Psychopharmcology* 146:101–7.

Di Monte, D. A., A. McCormack, G. Petzinger, A. M. Janson, M. Quik, and W. J. Langston. 2000. Relationship among nigrostriatal denervation, parkinsonism, and dyskinesias in the MPTP primate model. *Mov. Disord.* 15:459–66.

Dinges, D. F., and N. B. Kribbs. 1991. Performing while sleepy: Effects of experimentally induced sleepiness. In *Sleep, sleepiness and performance*, edited by T. H. Monk. New York: John Wiley & Sons. pp. 97–128.

Dittrich, A. 1998. The standardized psychometric assessment of altered states of consciousness (ASCs) in humans. *Pharmacopsychiatry* 31:80–4.

Dornan, W. A., J. L. Katz, and G. A. Ricaurte. 1991. The effects of repeated administration of MDMA on the expression of sexual behavior in the male rat. *Pharmacol. Biochem. Behav.* 39:813–6.

Dowling, G. P. 1990a. Human deaths and toxic reactions attributed to MDMA and MDEA. In *Ecstasy: The clinical, pharmacological and neurotoxicological effects of the drug MDMA*, edited by S. J. Peroutka. Norwell, Mass.: Kluwer Academic Publishers.

———. 1990b. On drug-related deaths database first results for England and Wales. *Health Statistics Quarterly.* 5:

Dowling, G. P., E. T. McDonough, and R. O. Bost. 1987. "Eve" and "ecstasy": A report of five deaths associated with the use of MDEA and MDMA. *JAMA* 257:1615–7.

Downing, J. 1986. The psychological and physiological effects of MDMA on normal volunteers. *J. Psychoactive Drugs* 18:335–40.

Drake, W. M., and P. A. Broadhurst. 1996. QT-interval prolongation with ecstasy. *S. Afr. Med. J.* 86(2):180–1.

Dworkin, R. H., and L. A. Opler. 1992. Simple schizophrenia, negative symptoms, and prefrontal hypodopaminergia. *Am. J. Psychiatry* 149(9):1284–5.

Dyck, R. J., R. C. Bland, S. C. Newman, and H. Orn. 1988. Suicide attempts and psychiatric disorders in Edmonton. *Acta Psychiatr. Scand. Suppl.* 338:64–71.

Dykhuizen, R. S., P. W. Brunt, P. Atkinson, J. G. Simpson, and C. C. Smith. 1995. Ecstasy induced hepatitis mimicking viral hepatitis. *Gut* 36:939–41.

Echeburúa, E., and P. de Corral. 1995. Trastorno de estrés postraumático. In *Manual de psicopatología*, edited by A. Belloch, B. Sandín, and F. Ramos. Madrid: McGraw Hill.

———. 1997. Avances en el tratamiento cognitivo conductual del trastorno de estrés postraumático. *Ansiedad y Estrés* 3(2–3):249–64.

Echeburúa, E., P. de Corral, B. Sarasua, and I. Zubizarreta. 1990. Tratamiento psicológico del estrés postraumático en víctimas de agresiones sexuales: Una revisión. *Análisis y Modificación de Conducta* 16(49):417–37.

Echeburúa, E., P. de Corral, I. Zubizarreta, and B. Sarasua. 1995. *Trastorno de estrés postraumático crónico en víctimas de agresiones sexuales*. La Coruña: Fundación Paideia.

Eisner, B. 1989. *Ecstasy: The MDMA story*. Berkeley, Calif.: Ronin Press.

Elayan, I., J. W. Gibb, G. R. Hanson, R. L. Foltz, H. K. Lim, and M. Johnson. 1992. Long-term alteration in the central monoaminergic systems of the rat by 2,4,5-trihydroxyamphetamine but not by 2-hydroxy-4,5-methylenedioxymethamphetamine or 2-hydroxy-4,5-methylenedioxyamphetamine. *Eur. J. Pharmacol.* 221:281–8.

Ellis, A. J., J. A. Wendon, B. Portman, and R. Williams. 1996. Acute liver damage and ecstasy ingestion. *Gut* 38:454–8.

Ellison, G. 1994. Stimulant-induced psychosis, the dopamine theory of schizophrenia, and the habenula. *Brain Res. Rev.* 19(2):223–39.

Evenden, J. L. 1999. Varieties of impulsivity. *Psychopharmacology* 146:348–61.

Everhart, E. T., P. Jacob III, P. Shwonek, M. Baggott, R. T. Jones, and J. Mendelson. 2000. Estimation of the metabolic disposition of MDMA and MDA enantiomers in humans. In *Problems of drug dependence*, edited by L. S. Harris. Washington D.C.: U.S. Government Printing Office.

Fahal, B. A., D. F. Sallomi, M. Yaqoob, and G. M. Bell. 1992. Acute renal failure after ecstasy. *Br. Med. J.* 305:29.

Fallon, J. K., A. T. Kicman, J. A. Henry, P. J. Milligan, D. A. Cowan, and A. J. Hutt. 1999. Stereospecific analysis and enantiomeric disposition of 3,4-methylenedioxy-methamphetamine (Ecstasy) in humans. *Clin. Chem.* 45:1058–69.

Faraj, B. A., Z. L. Olkowski, and R. T. Jackson. 1994. Active [³H]-dopamine uptake by human lymphocytes: Correlates with serotonin transporter activity. *Pharmacology* 48:320–7.

Farley, Christopher John. 2000. Rave New World. *Time*, 5 June.

Farré, M., P. N. Roset, A. Tomillero, et al. 2000. Repeated administration of ecstasy to humans: Preliminary findings. *Br. J. Clin. Pharmacol.* Special issue:111.

Feixas, G., and M. T. Miró. 1993. *Aproximaciones a la psicoterapia: Una introducción a los tratamientos psicológicos.* Barcelona: Paidós.

Finnegan, K. T., G. A. Ricaurte, L. D. Ritchie, I. Irwin, S. J. Peroutka, and J. W. Langston. 1988. Orally administered MDMA causes a long-term depletion of serotonin in rat brain. *Brain Res.* 447:141–4.

Fischer, C., G. Hatzidimitriou, J. Wlos, J. Katz, and G. Ricaurte. 1995. Reorganization of ascending 5-HT axon projections in animals previously exposed to recreational drug (±)3,4-methylenedioxymethamphetamine (MDMA, "Ecstasy"). *J. Neurosci.* 15:5476–85.

Fitzgerald, J. L., and J. J. Reid. 1990. Effects of methylenedioxymethamphetamine on the release of monoamines from rat brain slices. *Eur. J. Pharmacol.* 191:217–20.

Fleckenstein, A. E., H. M. Haughey, R. R. Metzger, et al. 1999. Differential effects of psychostimulants and related agents on dopaminergic and serotonergic transporter function. *Eur. J. Pharmacol.* 382:45–9.

Foa, E. B., B. O. Rothbaum, D. S. Siggs, and T. B. Murdock. 1991. Treatment of posttraumatic stress disorder in rape victims: A comparison between cognitive-behavioral procedures and counseling. *Jour. Cons. Clin. Psych.* 59:715–23.

Frederick, D. L., S. F. Ali, W. Slikker Jr., M. P. Gillam, R. R. Allen, and M. G. Paule. 1995. Behavioral and neurochemical effects of chronic methylenedioxymeth-amphetamine (MDMA) treatment in rhesus monkeys. *Neurotoxicol. Teratol.* 17:531–43.

Frederick, D. L., S. F. Ali, M. P. Gillam, J. Gossett, W. Slikker, and M. G. Paule. 1998. Acute effects of dexfenfluramine (d-FEN) and methylenedioxymethamphetamine (MDMA) before and after short-course, high-dose treatment. *Ann. N. Y. Acad. Sci.* 844:183–90.

Freedman, D. X., R. Gottlieb, and R. A. Lovell. 1970. Psychotomimetic drugs and brain 5-hydroxytryptamine metabolism. *Biochem. Pharmacol.* 19:1181–8.

Frei, E., A. Gamma, R. D. Pascual-Marqui, D. Hell, and F. X. Vollenweider. 2001. Localization of MDMA-induced electrical brain activity in healthy volunteers using low resolution brain electric tomography (LORETA). Submitted.

Frey, K., M. Kilbourn, and T. Robinson. 1997. Reduced striatal vesicular monoamine transporters after neurotoxic but not after behaviorally-sensitizing doses of methamphetamine. *Eur. J. Pharmacol.* 334:273–9.

Frith, C. M., and L. Chang. 1987. Toxicity of methylenedioxymethamphetamine (MDMA) in the dog and rat. *Fundam. Appl. Toxicol.* 9:110–9.

Fritschy, J. M., W. E. Lyons, M. E. Molliver, and R. Grzanna. 1988. Neurotoxic effects of *p*-chloroamphetamine on the serotoninergic innervation of the trigeminal motor nucleus: A retrograde transport study. *Brain Res.* 473:261–70.

Gaddum, J., and K. Hameed. 1954. Drugs which antagonize 5-hydroxytryptamine. *Br. J. Pharmacol.* 9:240–8.

Gamella, J., and A. Álvarez. 1999. *Las rutas del Éxtasis: Drogas de síntesis y nuevas culturas juveniles* (The route of Ecstasy: drugs of synthesis and new youth cultures). Barcelona: Ariel.

Gamma, A., E. Frei, D. Lehmann, R. D. Pascual-Marqui, D. Hell, and F. X. Vollenweider. 2000a. Mood state and brain electric activity in ecstasy users. *Neuroreport* 11:157–62.

Gamma, A., A. Buck, T. Berthold, M. E. Liechti, and F. X. Vollenweider. 2000b. 3,4-Methylenedioxymethamphetamine (MDMA) modulates cortical and limbic brain activity as measured by $[H_2O^{15}]$-PET in healthy humans. *Neuropsychopharmacology* 23:388–95.

Gamma, A., A. Buck, T. Berthold, and F. X. Vollenweider. 2001. No difference in brain activation during cognitive performance between Ecstasy (MDMA) user and controls: A $[H_2^{15}O]$-PET study. *J. Clin. Psychopharmacol.* 21:66–71.

Gartside, S. E., R. McQuade, and T. Sharp. 1996. Effects of repeated administration of 3,4-methylenedioxymethamphetamine on 5-hydroxytryptamine neuronal activity and release in the rat brain in vivo. *J. Pharmacol. Exp. Ther.* 279:277–83.

Gasser, P. 1994–95. Psycholytic therapy with MDMA and LSD in Switzerland. *Newsletter of the Multidisciplinary Association for Psychedelic Studies* 5 no. 3: 3–7.

———. 1996. Die psycholoytische Therapie in der Schweiz von 1988–1993. Eine Katamnestische Erhebung. *Shweiz. Arch. Neurol. Psychiat.* 2:59–65.

Gaston, T. R., and G. T. Rasmussen. 1972. Identification of 3,4-methylene-dioxymethamphetamine. *Microgram* 5:60–3.

Gelder, M., D. Gath, and R. Mayou. 1995. *Concise Oxford texbook of psychiatry*. Oxford: Oxford University Press. pp 149–50.

Geller, E., E. R. Ritvo, B. J. Freeman, and A. Yuwiler. 1982. Preliminary observations on the effect of fenfluramine on blood serotonin and symptoms in three autistic boys. *N. Engl. J. Med.* 37:165–9.

Gerra, G., A. Zaimovic, G. Giucastro, et al. 1998. Serotonergic function after (±)3,4-methylenedioxymethamphetamine ("Ecstasy") in humans. *Int. Clin. Psychopharmacol.* 13:1–9.

Gerra, G., A. Zaimovic, M. Ferri, et al. 2000. Long-lasting effects of (±)3,4-methylene-dioxymethamphetamine (ecstasy) on serotonin system function in humans. *Biol. Psychiatry* 47:127–36.

Gerson, S. C., and R. J. Baldessarini. 1980. Motor effects of serotonin in the central nervous system. *Life Sci.* 27:1435–51.

Geyer, M. A., and C. W. Callaway. 1994. Behavioral pharmacology of ring-substituted amphetamine analogs. In *Amphetamine and its analogs: Psychopharmacology, toxicology, and abuse*, edited by A. K. Cho and D. S. Segal. New York: Academic Press. pp 177–208.

Globus, M. Y., R. Busto, B. Lin, H. Schnippering, and M. D. Ginsberg. 1995. Detection of free radical activity during transient global ischemia and recirculation: Effects of intra-ischemic brain temperature modulation. *J. Neurochem.* 65:1250–6.

Goff, D. C., K. K. Midha, O. Sarid-Segal, J. W. Hubbard, and E. Amico. 1995. A placebo controlled trial of fluoxetine added to neuroleptic in patients with schizophrenia. *Psychopharmacol. Berl.* 117:417–23.

Gold, L. H., G. F. Koob, and M. A. Geyer. 1988. Stimulant and hallucinogenic behavioral profiles of 3,4-methylenedioxymethamphetamine and N-ethyl-3,4-methylenedioxyamphetamine in rats. *J. Pharmacol. Exp. Ther.* 247(2):547–55.

Goldberg, T. E., L. B. Bigelow, D. R. Weinberger, D. G. Daniel, and J. E. Kleinman. 1991. Cognitive and behavioral effects of coadministration of dextroamphetamine and haloperidol in schizophrenia. *Am. J. Psychiatry* 148:78–84.

Goldstein, L. B., and C. E. Hulsebosch. 1999. Amphetamine-facilitated poststroke recovery. *Stroke* 30(3):696–8.

Gollamudi, R., S. F. Ali, G. Lipe, et al. 1989. Influence of inducers and inhibitors on the metabolism in vitro and neurochemical effects in vivo of MDMA. *Neurotoxicology* 10:455–66.

González de Rivera, J. L. 1990. El síndrome de estrés post-traumático. *Psiquis* 11:11–24.

———. 1994. El síndrome post-traumático de estrés: Una revisión crítica. In *Psiquiatría legal y forense*, edited by S. Delgado. Madrid: Colex.

Gordon, C. J., and L. Fogelson. 1994. Metabolic and thermoregulatory responses of the rat maintained in acrylic or wire-screen cages: Implications for pharmacological studies. *Physiol. Behav.* 56:73–9.

Gordon, C. J., W. P. Watkinson, J. P. O'Callaghan, and D. B. Miller. 1991. Effects of 3,4-methylenedioxymethamphetamine on autonomic thermoregulatory responses of the rat. *Pharmacol. Biochem. Behav.* 38:339–44.

Gough, B., S. F. Ali, W. Slikker Jr., and R. R. Holson. 1991. Acute effects of 3,4-methylenedioxymethamphetamine (MDMA) on monoamines in rat caudate. *Pharmacol. Biochem. Behav.* 39:619–23.

Gouzoulis, E., and L. Hermle. 1994. Die Gefarhen von Ecstasy. *Nervenartz* 64:478–80.

Gouzoulis, E., D. Dorchardt, and L. Hermle. 1993. A case of toxic psychosis induced by "Eve" (3,4-methylene-dioxyethylamphetamine). *Arch. Gen. Psychiatry* 50:75.

Gouzoulis-Mayfrank, E., B. Thelen, E. Habermeyer, et al. 1999. Psychopathological, neuroendocrine and autonomic effects of 3,4-methylenedioxyethylamphetamine (MDE), psilocybin and d-methamphetamine in healthy volunteers. *Psychopharmacology* 142:41–50.

Gouzoulis-Mayfrank, E., J. Daumann, F. Tuchtenhagen, et al. 2000. Impaired cognitive performance in drug free users of recreational ecstasy (MDMA) [see Comments]. *J. Neurol. Neurosurg. Psychiatry* 68:719–25.

Graham, D. G., S. M. Tiffany, W. R. Bell Jr., and W. F. Gutknecht. 1978. Autoxidation versus covalent binding of quinones as the mechanism of toxicity of dopamine, 6-hydroxydopamine, and related compounds toward C1300 neuroblastoma cells in vitro. *Mol. Pharmacol.* 14:644–53.

Granoff, M. I., and C. R. Ashby Jr. 1998. The effect of the repeated administration of the compound 3,4-methylenedioxymethamphetamine on the response of rats to the

5-HT2A,C receptor agonist (±)-1-(2,5-dimethoxy-4-iodophenyl)-2-aminopropane (DOI). *Neuropsychobiology* 37:36–40.

Graumlich, J. F., T. M. Ludden, C. Conry-Cantilena, L. R. Cantilena Jr., Y. Wang, and M. Levine. 1997. Pharmacokinetic model of ascorbic acid in healthy male volunteers during depletion and repletion. *Pharmacol. Res.* 14:1133–9.

Graves, A. B., J. A. Mortimer, E. B. Larson, A. Wenzlow, J. D. Bowen, and W. C. McCormick. 1996. Head circumference as a measure of cognitive reserve: Association with severity of impairment in Alzheimer's disease. *Br. J. Psychiatry* 169:86–92.

Green, A. R., A. J. Cross, and G. M. Goodwin. 1995. Review of the pharmacology and clinical pharmacology of 3,4-methylenedioxymethamphetamine (MDMA or "Ecstasy"). *Psychopharmacology (Berlin)* 119:247–60.

Greer, G. 1985. Using MDMA in psychotherapy. *Adv. J. Inst. Adv. Health* 2:57–9.

Greer, G., and R. Tolbert. 1986. Subjective reports of the effects of MDMA in a clinical setting. *J. Psychoactive Drugs* 18(4):319–27.

———. 1990. The therapeutic use of MDMA. In: *Ecstasy: The clinical, pharmacological and neurotoxicological effects of the drug MDMA*, edited by S. J. Peroutka. Boston: Kluwer Academic Publishers.

———. 1998. A method of conducting therapeutic sessions with MDMA. *J. Psychoactive Drugs* 30(4):371–9.

———. 1979. *Psychedelic drugs reconsidered.* New York: Basic Books.

———. 1983. *Psychedelic reflections.* New York: Human Sciences Press.

———. 1985. What is MDMA? *Harvard Medical School Medical Health Letter.* 2(2): 8.

———. 1986. Can drugs be used to enhance the psychotherapeutic process? *Am. J. Psychother.* 40:393–404.

———. 1990. Testing psychotherapies and drug therapies: The case of psychedelic drugs. In: *Ecstasy: The clinical, pharmacological and neurotoxicological effects of the drug MDMA*, edited by S. J. Peroutka. Boston: Kluwer Academic Publishers.

Grob, C. S. 1998. MDMA research: preliminary investigations with human subjects. *Int. J. Drug Policy* 9:119–24.

———. 2000. Deconstructing Ecstasy: The politics of MDMA research. *Addiction Res.* 8:549–88.

Grob, C. S., G. Bravo, and R. Walsh. 1990. Second thoughts on 3,4-methylene-dioxymethamphetamine (MDMA) neurotoxicity. *Arch. Gen. Psychiatry* 47:288.

Grob, C. S., R. E. Poland, L. Chang, and T. Ernst. 1996. Psychobiologic effects of 3,4-methylenedioxymethamphetamine in humans: Methodological considerations and preliminary observations. *Behav. Brain Res.* 73:103–7.

Grob, C. S., Poland, R. E. 1997. MDMA. In: *Substance abuse: A comprehensive textbook*, 3rd ed., edited by J. H. Lowinson, P. Ruiz, R. B. Millman, and J. G. Langrod. Baltimore: Williams and Wilkins. pp. 269–75.

Grof, Stanislav. 1980. *LSD psychotherapy.* Pomona, Calif.: Hunter House.

Gudelsky, G. A. 1996. Effect of ascorbate and cysteine on the 3,4-methylenedioxy-methamphetamine-induced depletion of brain serotonin. *J. Neural Transm.* 103:1397–404.

Gudelsky, G. A., and J. F. Nash. 1996. Carrier-mediated release of serotonin by 3,4-methylenedioxymethamphetamine: Implications for serotonin-dopamine interactions. *J. Neurochem.* 66:243–49.

Gudelsky, G. A., B. K. Yamamoto, and J. F. Nash. 1994. Potentiation of 3,4-methylene-dioxymethamphetamine-induced dopamine release and serotonin neurotoxicity by 5-HT2 receptor agonists. *Eur. J. Pharmacol.* 264:325–30.

Guttman, E., and W. Sargant. 1937. Observations on benzedrine. *Br. Med. J.* 1:1013–5.

Gur, R. E., S. M. Resnick, and R. C. Gur, et al. 1989. Laterality and frontality of cerebral blood flow and metabolism in schizophrenia: Relationship to symptom specificity. *Psychiatry Res.* 27(3):325–34.

Haigler, H. J., and G. K. Aghajanian. 1973. Mescaline and LSD: Directed and indirect effects on serotonin-containing neurons in the brain. *Eur. J. Pharmacol.* 21:53–60.

Hall, F. S., A. C. Devries, G. W. Fong, S. Huang, and A. Pert. 1999. Effects of 5,7-dihydroxy-tryptamine depletion of tissue serotonin levels on extracellular serotonin in the striatum assessed with in vivo microdialysis: Relationship to behavior. *Synapse* 33:16–25.

Hardman, H. F., C. O. Haavik, and M. H. Seevers. 1973. Relationship of the structure of mescaline and behavior in five species of laboratory animals. *Toxicol. Appl. Pharmacol.* 25:299–309.

Haring, J. H., L. Meyerson, and T. L. Hoffman. 1992. Effects of para-chloroamphetamine upon the serotonergic innervation of the rat hippocampus. *Brain Res.* 577:253–60.

Harlow, D., and J. Beck. 1990. Survey of the clinical uses of MDMA. Paper presented at the MAPS International Conference on Psycholytic Psychotherapy, 29 November, in Bern, Switzerland.

Harries, D. P., and R. DeSilva. 1992. "Ecstasy" and intracerebral hemorrhage. *Scot. Med. J.* 37:150–2.

Harris, D., M. Baggott, R. T. Jones, and J. Mendelson. 2000. MDMA pharmacokinetics and physiological and subjective effects in humans. In *Problems of drug dependence*, edited by L. S. Harris. Washington, D.C.: U.S. Government Printing Office.

Harris Research Center. 1982. Young people's poll. January.

Hartley, D. E. 1985. Research on the therapeutic alliance in psychotherapy. *Ann. Rev. Psychiatry* 4:532–49.

Harvey, D. C., G. Lacan, S. P. Tanious, and W. P. Melega. 2000. Recovery from methamphetamine induced long-term nigrostriatal dopaminergic deficits without substantia nigra cell loss. *Brain Res.* 871:259–70.

Hatzidimitriou, G., U. D. McCann, and G. A. Ricaurte. 1999. Altered serotonin innervation patterns in the forebrain of monkeys treated with (±)3,4-methylene-dioxymethamphetamine seven years previously: factors influencing abnormal recovery. *J. Neurosci.* 19:5096–107.

Hayner, G. N., and H. McKinney. 1986. MDMA: The dark side of ecstasy. *J. Psychoactive Drugs* 18:341–7.

Heffernan, T. M., J. L. Ling, and A. B. Scholey. Prospective memory deficits in MDMA ("ecstasy") users. *Hum. Psychopharmacol.* (in press)

Hegadoren, K. M., G. B. Baker, and M. Bourin. 1999. 3,4-Methylenedioxy analogues of amphetamine: Defining the risks to humans. *Neurosci. Biobehav. Rev.* 23:539–53.

Heinz, A., and D. W. Jones. 2000. Serotonin transporters in ecstasy users [Letter; Comment]. *Br. J. Psychiatry* 176:193–5.

Hekmatpanah, C. R., and S. J. Peroutka. 1990. 5-Hydroxytryptamine uptake blockers attenuate the 5-hydroxytryptamine-releasing effect of 3,4-methylenedioxymethamphetamine and related agents. *Eur. J. Pharmacol.* 177:95–8.

Helzer, J. E., L. N. Robins, and L. McEvoy. 1987. Post-traumatic stress disorder in the general population: Findings of the epidemiologic catchment area survey. *N. Engl. J. Med.* 317(24):1630–4.

Hendin, H. 1982. *Suicide in America.* New York: W.W. Norton.

Henry, J. A. 1992. Ecstasy and the dance of death. *Br. Med. J.* 305:5–6.

Henry, J. A., K. J. Jeffreys, and S. Dawling. 1992. Toxicity and deaths from 3,4-methylenedioxymethamphetamine ("ecstasy"). *Lancet* 340:384–7.

Henry, J. A., J. K. Fallon, A. T. Kicman, A. J. Hutt, D. A. Cowan, and M. Forsling. 1998. Low-dose MDMA ("Ecstasy") induces vasopressin secretion. *Lancet* 351:1784.

Henry, W. P., H. H. Strupp, and T. E. Schacht. 1990. Patient and therapist introject, interpersonal process, and differential psychotherapy outcome. *J. Consult. Clin. Psychol.* 58(6):768–74.

Hermle, L., M. Spitzer, D. Borchardt, K. A. Kovar, and E. Gouzoulis. 1993. Psychological effects of MDE in normal subjects: Are entactogens a new class of psychoactive agents? *Neuropsychopharmacology* 8:171–6.

Hernández-Lopéz, C., M. Farré, P. N. Roset, et al. 2000. MDMA and alcohol interactions: Psychomotor and subjective effects and pharmacokinetics. *Br. J. Clin. Pharmacol.* Special issue:111.

Herning, R. I., D. E. King, W. E. Better, and J. L. Cadet. 1999. Neurovascular deficits in cocaine abusers. *Neuropsychopharmacology* 21:110–8.

Hervias, I., B. Lasheras, and N. Aguirre. 2000. 2-Deoxy-D-glucose prevents and nicotinamide potentiates 3,4-methylenedioxymethamphetamine-induced serotonin neurotoxicity. *J. Neurochem.* 75:982–90.

Hiramatsu, M., and A. K. Cho. 1990. Enantiomeric differences in the effects of 3,4-methylenedioxymethamphetamine on extracellular monoamines and metabolites in the striatum of freely-moving rats: An in vivo microdialysis study. *Neuropharmacology* 29:269–75.

Holden, R. M., and M. A. Jackson. 1996. Near-fatal hyponatraemic coma due to vasopressin over-secretion after "ecstasy" (3,4-MDMA). *Lancet* 347:1052.

Horan, B., E. L. Gardner, and C. R. Ashby Jr. 2000. Enhancement of conditioned place preference response to cocaine in rats following subchronic administration of 3,4-methylenedioxymethamphetamine (MDMA). *Synapse* 35:160–2.

Horton, A. A., and S. Fairhurst. 1987. Lipid peroxidation and mechanisms of toxicity. *Crit. Rev. Toxicol.* 18:27–79.

Huether, G., D. Zhou, and E. Ruther. 1997. Causes and consequences of the loss of serotonergic presynapses elicited by the consumption of 3,4-methylenedioxymethamphetamine (MDMA, "ecstasy") and its congeners. *J. Neural Transm.* 104:771–94.

Ings, R. M. 1990. Interspecies scaling and comparisons in drug development and toxicokinetics. *Xenobiotica* 20:1201–31.

Insel, T. R., G. Battaglia, J. N. Johannessen, S. Marra, and E. B. De Souza. 1989. 3,4-Methylenedioxymethamphetamine ("ecstasy") selectively destroys brain serotonin terminals in rhesus monkeys. *J. Pharmacol. Exp. Ther.* 249:713–20.

Iqbal, N., G. M. Asins, S. Wetzler, R. S. Kahn, S. Kay, and H. M. van Praag. 1991. The MCPP challenge test in schizophrenia: Hormonal and behavioral responses. *Biol. Psychiatry* 30:770–7.

Irwin, M. R., S. R. Marder, F. Fuentenbro, and A. Yuwiler A. 1987. L-5-Hydroxytryptophan attenuates positive psychotic symptoms induced by D-amphetamine. *Psychiatry Res.* 22:283–9.

Itil, T., A. Keskiner, N. Kiremitci, and J. M. Holden. 1967. Effect of phencyclidine in chronic schizophrenics. *Can. Pschiatr. Assoc. J.* 12:209–12.

Jacobsen, L. K., J. K. Staley, R. T. Malison, et al. 2000. Elevated central serotonin transporter binding availability in acutely abstinent cocaine-dependent patients. *Am. J. Psychiatry* 157:1134–40.

Janke, W., and G. Debus. 1978. *Die Eigenschaftswörterliste (EWL-K): Ein Verfahren zur Erfassung der Befindlichkeit.* Göttingen: Hogrefe.

Jansen, K. L. R. 1993. Non-medical use of ketamine. *Br. Med. J.* 306:601–2.

———. 1997. Adverse psychological effects associated with the use of Ecstasy (MDMA) and their treatment. In *Ecstasy reconsidered*, edited by N. Saunders. London: Neal's Yard Desk Top Publishing Studio. pp. 112–33.

———. 1998. Ecstasy (MDMA) dependence. *Drug Alcohol Depend.* 53(2):121–4.

———. 2000. A Review of the Nonmedical Use of Ketamine: Use, Uses, and Consequences. *J. Psychoactive Drugs* 32(4):419–433

———. *Ketamine: Dreams and Realities.* Sarasota, FL.: Multidisciplinary Association for Psychedelic Studies (available from www.maps.org).

Jansen, K. L. R., and A. R. Forrest. 1999. Toxic effect of MDMA on brain serotonin neurons [Letter]. *Lancet* 353(9160):1270–1.

Jayanthi, S., B. Ladenheim, A. M. Andrews, and J. L. Cadet. 1999. Overexpression of human copper/zinc superoxide dismutase in transgenic mice attenuates oxidative stress caused by methylenedioxymethamphetamine (Ecstasy). *Neuroscience* 91:1379–87.

Jensen, K. F., J. Olin, N. Haykal-Coates, J. O'Callaghan, D. B. Miller, and J. S. de Olmos. 1993. Mapping toxicant-induced nervous system damage with a cupric silver stain: A quantitative analysis of neural degeneration induced by 3,4-methylenedioxymethamphetamine. *NIDA Res. Monogr.* 136:133–49; discussion 150–4.

Johnson, M., I. Elayan, G. R. Hanson, R. L. Foltz, J. W. Gibb, and H. K. Lim. 1992. Effects of 3,4-dihydroxymethamphetamine and 2,4,5-trihydroxymethamphetamine, two metabolites of 3,4-methylenedioxymethamphetamine, on central serotonergic and dopaminergic systems. *J. Pharmacol. Exp. Ther.* 261:447–53.

Kahn, R. S., L. J. Siever, S. Gabriel, et al. 1992. Serotonin function in schizophrenia: Effects of meta-chlorophenylpiperazine in schizophrenic patients and healthy subjects. *Psychiatry Res.* 43:1–12.

Kalia, M., J. P. O'Callaghan, D. B. Miller, and M. Kramer. 2000. Comparative study of fluoxetine, sibutramine, sertraline and dexfenfluramine on the morphology of serotonergic nerve terminals using serotonin immunohistochemistry. *Brain Res.* 858:92–105.

Kalin, N. H., R. J. Davidson, W. Irwin, et al. 1997. Functional magnetic resonance imaging studies of emotional processing in normal and depressed patients: Effects of venlafaxine. *J. Clin. Psychiatry* 58:32–9.

Kalivas, P. W., P. Duffy, and S. R. White. 1998. MDMA elicits behavioral and neuro-chemical sensitization in rats. *Neuropsychopharmacology* 18:469–79.

Kapur, S., and G. Remington. 1996. Serotonin-dopamine interaction and its relevance to schizophrenia. *Am. J. Psychiatry* 153:466–76.

Karch, S. B. 1996. *Pathology of drug abuse.* 2d ed. Boca Raton, Fla.: CRC Press. pp. 249–53.

Kelland, M. D., A. S. Freeman, and L. A. Chiodo. 1989. (±)-3,4-Methylenedioxymeth-amphetamine-induced changes in the basal activity and pharmacological respon-siveness of nigrostriatal dopamine neurons. *Eur. J. Pharmacol.* 169:11–21.

———. 1990. Serotonergic afferent regulation of the basic physiology and pharmaco-logical responsiveness of nigrostriatal dopamine neurons. *J. Pharm. Exp. Ther.* 253:803–11.

Kemmerling, K., R. Haller, and H. Hinterhuber. 1996. Das neuropsychiatrische Risiko von 3,4-Methylenedioxymethamphetamin ("Ecstasy"). *Neuropsychiatrie* 10:94–102.

Kernberg, O. F., C. S. Burnstein, R. Coyne, D. A. Appelbaum, H. Horwitz, and T. J. Voth. 1972. Psychotherapy and psychoanalysis: Final report of the Menninger Foundation's Psychotherapy Research Project. *Bull. Menninger Clin.* 36:1–198.

Ketter, T. A., P. J. Andreason, M. S. George, et al. 1996. Anterior paralimbic mediation of procaine-induced emotional and psychosensory experiences. *Arch. Gen. Psychiatry* 53:59–69.

Khakoo, S. L., C. J. Coles, J. S. Armstrong, and R. E. Barry. 1995. Hepatotoxicity and accelerated fibrosis following 3,4-methylenedioxymethamphetamine ("ecstasy") usage. *J. Clin. Gastroenterol.* 20:244–7.

Kilpatrick, D. G. 1992a. Etiología y factores predictivos de estrés postraumático en víctimas de agresiones sexuales. In *Avances en el tratamiento psicológico de los trastornos de ansiedad*, edited by E. Echeburúa. Madrid: Pirámide.

————. 1992b. Tratamiento psicológico de las agresiones sexuales. In *Avances en el tratamiento psicológico de los trastornos de ansiedad*, edited by E. Echeburúa. Madrid: Pirámide.

Kish, S. J., Y. Furukawa, L. Ang, S. P. Vorce, and K. S. Kalasinsky. 2000. Striatal serotonin is depleted in brain of a human MDMA (Ecstasy) user. *Neurology* 55:294–6.

Klein, Joe. 1985. The drug the call Ecstasy. *New York*, 20 May.

Kleven, M. S., W. L. Woolverton, and L. S. Seiden. 1989. Evidence that both intragastric and subcutaneous administration of methylenedioxymethamphetamine (MDMA) produce serotonin neurotoxicity in rhesus monkeys. *Brain Res.* 488:121–5.

Klugman, A., S. Hardy, T. Baldeweg, and J. Gruzelier. 1999. Letter to the *Lancet* in response to McCann et al. (1999) *Lancet* 353:1269.

Knable, M. B., and D. R. Weinberger. 1997. Dopamine, the prefrontal cortex and schizophrenia. *J. Psychopharmacol.* 11(2):123–31.

Koreen, A. R., S. G. Siris, M. Chakos, J. Alvir, D. Mayerhoff, and J. Lieberman. 1993. Depression in first episode schizophrenia. *Am. J. Psychiatry* 150:1643–8.

Koss, M. P. 1983. The scope of rape: Implications for the clinical treatment of victims. *Clin. Psychologist* 38:88–91.

Kretsch, M. J., M. W. Green, A. K. Fong, N. A. Elliman, and H. L. Johnson. 1997. Cognitive effects of a long-term weight reducing diet. *Int. J. Obes. Relat. Metab. Disord.* 21:14–21.

Krystal, J. H., J. P. Seibyl, L. P. Price, S. W. Woods, G. R. Heninger, and D. S. Charney. 1991. MCPP effects in schizophrenic patients before and after typical and atypical neuroleptic treatment. *Schizophr. Res.* 4:350–9.

Krystal, J. H., L. H. Price, C. Opsahl, G. A. Ricaurte, and G. R. Heninger. 1992. Chronic 3,4-methylenedioxymethamphetamine (MDMA) use: Effects on mood and neuropsychological function? *Am. J. Drug Alcohol Abuse* 18(3):331–41.

Kuikka, J. T., and A. K. Ahonen. 1999. Toxic effect of MDMA on brain serotonin neurons [Letter; Comment]. *Lancet* 353:1269; discussion 1270–1.

Lahti. A. C., B. Koffel, D. LaPorte, and C. A. Tamminga. 1995. Subanesthetic doses of ketamine stimulate psychosis in schizophrenia. *Neuropsychopharmacology.* 13:9–19.

Lamb, R. J., and R. R. Griffiths. 1987. Self-injection of d,1-3,4-methylene-dioxymethamphetamine (MDMA) in the baboon. *Psychopharmacology* 91:268–72.

Langston, J. W., P. Ballard, J. W. Tetrud, and I. Irwin. 1983. Chronic parkinsonism in humans due to a product of meperidine-analog synthesis. *Science* 219:979–80.

Lapin, I. P., and G. F. Oxenburg. 1969. Intensification of the central serotonergic process as a possible determinant for the thymoleptic effect. *Lancet* 1:132–36.

Laruelle, M., A. Abi-Dargham, M. F. Casanova, R. Toti, D. R. Weinberger, and J. E. Kleinman. 1993. Selective abnormalities of prefrontal serotonergic receptors in schizophrenia: A postmortem study. *Arch. Gen. Psychiatry* 50:810–8.

Laruelle, M. A. Abi-Dargham, C. H. van Dyck, W. Rosenblatt, Y. Zea-Ponce, S. S. Zoghbi, R. M. Baldwin, D. S. Charney, P. B. Hoffer, H. F. Kung. 1995. SPECT imaging of striatal dopamine release after amphetamine challenge. *J. Nuc. Med.* 36:1182–1190.

Lauerma, H., M. Wuorela, and M. Halme. 1998. Interaction of serotonin reuptake inhibitor and 3,4-methylenedioxymethamphetamine? [Letter]. *Biol. Psychiatry* 43:929.

Laviola, G., W. Adriani, M. L. Terranova, and G. Gerra. 1999. Psychobiological risk factors for vulnerability to psychostimulants in human adolescents and animal models. *Neurosci. Biobehav. Rev.* 23:993–1010.

LaVoie, M. J., and T. G. Hastings. 1999. Dopamine quinone formation and protein modification associated with the striatal neurotoxicity of methamphetamine: Evidence against a role for extracellular dopamine. *J. Neurosci.* 19:1484–91.

Lawn, J. C. 1986. Schedules of controlled substances: scheduling of 3,4-methylenedioxymethamphetamine (MDMA) into schedule I. *Fed. Reg.* 51:36552–60.

Le Doux, J. E. 1995. Emotion: Clues from the brain. *Ann. Rev. Psychol.* 46:209–35.

Lee, M. S., Y. K. Kim, S. K. Lee, and K. Y. Suh. 1998. A double-blind study of adjunctive sertraline in haloperidol-stabilized patients with chronic schizophrenia. *J. Clin. Psychopharmacol.* 18:399–403.

Le Poul, E., C. Boni, N. Hanoun, et al. 2000. Differential adaptation of brain 5-HT1A and 5-HT1B receptors and 5-HT transporter in rats treated chronically with fluoxetine. *Neuropharmacology* 39:110–22.

Lesch, K. P., M. Wiesmann, A. Hoh, et al. 1992. 5-HT1A receptor-effector system responsivity in panic disorder. *Psychopharmacology (Berlin)* 106:111–7.

Lester, S., M. Baggott, S. Welm, et al. 2000. The cardiovascular effects of Ecstasy, 3-4-methylenedioxymethamphetamine (MDMA). *Ann. Intern. Med.* 133(12):969–73.

Lew, R., K. E. Sabol, C. Chou, G. L. Vosmer, J. Richards, and L. S. Seiden. 1996. Methylenedioxymethamphetamine-induced serotonin deficits are followed by partial recovery over a 52-week period. II. Radioligand binding and autoradiography studies. *J. Pharmacol. Exp. Ther.* 276:855–65.

Leysen, J. E., P. M. Janssen, A. Schotte, W. H. Luyten, and A. A. Megens. 1993. Interaction of antipsychotic drugs with neurotransmitter receptor sites in vitro and in vivo in relation to pharmacological and clinical effects: Role of 5HT2 receptors. *Psychopharmacology* 112:S40–54.

Li, A. A., G. J. Marek, G. Vosmer, and L. S. Seiden. 1989. Long-term central 5-HT depletions resulting from repeated administration of MDMA enhances the effects of single administration of MDMA on schedule-controlled behavior of rats. *Pharmacol. Biochem. Behav.* 33:641–8.

Lieberman, J. A., J. M. Kane, and J. Alvir. 1987. Provocative tests with psychostimulant drugs in schizophrenia. *Psychopharmacology* 91:415–33.

Lieberman, J. A., B. J. Kinon, and A. D. Loebel. 1990. Dopaminergic mechanism in idiopathic and drug-induced psychosis. *Schizophr. Bull.* 16:97–109

Liechti, M. E., and F. X. Vollenweider. 2000a. Acute psychological and physiological effects of MDMA ("Ecstasy") after haloperidol pretreatment in normal healthy humans. *Eur. Neuropsychopharmacol.* 22:513–21 (in press).

———. 2000b. The serotonin uptake inhibitor citalopram reduces acute cardiovascular and vegetative effects of MDMA ("Ecstasy") in healthy volunteers. *J. Psychopharmacol.* 14(3):269–74.

Liechti, M. E., C. Baumann, A. Gamma, and F. X. Vollenweider. 2000a. Acute psychological effects of 3,4-methylenedioxymethamphetamine (MDMA, "Ecstasy") are attenuated by the serotonin uptake inhibitor citalopram. *Neuropsychopharmacology* 22:513–21.

Liechti, M. E., M. Saur, A. Gamma, D. Hell, and F. X. Vollenweider. 2000b. Psychological and physiological effects of MDMA ("Ecstasy") after pretreatment with the 5-HT2 antagonist ketanserin in healthy humans. *Neuropsychopharmacology* 23(4):396–405.

Liechti, M. E., A. Gamma, and F. X. Vollenweider. 2001a. Gender differences in the subjective effects of MDMA. *Psychopharmacology (Berlin)* 154(2):161–68.

Liechti, M. E., M. A. Geyer, D. Hell, and F. X. Vollenweider. 2001b. Effects of MDMA (Ecstasy) on prepulse inhibition and habituation of startle in humans after pretreatment with citalopram, haloperidol, or ketanserin. *Neuropsychopharmacology* 24:240–52.

Liester, M. B., C. S. Grob, G. L. Bravo, and R. N. Walsh. 1992. Phenomenology and sequelae of 3,4-methylenedioxymethamphetamine use. *J. Nerv. Ment. Dis.* 180:345–52.

Lin, J. H. 1998. Applications and limitations of interspecies scaling and in vitro extrapolation in pharmacokinetics. *Drug Metab. Dispos.* 26:1202–12.

Little, K. Y., D. P. McLaughlin, L. Zhang, et al. 1998. Cocaine, ethanol, and genotype effects on human midbrain serotonin transporter binding sites and mRNA levels. *Am. J. Psychiatry* 155:207–13.

Liu, B. A., N. Mittmann, S. R. Knowles, et al. 1996. Hyponatremia and the syndrome of inappropriate secretion of antidiuretic hormone associated with the use of selective serotonin reuptake inhibitors: A review of spontaneous reports. *Can. Med. Assoc. J.* 155:519–27.

Logan, A. S. C., B. Stickle, N. O'Keefe, and H. Hewitson. 1993. Survival following "Ecstasy" ingestion with a peak temperature of 42 degrees Celsius. *Anesthesia* 48:1017–8.

Logan, B. J., R. Laverty, W. D. Sanderson, and Y. B. Yee. 1988. Differences between rats and mice in MDMA (methylenedioxymethamphetamine) neurotoxicity. *Eur. J. Pharmacol.* 152:227–34.

Lucki, I. 1998. The spectrum of behaviors influenced by serotonin. *Biol. Psychiatry* 44:151–62.

Lukas, S. E. 1985. Amphetamines: Danger in the fast lane. *The encyclopaedia of psychoactive drugs*. New York: Chelsea House Publishers.

Lyness, W. H., N. M. Friedle, and K. E. Moore. 1981. Increased self-administration of *d*-amphetamine after destruction of 5-hydroxytryptaminergic (serotonergic) nerves. *Pharmacol. Biochem. Behav.* 12:937–41.

Maes, M., and H. Meltzer. 1995. The serotonin hypothesis of major depression. In *Psychopharmacology: The fourth generation of progress*, edited by F. E. Bloom and D. J. Kupfer. New York: Raven Press. pp. 933–44.

Mahmood, I. 1999. Allometric issues in drug development. *J. Pharm. Sci.* 88:1101–6.

Malberg, J. E., and L. S. Seiden. 1998. Small changes in ambient temperature cause large changes in 3,4-methylenedioxymethamphetamine (MDMA)-induced serotonin neurotoxicity and core body temperature in the rat. *J. Neurosci.* 18:5086–94.

Malberg, J. E., K. E. Sabol, and L. S. Seiden. 1996. Co-administration of MDMA with drugs that protect against MDMA neurotoxicity produces different effects on body temperature in the rat. *J. Pharmacol. Exp. Ther.* 278:258–67.

Malhotra, A. K., D. A. Pinals, C. M. Adler et al. 1997. Ketamine-induced exacerbation of psychotic symptoms and cognitive impairment in neuroleptic-free schizophrenics. *Neuropsychopharacology.* 17: 141–50.

Mandel, W. 1984. The yuppie psychedelic. *San Francisco Chronicle,* 10 June.

Mann, J. J. 1987. Psychobiologic predictors of suicide. *J. Clin. Psychiatry* 48:39–43.

———. 1995. Violence and aggression. In *Psychopharmacology: The fourth generation of progress,* edited by F. E. Bloom and D. J. Kupfer. New York: Raven Press.

Mann, J. J., Y. Y. Huang, and M. D. Underwood. 2000. A serotonin transporter gene promoter polymorphism (5-HTTLPR) and prefrontal cortical binding in major depression and suicide. *Arch. Gen. Psychiatry* 57(8):729–38.

Marchant, N. C., M. A. Breen, D. Wallace, et al. 1992. Comparative biodisposition and metabolism of ^{14}C-(±)-fenfluramine in mouse, rat, dog and man. *Xenobiotica* 22:1251–66.

Marston, H. M., M. E. Reid, J. A. Lawrence, H. J. Olverman, and S. P. Butcher. 1999. Behavioural analysis of the acute and chronic effects of MDMA treatment in the rat. *Psychopharmacology (Berlin)* 144:67–76.

Mas, M., M. Farré, R. de la Torre, et al. 1999. Cardiovascular and neuroendocrine effects and pharmacokinetics of 3,4-methylenedioxymethamphetamine in humans. *J. Pharmacol. Exp. Ther.* 290:136–45.

Mathers, D. C., and A. H. Ghodse. 1992. Cannabis and psychotic illness. *Br. J. Psychiatry* 161:648–53.

Matthew, R. J., and W. H. Wilson. 1989. Changes in cerebral blood flow and mental state after amphetamine challange in schizophrenic patients. *Neuropsychobiology* 21:117–23.

Maxwell, D. L., M. I. Polkey, and J. A. Henry. 1993. Hyponatremia and catatonic stupor after taking "ecstasy." *Br. Med. J.* 307:1399.

McBean, D. E., J. Sharkey, I. M. Ritchie, and P. A. Kelly. 1990. Evidence for a possible role for serotonergic systems in the control of cerebral blood flow. *Brain Res.* 537:307–10.

McCann, U. D., and G. A. Ricaurte. 1991a. Lasting neuropsychiatric sequelae of (±)3,4-methylenedioxymethamphetamine ("Ecstasy") in recreational users. *J. Clin. Psychopharmacol.* 11:302–5.

———. 1991b. Major metabolites of (±)3,4-methylenedioxyamphetamine (MDA) do not mediate its toxic effects on brain serotonin neurons. *Brain Res.* 545:279–82.

McCann, U. D., A. Ridenour, Y. Shaham, and G. A. Ricaurte. 1994. Serotonin neurotoxicity after (±)3,4 methylenedioxymethamphetamine (MDMA; "Ecstasy"): A controlled study in humans. *Neuropsychopharmacology* 10:129–38.

McCann, U. D., S. O. Slate, and G. A. Ricaurte. 1996. Adverse reactions with 3,4-methylenedioxymethamphetamine (MDMA; "Ecstasy"). *Drug Saf.* 15:107–15.

McCann, U. D., Z. Szabo, U. Scheffel, R. F. Dannals, and G. A. Ricaurte. 1998. Positron emission tomographic evidence of toxic effect of MDMA ("Ecstasy") on brain serotonin neurons in human beings [see Comments]. *Lancet* 352:1433–7.

McCann, U. D., V. Eligulashvili, M. Mertl, D. L. Murphy, and G. A. Ricaurte. 1999a. Altered neuroendocrine and behavioral responses to *m*-chlorophenylpiperazine in 3,4-methylenedioxymethamphetamine (MDMA) users. *Psychopharmacology (Berlin)* 147:56–65.

McCann, U. D., M. Mertl, V. Eligulashvili, and G. A. Ricaurte. 1999b. Cognitive performance in (±)3,4-methylenedioxymethamphetamine (MDMA, "ecstasy") users: A controlled study. *Psychopharmacology (Berlin)* 143:417–25.

McElhatton, P. R., D. N.Bateman, and C. Evans et al. 1999. Congenital anomalies after prenatal ecstasy exposure. *Lancet* 354:1441–2.

McGuire, P. 2000. Long term psychiatric and cognitive effects of MDMA use. *Toxicol. Lett.* 112–113:153–6.

McGuire, P., and T. Fahy. 1991. Chronic paranoid psychosis after misuse of MDMA ("Ecstasy") [see Comments]. *Br. Med. J.* 302:697.

———. 1992. Flashbacks following MDMA. *Br. J. Psychiatry* 160:276.

McGuire, P., H. Cope, and T. Fahy. 1994. Diversity of psychopathology associated with the use of 3,4-methylenedioxymethamphetamine (Ecstasy) *Br. J. Psychiatry* 165:391–5.

McKenna, D. J., and S. J. Peroutka. 1990. Neurochemistry and neurotoxicity of 3,4-methylenedioxymethamphetamine (MDMA, "Ecstasy"). *J. Neurochem.* 54:14–22.

McKenna, T. K., and D. J. McKenna. 1975. *The Invisible Landscape.* New York: Seabury Press.

McKetin, R., and N. Solowij. 1999. Event-related potential indices of auditory selective attention in dependent amphetamine users. *Biol. Psychiatry* 45:1488–97.

McMiller, P., and M. Plant. 1996. Drinking, smoking, and illicit drug use among 15 and 16 year olds in the United Kingdom. *Br. Med. J.* 313:394–7.

McNamara, M. G., J. P. Kelly, and B. E. Leonard. 1995. Some behavioural and neurochemical aspects of subacute (±)3,4-methylenedioxymethamphetamine administration in rats. *Pharmacol. Biochem. Behav.* 52:479–84.

Meichenbaum, D. 1994. Tratamiento de clientes con trastornos de estrés post-traumático: Un enfoque cognitivo conductual. *Rev. Psicoterapia* 5(17):5–84.

Meltzer, C. C., G. Smith, S. T. DeKosky, et al. 1998. Serotonin in aging, late-life depression, and Alzheimer's disease: The emerging role of functional imaging [see Comments]. *Neuropsychopharmacology* 18:407–30.

Meltzer, H. Y. 1990. Role of serotonin in depression. *Ann. N. Y. Acad. Sci.* 600:486–500.

Meltzer, H. Y., and G. Okayli. 1995. Reduction of suicidality during clozapine treatment of neuroleptic-resistant schizophrenia: Impact on risk-benefit assessment. *Am. J. Psychiatry* 152:183–90.

Meltzer, H. Y., and S. M. Stahl. 1976. The dopamine hypothesis of schizophrenia: A review. *Schizophr. Bull.* 2:19–76.

Meltzer, H. Y., R. G. Fessler, M. Simonovic, and V. S. Fang. 1978. The effect of mescaline, 3,4-dimethoxyphenethylamine and 2,5-dimethoxy-4-methyl-amphetamine on rat plasma prolactin: Evidence for serotonergic mediation. *Life Sci.* 23:1185–92.

Meltzer, H., S. Matsubara, and J. Lee. 1989. Classification of typical and atypical antipsychotic drugs on the basis of dopamine D-1, D-2, and serotonin 2 pKi values. *J. Pharmacol. Exp. Ther.* 251:238–46.

Metzger, R. R., G. R. Hanson, J. W. Gibb, and A. E. Fleckenstein. 1998. 3,4-Methylenedioxymethamphetamine-induced acute changes in dopamine transporter function. *Eur. J. Pharmacol.* 349:205–10.

Metzner, R., and S. Adamson. 1988. The nature of the MDMA experience and its role in healing, psychotherapy, and spiritual practice. *ReVision* 10, no. 4.

Meyerson, A. 1936. Effect of benzedrine sulfate on mood and fatigue in normal and neurotic persons. *Arch. Neurol. Psychiatry* 816–22.

Miller, D. B., and J. P. O'Callaghan. 1994. Environment-, drug- and stress-induced alterations in body temperature affect the neurotoxicity of substituted amphet-amines in the C57BL/6J mouse. *J. Pharmacol. Exp. Ther.* 270:752–60.

Miller, N. S., M. S. Gold, and D. E. Smith, eds. 1997. Ecstasy. In *Manual of therapeutics for addiction.* "Intoxication and Withdrawal from Marijuana, LSD, and MDMA" by M. Gold. New York: John Wiley and Sons. pp. 52–4.

Milroy, C. M. 1999. Ten years of ecstasy. *J. R. Soc. Med.* 92:68–72.

Milroy, C. M., J. C. Clark, and A. R. W. Forrest. 1996. Pathology of deaths associated with "ecstasy" and "eve" misuse. *J. Clin. Pathol.* 49:149–53.

Molliver, M. E., L. A. Mamounas, and M. A. Wilson. 1989. Effects of neurotoxic amphet-amines on serotonergic neurons: Immunocytochemical studies. In: *Pharmacology and toxicology of amphetamine and related designer drugs,* edited by K. Asghar and E. De Souza. NIDA Research Monograph no. 94. Baltimore, Md.: NIDA, pp. 270–304.

Montgomery, H., and S. Myerson. 1997. 3,4-Methylenedioxymethamphetamine (MDMA, or "ecstasy") and associated hypoglycemia. *Am. J. Emerg. Med.*15:218.

Mordenti, J., and W. Chappell. 1989. The use of interspecies scaling in toxicokinetics. In *Toxicokinetics in new drug development,* edited by A. Yacobi, J. Kelly, and V. Batra. New York: Pergamon Press. pp. 42–96.

Morgan, A. E., B. Horan, S. L. Dewey, and C. R. Ashby Jr. 1997. Repeated administra-tion of 3,4-methylenedioxymethamphetamine augments cocaine's action on dopamine in the nucleus accumbens: A microdialysis study. *Eur. J. Pharmacol.* 331:R1–3.

Morgan, M. J. 1998. Recreational use of "ecstasy" (MDMA) is associated with elevated impulsivity. *Neuropsychopharmacology* 19:252–64.

———. 1999. Memory deficits associated with recreational use of "ecstasy" (MDMA). *Psychopharmacology (Berlin)* 141:30–6.

———. 2000. Ecstasy (MDMA): A review of its possible persistent psychological effects. *Psychopharmacology (Berlin)* 152:230–48.

Mossner, R., H. Westphal, and K. P. Lesch. 1998. Altered brain serotonin homeostasis and locomotor insensitivity to 3,4-methylenedioxymethamphetamine ("Ecstasy") in serotonin transporter-deficient mice. *Mol. Pharmacol.* 53:649–55.

Mueller, P. D., and W. S. Korey. 1998. Death by "ecstasy": The serotonin syndrome? *Ann. Emerg. Med.* 32:377–80.

Mulan, S., and W. Penfield. 1959. Illusions of comparative interpretation and emotion. *Arch. Neurol. Psychiatry* 81:269–84.

Murphy, D. L., E. A. Mueller, N. A. Garrick, and C. S. Aulakh. 1986. Use of serotonergic agents in the clinical assessment of central serotonin function. *J. Clin. Psychiatry* 47:9–15.

Murphy, D. L., K. P. Lesch, C. S. Aulakh, et al. 1991. Serotonin-selective arylpiperizines with neuroendocrine, behavioral, temperature, and cardiovascular effects in humans. *Pharmacol. Rev.* 43:527–52.

Naranjo, C. 1973. *The healing journey: New approaches to consciousness.* New York: Random House.

Naranjo, C., A. Shulgin, and T. Sargent. 1967. Evaluation of 3,4- methylenedioxy-amphetamine (MDA) as an adjunct to psychotherapy. *Med. Pharmacol. Exp.* 17:359–64.

Nash, J. F. 1990. Ketanserin pretreatment attenuates MDMA-induced dopamine release in the striatum as measured by in vivo microdialysis. *Life Sci.* 47:2401–8.

Nash, J. F., and J. Brodkin. 1991. Microdialysis studies on 3,4-methylenedioxy-methamphetamine-induced dopamine release: Effect of dopamine uptake inhibitors. *J. Pharmacol. Exp. Ther.* 259:820–5.

Nash, J. F., H. Y. Meltzer, and G. A. Gudelsky. 1990. Effect of 3,4-methylenedioxy-methamphetamine on 3,4-dihydroxyphenylalanine accumulation in the striatum and nucleus accumbens. *J. Neurochem.* 54:1062–7.

Nencini, P., W. L. Woolverton, and L. S. Seiden. 1988. Enhancement of morphine-induced analgesia after repeated injections of methylenedioxymethamphetamine. *Brain Res.* 457:136–42.

Netter, P., J. Hennig, and I. S. Roed. 1996. Serotonin and dopamine as mediators of sensation seeking behavior. *Neuropsychobiology* 34:155–65.

Neylan, T. C. 1999. Frontal lobe function: Mr. Phineas Gage's famous injury. *J. Neuro. Clin. Neurosci.*

Nichols, D. E. 1986. Differences between the mechanisms of action of MDMA, MBDB, and the classic hallucinogens: Identification of a new therapeutic class—entactogens. *J. Psychoactive Drugs* 18(4): 305–13.

Nichols, D. E., and R. Oberlender. 1989. Structure-activity relationships of MDMA-like substances. In: *Pharmacology and toxicology of amphetamine and related designer drugs,* edited by K. Asghar and E. De Souza, NIDA Research Monograph, no. 94. Baltimore, Md.: NIDA. pp. 1–29.

Nichols, D. E., and R. Oberlender. 1990. Structure-activity relationships of MDMA and related compounds: A new class of psychoactive agents? In *Ecstasy: The clinical, pharmacological and neurotoxicological effects of the drug MDMA,* edited by S. J. Peroutka. Boston: Kluwer Academic Publishers. pp. 105–31.

Nichols, D. E., D. H. Lloyd, A. J. Hoffman, M. B. Nichols, and G. K. W. Yim. 1982. Effects of certain hallucinogenic amphetamine analogues on the release of (3H) serotonin from rat brain synaptosomes. *J. Med. Chem.* 25:530–5.

Nichols, D. E., R. Yensen, and R. Metzner. 1993.The great entactogen empathogen debate. *MAPS Bulletin.* 4: 47–49.

Nimmo, S. M., B. W. Kennedy, W. M. Tullett, A. S. Blyth, and J. R. Dougall. 1993. Drug-induced hyperthermia. *Anaesthesia* 48:892–5.

Nobler, M. S., J. J. Mann, and H. A. Sackeim. 1999. Serotonin, cerebral blood flow, and cerebral metabolic rate in geriatric major depression and normal aging. *Brain Res. Rev.* 30:250–63.

Nuñez-Dominguiez, L. A. 1994. Psychosis because of ecstasy. *Addicciones* 6(3):301–7.

Obradovic, T., K. M. Imel, and S. R. White. 1998. Repeated exposure to methylenedioxymethamphetamine (MDMA) alters nucleus accumbens neuronal responses to dopamine and serotonin. *Brain Res.* 785:1–9.

Obrocki, J., R. Buchert, O. Vaterlein, R. Thomasius, W. Beyer, and T. Schiemann. 1999. Ecstasy: Long-term effects on the human central nervous system revealed by positron emission tomography [see Comments]. *Br. J. Psychiatry* 175:186–8.

O'Callaghan, J. P., and D. B. Miller. 1993. Quantification of reactive gliosis as an approach to neurotoxicity assessment. *NIDA Res. Monogr.* 136:188–212.

———. 2001. Neurotoxic effects of substituted amphetamines in rats and mice: Challenges to the current dogma. In: *Handbook of neurotoxicology*, edited by E. Massaro and P. A. Broderick. New York: Humana Press.

O'Hearn, E., G. Battaglia, E. B. De Souza, M. J. Kuhar, and M. E. Molliver. 1988. Methylenedioxyamphetamine (MDA) and methylenedioxymethamphetamine (MDMA) cause selective ablation of serotonergic axon terminals in forebrain: Immunocytochemical evidence for neurotoxicity. *J. Neurosci.* 8:2788–803.

O'Malley, S., M. Adamse, R. K. Heaton, and F. H. Gawin. 1992. Neuropsychological impairment in chronic cocaine abusers. *Am. J. Drug Alcohol Abuse* 18:131–44.

Ornstein, T. J., J. L. Iddon, A. M. Baldacchino, et al. 2000. Profiles of cognitive dysfunction in chronic amphetamine and heroin abusers. *Neuropsychopharmacology* 23:113–26.

Ortuño, J., N. Pizarro, M. Farré, et al. 1999. Quantification of 3,4-methylenedioxymethamphetamine and its metabolites in plasma and urine by gas chromatography with nitrogen-phosphorous detection. *J. Chromatogr. B. Biomed. Sci.* 723:221–32.

O'Shea, E., R. Granados, B. Esteban, M. I. Colado, and A. R. Green. 1998. The relationship between the degree of neurodegeneration of rat brain 5-HT nerve terminals and the dose and frequency of administration of MDMA ("ecstasy"). *Neuropharmacology* 37:919–26.

Pacifici, R., P. Zuccaro, M. Farré, et al. 1999. Immunomodulating properties of MDMA alone and in combination with alcohol: A pilot study. *Life Sci.* 65:309–16.

———. 2000. Immunomodulating activity of MDMA. *Ann. N. Y. Acad. Sci.* 914:215–24.

———. 2001. Acute effects of MDMA alone and in combination with ethanol on the immune system in humans. *J. Pharmacol. Exp. Ther.* 296:207–215.

Padkin, A. 1994. Treating MDMA ("ecstasy") toxicity. *Anaesthesia* 49:259.

Pallanti, S., and D. Mazzi. 1992. MDMA (Ecstasy) precipitation of panic disorder. *Biol. Psychiatry* 32:91–5.

Parrott, A. C. 2000. Human research on MDMA (3,4-methylenedioxymethamphetamine) neurotoxicity: Cognitive and behavioural indices of change. *Neuropsychobiology* 42:17–24.

Parrott, A. C., and J. Lasky. 1998. Ecstasy (MDMA) effects upon mood and cognition: Before, during and after a Saturday night dance. *Psychopharmacology (Berlin)* 139(3):261–8.

Parrott, A. C., A. Lees, N. J. Garnham, M. Jones, and K. Wesnes. 1998. Cognitive performance in recreational users of MDMA "ecstasy": Evidence for memory deficits. *J. Psychopharmacol.* 12:79–83.

Patterson, E. W., G. Myers, and D. M. Gallant. 1988. Patterns of substance abuse on a college campus: A 14-year comparison study. *Am. J. Drug Alcohol Abuse* 14(2):237–46.

Perls, F. 1969. *Gestalt therapy verbatim.* Laffayete, Calif.: Real People Press.

Peroutka, S. J. 1987. Incidence of recreational abuse of 3,4-methylenedioxymethamphetamine (MDMA, Ecstasy) on an undergraduate campus. *N. Engl. J. Med.* 317:1542–3.

———. 1990. Recreational use of MDMA. In: *Ecstasy: the clinical, pharmacological and neurotoxicological effects of the drug MDM,* edited by S. J. Peroutka. Boston: Kluwer Academic Publishers. pp. 53–63.

Peroutka, S. J., N. Pascoe, and K. F. Faull. 1987. Monoamine metabolites in the cerebral spinal fluid of recreational users of 3,4-methylenedioxymethamphetamine (MDMA; "Ecstasy"). *Res. Commun. Substance Abuse* 8:125–38.

Peroutka, S. J., H. Newman, and H. Harris. 1988. Subjective effects of 3,4- methylenedioxymethamphetamine in recreational users. *Neuropsychopharmacology* 1:273–7.

Poblete, J. C., and E. C. Azmitia. 1995. Activation of glycogen phosphorylase by serotonin and 3,4-methylenedioxymethamphetamine in astroglial-rich primary cultures: Involvement of the 5-HT2A receptor. *Brain Res.* 680:9–15.

Poch, J., and A. Ávila. 1998. *Investigación en psicoterapia: La contribución psicoanalítica.* Barcelona: Paidós.

Poland, R. E. 1990. Diminished corticotropin and enhanced prolactin responses to 8-hydroxy-2(di-n-propylamino)tetralin in methylenedioxymethamphetamine pretreated rats. *Neuropharmacology* 29:1099–101.

Poland, R. E., P. Lutchmansingh, J. T. McCracken, et al. 1997. Abnormal ACTH and prolactin responses to fenfluramine in rats exposed to single and multiple doses of MDMA. *Psychopharmacology (Berlin)* 131:411–9.

Poole, R., and C. Brabbins. 1996. Drug induced psychosis. *Br. J. Psychiatry* 168:135–8.

Pope, H. G. Jr., and D. Yurgelun-Todd. 1996. The residual cognitive effects of heavy marijuana use in college students [see Comments]. *JAMA* 275:521–7.

Post-traumatic stress disorder. 1996. *Harvard Mental Health Letter,* June–July.

President of the Council. 1998. Tackling drugs to build a better Britain: The government's ten year strategy for tackling drugs misuse. London: Her Majesty's Stationary Office.

Price, L. H., G. A. Ricaurte, J. H. Krystal, and G. R. Heninger. 1989. Neuroendocrine and mood responses to intravenous L-tryptophan in 3,4-methylenedioxymethamphetamine (MDMA) users: Preliminary observations [see Comments]. *Arch. Gen. Psychiatry* 46:20–2.

Price, L. H., J. H. Krystal, and G. R. Heninger. 1990. In reply [to Grob et al. 1990]. *Arch. Gen. Psychiatry* 47:289.

Ramamoorthy, S., E. Giovanetti, Y. Qian, and R. D. Blakely. 1998. Phosphorylation and regulation of antidepressant-sensitive serotonin transporters. *J. Biol. Chem.* 273:2458–66.

Ramsey, M., B. Partridge, and C. Byron. 1999. Drug misuse declared in 1998: Key results from the British Crime Survey. *Res. Find.* 93:1–4.

Randall, T. 1992. Ecstasy-fueled "rave" parties become dances of death for English youths. *JAMA* 268:1505–6.

Rao, M. L., and H. J. Moller. 1994. Biochemical findings of negative symptoms in schizophrenia and their putative relevance to pharmacologic treatment. *Neuropsychobiology* 30:160–72.

Redfearn, P. J., N. Agrawal, and L. H. Mair. 1998. An association between the regular use of 3,4-methlenedioxymethamphetamine (ecstasy) and excessive wear of the teeth. *Addiction* 93(5):745–8.

Reneman, L., J. Booij, B. Schmand, W. van den Brink, and B. Gunning. 2000a. Memory disturbances in "Ecstasy" users are correlated with an altered brain serotonin neurotransmission. *Psychopharmacology (Berlin)* 148:322–4.

Reneman, L., J. B. Habraken, C. B. Majoie, J. Booij, and G. J. den Heeten. 2000b. MDMA ("Ecstasy") and its association with cerebrovascular accidents: Preliminary findings. *Am. J. Neuroradiol.* 21:1001–7.

Reynolds, S. 1998. *Generation Ecstasy: Into the world of techno culture.* London: Little, Brown, and Company.

Riba, J., and M. Barbanoj. 1998. A pharmacological study of ayahuasca in healthy volunteers. *MAPS Bull.* 8(3):2–15.

Ricaurte, G. A., and U. D. McCann. 1992. Neurotoxic amphetamine analogues: Effects in monkeys and implications for humans. *Ann. N. Y. Acad. Sci.* 648:371–82.

Ricaurte, G. A., L. E. DeLanney, I. Irwin, and J. W. Langston. 1988a. Toxic effects of MDMA on central serotonergic neurons in the primate: Importance of route and frequency of drug administration. *Brain Res.* 446:165–8.

Ricaurte, G. A., L. E. DeLanney, S. G. Wiener, I. Irwin, and J. W. Langston. 1988b. 5-Hydroxyindoleacetic acid in cerebrospinal fluid reflects serotonergic damage induced by 3,4-methylenedioxymethamphetamine in CNS of non-human primates. *Brain Res.* 474:359–63.

Ricaurte, G. A., L. S. Forno, M. A. Wilson, et al. 1988c. (±)3,4-Methylenedioxy-methamphetamine selectively damages central serotonergic neurons in nonhuman primates. *JAMA* 260:51–5.

Ricaurte, G. A., K. T. Finnegan, I. Irwin, and J. W. Langston. 1990. Aminergic metabolites in cerebrospinal fluid of humans previously exposed to MDMA: preliminary observations. *Ann. N. Y. Acad. Sci.* 600:699–708; discussion 708–10.

Ricaurte, G. A., A. L. Martello, J. L. Katz, and M. B. Martello. 1992. Lasting effects of (±)-3,4-methylenedioxymethamphetamine (MDMA) on central serotonergic neurons in nonhuman primates: Neurochemical observations. *J. Pharmacol. Exp. Ther.* 261:616–22.

Ricaurte, G. A., A. L. Markowska, G. L. Wenk, G. Hatzidimitriou, J. Wlos, and D. S. Olton. 1993. 3,4-Methylenedioxymethamphetamine, serotonin and memory [published erratum appears in *J. Pharmacol. Exp. Ther.* 1994; 268(1):529]. *J. Pharmacol. Exp. Ther.* 266:1097–105.

Ricaurte, G. A., J. Yuan, and U. D. McCann. 2000. (±)3,4-Methylenedioxymeth-amphetamine ("Ecstasy")-induced serotonin neurotoxicity: studies in animals. *Neuropsychobiology* 42:5–10.

Riedel, W. J., T. Klaassen, N. E. Deutz, A. van Someren, and H. M. van Praag. 1999. Tryptophan depletion in normal volunteers produces selective impairment in memory consolidation. *Psychopharmacology (Berlin)* 141:362–9.

Riedlinger, J. E. 1985. The scheduling of MDMA: A pharmacist's perspective. *J. Psychoactive Drugs* 17(3):167–71.

Ritvo, E. R., B. J. Freeman, E. Geller, and A. Yuwiler. 1983. Effects of fenfluramine on 14 outpatients with the syndrome of autism. *J. Am. Acad. Child Psychiatry* 22:549–58.

Robinson, T. E., E. Castaneda, and I. Q. Whishaw. 1993. Effects of cortical serotonin depletion induced by 3,4-methylenedioxymethamphetamine (MDMA) on behavior, before and after additional cholinergic blockade. *Neuropsychopharmacology* 8:77–85.

Rochester, J. A, and J. T. Kirchner. 1999. Ecstasy (3,4-methylenedioxymethamphet-amine): History, neurochemistry, and toxicology. *J. Am. Board Fam. Pract.* 12:137–42.

Rodgers, J. 2000. Cognitive performance amongst recreational users of "ecstasy." *Psychopharmacology (Berlin)* 151:19–24.

Rof Carballo, J., and A. González Morado. 1958. Experiencia clínica con la dietilamida del ácido lisérgico (DAL). *Boletín del Instituto de Patología Médica*, 8(10):271–280.

Rosenbaum, M., and R. Doblin. 1991. Why MDMA should not have been made illegal. In *The drug legalization debate*, edited by J. Inciardi. Newbury Park, Calif.: Sage. p. 15.

Rossman, Martin. 1987. *Healing yourself.* New York: Walker.

Rudnick, G., and S. C. Wall. 1992. The molecular mechanism of "ecstasy" [3,4-methylenedioxymethamphetamine (MDMA)]: Serotonin transporters are targets for MDMA-induced serotonin release. *Proc. Natl. Acad. Sci. U. S. A.* 89:1817–21.

Ruiz-Ogara, C., J. L. Martí-Tusquets, and E. González-Monclús. 1956. Psicosis lisérgica. *Revista de Psiquiatría y Psicología Médica*, 2(6):566–590.

Rutty, G. N., and C. M. Milroy. 1997. The pathology of ring-substituted amphetamine analogue 3,4-methylenedioxymethylamphetamine (MDMA, "Ecstasy"). *J. Pathol.* 181:255–6.

Sabol, K. E., and L. S. Seiden. 1998. Reserpine attenuates D-amphetamine and MDMA-induced transmitter release in vivo: a consideration of dose, core temperature and dopamine synthesis. *Brain Res.* 806:69–78.

Sabol, K. E., R. Lew, J. B. Richards, G. L. Vosmer, and L. S. Seiden. 1996. Methylenedioxymethamphetamine-induced serotonin deficits are followed by partial recovery over a 52-week period. I. Synaptosomal uptake and tissue concentrations. *J. Pharmacol. Exp. Ther.* 276:846–4.

Sanders-Bush, E., and P. J. Conn. 1987. Neurochemistry of serotonin neuronal systems: Consequences of serotonin receptor activation. In *Psychopharmacology: The third generation of progress*, edited by H. Y. Meltzer. New York: Raven Press. pp. 95–103.

Sanfilipo, M., A. Wolkin, B. Angrist, et al. 1996. Amphetamine and negative symptoms of schizophrenia. *Psychopharmacology* 123:211–4.

Sarró, R. 1956. Fármacos y psiquiatría. *Med. Clín.* 26(3):184–7.

Satchell, S. C., and M. Connaughton. 1994. Inappropriate antidiuretic hormone secretion and extreme rises in serum creatinine kinase following MDMA ingestion. *Br. J. Hosp. Med.* 51:495.

Sato, M. 1992. A lasting vulnerability to psychosis in patients with previous metamphetamine psychosis. In *The neurobiology of drug and alcohol addiction*, edited by P. H. Kalivas and H. H. Samson. *Ann. N. Y. Acad. Sci.* 654:160–70.

Saunders, N. 1993. *E for ecstasy.* London: W. B. Saunders.

———. 1995. *Ecstasy and the dance culture.* London: Neal's Yard Desk Top Publishing Studio. p. 121.

Saunders, N. E., ed. 1997. *Ecstasy reconsidered.* London: Neal's Yard Desk Top Publishing Studio.

Scallet, A. C., G. W. Lipe, S. F. Ali, R. R. Holson, C. H. Frith, and W. Slikker Jr. 1988. Neuropathological evaluation by combined immunohistochemistry and degeneration-specific methods: Application to methylenedioxymethamphetamine. *Neurotoxicology* 9:529–37.

Scanzello, C. R., G. Hatzidimitriou, A. L. Martello, J. L. Katz, and G. A. Ricaurte. 1993. Serotonergic recovery after (±)3,4-(methylenedioxy) methamphetamine injury: Observations in rats. *J. Pharmacol. Exp. Ther.* 264:1484–91.

Schechter, M. D. 1991. Effect of MDMA neurotoxicity upon its conditioned place preference and discrimination. *Pharmacol. Biochem. Behav.* 38:539–44.

———. 1997. Serotonergic mediation of fenfluramine discriminative stimuli in fawn-hooded rats. *Life Sci.* 60(6):PL83–90.

Scheffel, U., J. R. Lever, M. Stathis, and G. A. Ricaurte. 1992. Repeated administration of MDMA causes transient down regulation of serotonin 5-HT2 receptors. *Neuropharmacology* 31:881–93.

Scheffel, U., Z. Szabo, W. B. Mathews, et al. 1998. In vivo detection of short- and long-term MDMA neurotoxicity: A positron emission tomography study in the living baboon brain. *Synapse* 29:183–92.

Schifano, F. 1991. Chronic atypical psychosis associated with MDMA (Ecstasy) abuse. *Lancet* 338:1335.

———. 2000. Potential human neurotoxicity of MDMA ("Ecstasy"): Subjective self-reports, evidence from an Italian drug addiction centre and clinical case studies. *Neuropsychobiology* 42:25–33.

Schifano, F., and G. Magni. 1994. ("Ecstasy") abuse: Psychopathological features and craving for chocolate—a case series. *Biol. Psychiatry* 36(11):763–7.

Schlaepfer, T. E., G. D. Pearlson, D. F. Wong, S. Marenco, and R. F. Dannals. 1997. PET study of competition between intravenous cocaine and [^{11}C]raclopride at dopamine receptors in human subjects. *Am. J. Psychiatry.* 154:1209–13.

Schmidt, C. J. 1987. Neurotoxicity of the psychedelic amphetamine methylenedioxymethamphetamine. *J. Pharmacol. Exp. Ther.* 240:1–7.

Schmidt, C. J., and J. H. Kehne. 1990. Neurotoxicity of MDMA: neurochemical effects. *Ann. N. Y. Acad. Sci.* 600:665–80; discussion 680–1.

Schmidt, C. J., and V. L. Taylor. 1988. Direct central effects of acute methylenedioxymethamphetamine on serotonergic neurons. *Eur. J. Pharmacol.* 156:121–31.

———. 1990. Reversal of the acute effects of 3,4-methylenedioxymethamphetamine by 5-HT uptake inhibitors. *Eur. J. Pharmacol.* 181:133–6.

Schmidt, C. J., L. Wu, and W. Lovenberg. 1986. Methylenedioxymethamphetamine: A potentially neurotoxic amphetamine analogue. *Eur. J. Pharmacol.*124:175–8.

Schmidt, C. J., J. A. Levin, and W. Lovenberg. 1987. In vitro and in vivo neurochemical effects of methylenedioxymethamphetamine on striatal monoamine systems in the rat brain. *Biochem. Pharmacol.* 36:747–55.

Schmidt, C. J., C. K. Black, G. M. Abbate, and V. L. Taylor. 1990a. MDMA-induced hyperthermia and neurotoxicity are independently mediated by 5-HT2 receptors. *Brain Res.* 529:85–90.

Schmidt, C. J., C. K. Black, and V. L. Taylor. 1990b. Antagonism of the neurotoxicity due to a single administration of methylenedioxymethamphetamine. *Eur. J. Pharmacol.* 181:59–70.

Schmidt, C. J., V. L. Taylor, G. M. Abbate, and T. R. Nieduzak. 1991. 5-HT2 antagonists stereoselectively prevent the neurotoxicity of 3,4-methylenedioxymethamphetamine by blocking the acute stimulation of dopamine synthesis: reversal by L-dopa. *J. Pharmacol. Exp. Ther.* 256:230–5.

Schneider, F., R. E. Gur, L. H. Mozley, et al. 1995. Mood effects on limbic blood flow correlate with emotional self-rating: A PET study with oxygen-15 labeled water. *Psychiatry Res. Neuroimaging* 61:265–83.

Screaton, G. R., H. S. Cairns, M. Sarner, M. Singer, A. Thrasher, and S. L. Cohen. 1992. Hyperpyrexia and rhabdomyolysis after MDMA ("ecstasy") abuse. *Lancet* 339:677–8.

Seeman, P., T. Lee, M. Chau-Wong, and K. Wong. 1976. Antipsychotic drug doses and neuroleptic/dopamine receptors. *Nature* 261:717–9.

Seiden, L. S., and K. E. Sabol. 1996. Methamphetamine and methylenedioxymethamphetamine neurotoxicity: Possible mechanisms of cell destruction. *NIDA Res. Monogr.* 163:251–76.

Semple, D. M., K. P. Ebmeier, M. F. Glabus, R. E. O'Carroll, and E. C. Johnstone. 1999. Reduced in vivo binding to the serotonin transporter in the cerebral cortex of MDMA ("ecstasy") users. *Br. J. Psychiatry* 175:63–9.

Series, H. G., P. J. Cowen, and T. Sharp. 1994. *p*-Chloroamphetamine (PCA), 3,4-methylenedioxy-methamphetamine (MDMA) and d-fenfluramine pretreatment attenuates d-fenfluramine-evoked release of 5-HT in vivo. *Psychopharmacology (Berlin)* 116:508–14.

Shankaran, M., and G. A. Gudelsky. 1999. A neurotoxic regimen of MDMA suppresses behavioral, thermal and neurochemical responses to subsequent MDMA administration. *Psychopharmacology (Berlin)* 147:66–72.

Shankaran, M., B. K. Yamamoto, and G. A. Gudelsky. 1999a. Involvement of the serotonin transporter in the formation of hydroxyl radicals induced by 3,4-methylenedioxymethamphetamine. *Eur. J. Pharmacol.* 385:103–10.

———. 1999b. Mazindol attenuates the 3,4-methylenedioxymethamphetamine-induced formation of hydroxyl radicals and long-term depletion of serotonin in the striatum. *J. Neurochem.* 72:2516–22.

Shapiro, H. 1996. *Drug deaths*. Druglink Factsheet no. 19, ISDD. London: Waterbridge House.

Shapiro, Y., A. Magazanik, R. Udassin, G. Ben-Baruch, E. Shvartz, and Y. Shoenfeld. 1979. Heat intolerance in former heatstroke patients. *Ann. Intern. Med.* 90:913–6.

Sharkey, J., D. E. McBean, and P. A. Kelly. 1991. Alterations in hippocampal function following repeated exposure to the amphetamine derivative methylenedioxymethamphetamine ("Ecstasy"). *Psychopharmacology (Berlin)* 105:113–8.

Sherlock, K., K. Wolff, A. W. Hay et al. 1999. Analysis of illicit ecstasy tablets: Implications for clinical management in the accident and emergency department. *J. Accid. Emerg. Med.* 16(3):194–7.

Shulgin, A. T. 1986. The background and chemistry of MDMA. *J. Psychoactive Drugs* 18:291–304.

Shulgin, A. T. 1990. History of MDMA. In *Ecstasy: The clinical, pharmacological and neurotoxicological effects of the drug MDMA*, edited by S. J. Peroutka. Boston: Kluwer Academic Publishers. pp. 1–20.

Shulgin, A. T., and D. E. Nichols. 1978. Characterization of three new psychotomimetics. In *The psychopharmacology of hallucinogens*, edited by R. C. Stillman and R. E. Willette. New York: Pergamon Press.

Shulgin, A. T., and T. Sargent. 1967. Evaluation of 3,4-methylenedioxyamphetamine (MDA) as an adjunct to psychotherapy. *Med. Pharmacol. Exp.*17:359–64.

Shulgin, A., and A. Shulgin. 1991. *PIHKAL: A chemical love story*. Berkeley: Transform Press.

Shulgin, A. T., T. Sargent, and C. Naranjo. 1969. Structure-activity relationships of one-ring psychotomimetics. *Nature* 221:537–541.

Shulgin, A. T., T. Sargent, and C. Naranjo. 1973. Animal pharmacology and human psychopharmacology of 3-methoxy-4,5-methylenedioxyphenylisopropylamine (MMDA). *Pharmacology* 10:12–8.

Siegel, B. V. Jr., R. L. Trestman, S. O'Flaithbhearthaigh, et al. 1996. D-amphetamine challenge effects on Wisconsin Card Sort Test: Performance in schizotypal personality disorder. *Schizophr. Res.* 20(1–2):29–32.

Siegel, R. K. 1985. Written testimony submitted on behalf of Drug Enforcement Administration, United States Department of Justice, Drug Enforcement Administration Law Hearings, docket no. 84–48.

Silver, H., and A. Nassar. 1992. Fluvoxamine improves negative symptoms in treated chronic schizophrenia. *Pharmacopsychiatry* 25:245.

Silver, H., and N. Shmugliakov. 1998. Augmentation with fluvoxamine but not maprotiline improves negative symptoms in treated schizophrenia. *J. Clin. Psychopharmacol.* 18:208–11.

Simpson, D. L., and B. H. Rumack. 1981. Methylenedioxyamphetamine: Clinical description of overdose, death, and review of pharmacology. *Arch. Intern. Med.* 141:1507–9.

Singarajah, C., and N. G. Lavies. 1992. An overdose of ecstasy: A role for dantrolene. *Anaesthesia* 47:686–7.

Slikker, W. Jr., S. F. Ali, A. C. Scallet, C. H. Frith, G. D. Newport, and J. R. Bailey. 1988. Neurochemical and neurohistological alterations in the rat and monkey produced by orally administered methylenedioxymethamphetamine (MDMA). *Toxicol. Appl. Pharmacol.* 94:448–57.

Slikker, W. Jr., R. R. Holson, S. F. Ali, et al. 1989. Behavioral and neurochemical effects of orally administered MDMA in the rodent and nonhuman primate. *Neurotoxicology* 10:529–42.

Smilkstein, M. J., S. C. Smolinske, and B. H. Rumack. 1987. A case of MAO inhibitor/ MDMA interaction: Agony after ecstasy. *Clin. Toxicol.* 25:149–59.

Snyder, S. H. 1973. Amphetamine psychosis: A "model" schizophrenia mediated by catecholamines. *Am. J. Psychiatry* 130:61–7.

Solowij, N., W. Hall, and N. Lee. 1992. Recreational MDMA use in Sydney: A profile of "Ecstacy" users and their experiences with the drug. *Br. J. Addict.* 87:1161–72.

Soper, H. V., R. O. Elliot Jr., A. A. Rejzer, et al. 1990. Effects of fenfluramine on neuropsychological and communicative functioning in treatment refractory schizophrenic patients. *J. Clin. Psychopharmacol.* 10:168–75.

Spatt, J., B. Glawar, and B. Mamoli. 1997. A pure amnestic syndrome after MDMA ("Ecstasy") ingestion. *J. Neurol. Neurosurg. Psychiatry* 62(4):418–9.

Spiegel, R., and H.-J. Aebi. 1983. *Psychopharmacology: An introduction.* New York: John Wiley & Sons.

Spigset, O., and T. Mjorndal. 1997. The effect of fluvoxamine on serum prolactin and serum sodium concentrations: Relation to platelet 5HT2A receptor status. *J. Clin. Psychopharmacol.* 17:292–7.

Spina, E., P. DeDomenico, C. Ruello, et al. 1994. Adjunctive fluoxetine in the treatment of negative symptoms in chronic schizophrenic patients. *Int. Clin. Psychopharmacol.* 9:281–5.

Sprague, J. E., and D. E. Nichols. 1995a. Inhibition of MAO-B protects against MDMA-induced neurotoxicity in the striatum. *Psychopharmacology (Berlin)* 118:357–9.

———. 1995b. The monoamine oxidase-B inhibitor L-deprenyl protects against 3,4-methylenedioxymethamphetamine-induced lipid peroxidation and long-term serotonergic deficits. *J. Pharmacol. Exp. Ther.* 273:667–73.

Sprague, J. E., S. L. Everman, and D. E. Nichols. 1998. An integrated hypothesis for the serotonergic axonal loss induced by 3,4-methylenedioxymethamphetamine. *Neurotoxicology* 19:427–41.

Sprague, J. E., T. Worst, A. Kanthasamy, D. E. Nichols, and M. D. Kane. 1999. Effects of antisense oligonucleotide alteration of MAO-B gene expression on MDMA-induced serotonergic neurotoxicity. Paper presented at the Society for Neuroscience, Miami, Florida. [Abstract] p. 836.

Stafford, P. 1992. *Psychedelics encyclopedia.* 3d ed., expanded. Berkeley, Calif.: Ronin Publishing.

Stahl, S. M., S. B. Uhr, and P. A. Berger. 1985. Pilot study on the effects of fenfluramine on negative symptoms in twelve schizophrenic inpatients. *Biol. Psychiatry* 20:1098–102.

Steele, T. D., W. K. Brewster, M. P. Johnson, D. E. Nichols, and G. K. Yim. 1991. Assessment of the role of alpha-methylepinine in the neurotoxicity of MDMA. *Pharmacol. Biochem. Behav.* 38:345–51.

Steele, T. D., U. D. McCann, and G. A. Ricaurte. 1994. 3,4-Methylenedioxymethamphetamine (MDMA, "Ecstasy"): pharmacology and toxicology in animals and humans. *Addiction* 89:539–51.

Stein, M. B., C. Hanna, C. Koverola, M. Torchia, and B. McClarty. 1997. Structural brain changes in PTSD: Does trauma alter neuroanatomy? *Ann. N. Y. Acad. Sci.* 821:76–82.

Stern, R. A., S. G. Silva, N. Chaisson, and D. L. Evans. 1996. Influence of cognitive reserve on neuropsychological functioning in asymptomatic human immunodeficiency virus-1 infection. *Arch. Neurol.* 53:148–53.

Sternbach, H. 1991. The serotonin syndrome. *Am. J. Psychiatry* 148:705–13.

Stol, W. 1947. Lysergaure-diatheyl-amid, ein Phantastidum aus der Mutterkorngruppe. [LSD, a hallucinatory agent from the ergot group]. *Schweitz. Arch. Neut.* 60.

Stolaroff, M. J. 1997. *The secret chief: Conversations with a pioneer of the underground psychedelic therapy movement.* Charlotte, N.C.: MAPS.

Stone, A. A., C. A. Macro, C. E. Cruise, D. A. Cox, and J. M. Neale. 1996. Are stress-induced immunological changes mediated by mood? A closer look at how both desirable and undesirable daily events influence salivary IGA antibody. *Int. J. Behav. Med.* 3:1–13.

Stone, D. M., D. C. Stahl, G. R. Hanson, and J. W. Gibb. 1986. The effects of 3,4-methylenedioxymethamphetamine (MDMA) and 3,4-methylenedioxyamphetamine (MDA) on monoaminergic systems in the rat brain. *Eur. J. Pharmacol.* 128:41–8.

Stone, D. M., G. R. Hanson, and J. W. Gibb. 1987a. Differences in the central serotonergic effects of methylenedioxymethamphetamine (MDMA) in mice and rats. *Neuropharmacology* 26:1657–61.

Stone, D. M., K. M. Merchant, G. R. Hanson, and J. W. Gibb. 1987b. Immediate and long-term effects of 3,4-methylenedioxymethamphetamine on serotonin pathways in brain of rat. *Neuropharmacology* 26:1677–83.

Stone, D. M., M. Johnson, G. R. Hanson, and J. W. Gibb. 1988. Role of endogenous dopamine in the central serotonergic deficits induced by 3,4-methylenedioxymethamphetamine. *J. Pharmacol. Exp. Ther.* 247:79–87.

Stone, D. M., G. R. Hanson, and J. W. Gibb. 1989a. In vitro reactivation of rat cortical tryptophan hydroxylase following in vivo inactivation by methylenedioxymethamphetamine. *J. Neurochem.* 53:572–81.

Stone, D. M., M. Johnson, G. R. Hanson, and J. W. Gibb. 1989b. Acute inactivation of tryptophan hydroxylase by amphetamine analogs involves the oxidation of sulfhydryl sites. *Eur. J. Pharmacol.* 172:93–7.

Strassman, R. J. 1984. Adverse reactions to psychedelic drugs: A review of the literature. *J. Nerv. Ment. Dis.* 172(10):577–95.

Strupp, H. H. 1993. The Vanderbilt psychotherapy studies: A synopsis. *J. Consult. Clin. Psychol.* 61(3):431–3.

Styk, J., and S. Styk. 1999. Review of clinical issues in MDMA-assisted psychotherapy, based on their use of MDMA with patients from 1988–1993 in Switzerland. Paper presented at MAPS MDMA Conference, August 30 to September, Dead Sea, Israel. (The transcript of this lecture can be found at www.maps.org.)

Suicide: Part I. 1986. *Harvard Medical School Medical Health Letter,* 2(8): 1–4.

Swiss court downgrades ecstasy drug. 1999. *Associated Press,* 21 June.

Tagaya, M., K. F. Liu, B. Copeland, et al. 1997. DNA scission after focal brain ischemia: Temporal differences in two species. *Stroke* 28:1245–54.

Talley, P. F., H. H. Strupp, and L. C. Morey. 1990. Matchmaking in psychotherapy: Patient-therapist dimensions and their impact on outcome. *J. Consult. Clin. Psychol.* 58(2):182–8.

Tehan, B., R. Hardern, and A. Bodenham. 1993. Hyperthermia associated with 3,4-methylenedioxylmethamphetamine ("Eve"). *Anaesthesia* 48:507–10.

Thakore, J. H., C. Berti, and T. G. Dinan. 1996. An open trial of adjunctive sertraline in the treatment of chronic schizophrenia. *Acta Psychiatr. Scand.* 94:194–7.

Tork, I. 1991. Anatomy of the serotonergic system. *Ann. N. Y. Acad. Sci.* 600:9–34.

Tuchtenhagen, F., J. Daumann, C. Norra, et al. 2000. High intensity dependence of auditory evoked dipole source activity indicates decreased serotonergic activity in abstinent ecstasy (MDMA) users. *Neuropsychopharmacology* 22:608–17.

Tucker, G. T., M. S. Lennard, S. W. Ellis et al. 1994. The demethylation of methlenedioxymethamphetamine ("ecstasy") by debrisoquine hydroxylase. *Biochem. Pharmacol.* 47(7):1151–6.

Turek, I. S., R. A. Soskin, and A. A. Kurland. 1974. Methylenedioxyamphetamine (MDA) subjective effects. *J. Psychedelic Drugs* 6:7–14.

U.S. Department of Health and Human Services. National Household Survey on Drug Abuse. 1996, 1997, 1998.

Vander Borght, T., M. Kilbourn, T. Desmond, D. Kuhl, and K. Frey. 1995. The vesicular monoamine transporter is not regulated by dopaminergic drug treatments. *Eur. J. Pharmacol.* 294:577–83.

van der Kolk, B. A. 1997. The psychobiology of posttraumatic stress disorder. *J. Clin. Psychiatry* 58(suppl 9):16–24.

van der Kolk, B. A., O. van der Hart, and J. Burbridge. 1995. *Approaches to the treatment of PTSD.* Lutherville, Md.: Bookshelf.

van Dyck, C. H., R. T. Malison, J. P. Seibyl, et al. 2000. Age-related decline in central serotonin transporter availability with [123I]beta-CIT SPECT. *Neurobiol. Aging* 21:497–501.

van Kammen, D. P., and J. J. Boronow. 1988. Dextro-amphetamine diminishes negative symptoms in schizophrenia. *Int. Clin. Psychopharmacol.* 3:111–21.

van Praag, H. M. 1962. A critical investigation of the significance of MAO inhibition as a therapeutic principle in the treatment of depression. Thesis, University of Utrecht.

van Praag, H. M. 1981. Management of depression with serotonin precursors. *Biol. Psychiatry* 16:291–310.

———. 1982. Depression, suicide and the metabolism of serotonin in the brain. *J. Affect. Disord.* 4:275–90.

van Praag, H. M. 1994. 5-HT-related, anxiety- and/or aggression-driven depression. *Int. Clin. Psychopharmacol.* 1:5–6.

Verkes, R. J., H. J. Gijsman, M. S. M. Pieters, et al. 2000. Cognitive performance and serotonergic function in users of ecstasy. *Psychopharmacology (Berlin)* 153:196–202.

Virden, T. B., and L. E. Baker. 1999. Disruption of the discriminative stimulus effects of S(+)-3,4-methylenedioxymethamphetamine (MDMA) by (±)-MDMA neurotoxicity: protection by fluoxetine. *Behav. Pharmacol.* 10:195–204.

Volkow, N. D., G. J. Wang, M. W. Fischman, et al. 1997. Relationship between subjective effects of cocaine and dopamine transporter occupancy. *Nature* 386:827–30.

Vollenweider, F. X., A. Gamma, M. Liechti, and T. Huber. 1998a. Psychological and cardiovascular effects and short-term sequelae of MDMA ("Ecstasy") in MDMA-naive healthy volunteers. *Neuropsychopharmacology* 19:241–51.

Vollenweider, F. X., M. F. I. Vollenweider-Scherpenhuyzen, A. Babler, H. Vogel, and D. Hell. 1998b. Psilocybin induces schizophrenia-like psychosis in humans via a serotonin-2 agonist action. *NeuroReport* 9:3897–902.

Vollenweider, F. X., A. Gamma, M. Liechti, and T. Huber. 1999a. Is a single dose of MDMA harmless? [Letter]. *Neuropsychopharmacology* 21:598–600.

Vollenweider, F. X., S. Remensberger, D. Hell, and M. A. Geyer. 1999b. Opposite effects of 3,4-methylenedioxymethamphetamine (MDMA) on sensorimotor gating in rats versus healthy humans. *Psychopharmacology* 143(4):365–72.

Wareing, M., J. E. Fisk, and P. N. Murphy. 2000. Working memory deficits in current and previous users of MDMA ("ecstasy"). *Br. J. Psychol.* 91:181–8.

Watson, L., and J. Beck. 1991. New Age seekers: MDMA use as an adjunct to spiritual pursuit. *J. Psychoactive Drugs* 23:261–70.

Webb, C., and V. Williams. 1993. Ecstasy intoxication: Appreciation of complications and the role of dantrolene. *Anaesthesia* 48:542–3.

Weil, Andrew, and Winifred Rosen. *From chocolate to morphine.* Boston: Houghton Mifflin, 1983.

Whitaker-Azmita, P. M., and T. A. Aronson. 1989. "Ecstasy" (MDMA)–induced panic. *Am. J. Psychiatry* 146:119.

Williams, H., D. Meager, and P. Galligan. 1993. MDMA (Ecstasy): A case of possible drug induced psychosis. *Ir. J. Psychol. Med.* 162:43–4.

Williams, H., L. Dratcu, R. Taylor, M. Roberts, and A. Oyefeso. 1998. "Saturday night fever": Ecstasy related problems in a London accident and emergency department. *J. Accid. Emerg. Med.* 15(5):322–6.

Williamson, S., M. Gossop, B. Powis, P. Griffiths, J. Fountain, and J. Strang. 1997. Adverse effects of stimulant drugs in a community sample of drug users. *Drug Alcohol Depend.* 44:87–94.

Wilson, J. M., K. S. Kalasinsky, A. I. Levey, et al. 1996. Striatal dopamine nerve terminal markers in human, chronic methamphetamine users. *Nat. Med.* 2:699–703.

Wilson, M. A., and M. E. Molliver. 1994. Microglial response to degeneration of serotonergic axon terminals. *Glia* 11:18–34.

Wilson, M. A., G. A. Ricaurte, and M. E. Molliver. 1989. Distinct morphologic classes of serotonergic axons in primates exhibit differential vulnerability to the psychotropic drug 3,4-methylenedioxymethamphetamine. *Neuroscience* 28:121–37.

Windhaber, J., D. Maierhofer, and K. Dantendorfer. 1998. Panic disorder induced by large doses of 3,4-methylenedioxymethamphetamine resolved by paroxetine. *J. Clin. Psychopharmacol.* 18(1):95–6.

Winslow, J. T., and T. R. Insel. 1990. Serotonergic modulation of rat pup ultrasonic vocal development: studies with 3,4-methylenedioxymethamphetamine. *J. Pharmacol. Exp. Ther.* 254:212–20.

Winstock, A. R. 1991. Chronic paranoid psychosis after misuse of 3,4-methylenedioxymethamphetamine. *Br. Med. J.* 302:1150–1.

Winter, J. C. 1975. Blockade of the stimulus properties of mescaline by a serotonin antagonist. *Archiv. Int. Pharmacodyn. Ther.* 214:250–3.

Wodarz, N., and J. Boning. 1993. Ecstasy-induziertes psychotisches Depersonalisation Syndrom. *Nervenartz* 64:478–80.

Wollina, U., H. J. Kammler, N. Hesselbarth et al. 1998. Ecstasy pimples: A new facial dermatosis. *Dermatology* 197(2):171–3.

World Health Organization 1958. *Ataractic and hallucinogenic drugs in psychiatry: Report of a study group.* Technical Report Series, no. 152. Geneva: World Health Organization.

World Health Organization. 1985. Expert Committee on Drug Dependence. Twenty-second report, series 729. Geneva: World Health Organization. pp. 24–25.

World Health Organization. 1992. The ICD-10 classification of mental and behavioral disorders: Clinical descriptions and diagnostic guidelines. Geneva: World Health Organization. pp. 70–83.

Wu, D., S. V. Otton, T. Inaba, W. Kalow, and E. M. Sellers. 1997. Interactions of amphetamine analogs with human liver CYP2D6. *Biochem. Pharmacol.* 53:1605–12.

Yamamoto, B. K., and L. J. Spanos. 1988. The acute effects of methylenedioxymethamphetamine on dopamine release in the awake-behaving rat. *Eur. J. Pharmacol.* 148:195–203.

Yeh, S. Y. 1999. *N*-tert-butyl-alpha-phenylnitrone protects against 3,4-methylenedioxymethamphetamine-induced depletion of serotonin in rats. *Synapse* 31:169–77.

Young, F. 1986. Opinion and recommended ruling, findings of fact, conclusions of law, and decision of administrative law judge. Submitted in the matter of MDMA scheduling, docket no. 84-48, 22 May. erowid.org/chemicals/mdma/mdma_law2.shtml

Zhao, Z. Y., N. Castagnoli Jr., G. A. Ricaurte, T. Steele, and M. Martello. 1992. Synthesis and neurotoxicological evaluation of putative metabolites of the serotonergic neurotoxin 2-(methylamino)-1-[3,4-(methylenedioxy)phenyl] propane [methylenedioxymethamphetamine]. *Chem. Res. Toxicol.* 5:89–94.

Zuckerman, M. 1996. The psychobiological model for impulsive unsocialized sensation seeking: A comparative approach. *Neuropsychobiology* 34:125–9.

CONTRIBUTORS

Matthew Baggot matt@baggot.net
Mr. Baggott has conducted psychopharmacology research for over a decade, most recently at the University of California, San Francisco. He has published on the pharmacology of entactogens, psychostimulants, and opiates.

Katherine Bonson, Ph.D. kbonson@codon.nih.gov
Dr. Bonson is a Team Pharmacologist with the Controlled Substances Staff of the Food and Drug Administration. She has studied the effects of drugs on serotonergic systems of the brain at the National Institute of Mental Health, the National Institute on Drug Abuse and Johns Hopkins University. Dr. Bonson's statements are those of an individual pharmacologist and do not represent official FDA positions.

José Carlos Bouso
Mr. Bouso is a psychologist and Ph.D. candidate at the Universidad Autónoma de Madrid. He is currently conducting the first officially authorized MDMA/PTSD psychotherapy study at the Psychiatric Hospital of Madrid.

Gary Bravo M.D. glbravo@aol.com.
Dr. Bravo is a staff psychiatrist for Sonoma County Mental Health in Santa Rosa, California. While on the clinical faculty at the University of California-Irvine, he wrote about the effects of MDMA and worked with Dr. Charles Grob on the first federally-approved MDMA protocol. He has also written articles on psychedelics and psychiatry, and transpersonal psychology.

Rick Doblin, Ph.D. rick@maps.org
Dr. Doblin is the president of MAPS, Multidisciplinary Association for Psychedelic Studies (www.maps.org). He founded MAPS in 1986 in order to develop MDMA into an FDA-approved prescription medicine. He received his Ph.D. in public policy from the Kennedy School of Government, Harvard University.

Alex Gamma, Ph.D. gamma@bli.unizh.ch
Dr. Gamma is a biologist specializing in neuropsychopharmacology and a research assistant at the University Hospital of Psychiatry, Zurich, Switzerland. For the past five years, he has been conducting basic experimental research into the acute effects of MDMA in healthy subjects, as well as clinical studies in long-term Ecstasy users.

George R. Greer, M.D. george@newmexico.com
Dr. Greer, M.D. worked with his wife Requa Tolbert, a psychiatric nurse, to administer MDMA over 100 times to 80 people as part of his clinical psychiatric practice from 1980 to 1985. Their review of this work remains the largest published study of the therapeutic use of MDMA to date. Dr. Greer is a fellow of the American Psychiatric Association and is the Medical Director of Heffter Research Institute.

Charles S. Grob, M.D.
Dr. Grob conducted the first FDA approved research study examining the effects of MDMA on human volunteers. He has written extensively on the history of MDMA and the putative MDMA treatment paradigm and has provided a critical analysis of the neurotoxicity hypothesis. He is Professor of Psychiatry at the UCLA School of Medicine and currently serves as Director of the Division of Child and Adolescent Psychiatry, Harbor-UCLA Medical Center.

Professor John A Henry, M.D.
Professor Henry spent fifteen years as Consultant Physician at Guy's Hospital and the National Poisons Information Service, London. He was the first to describe hepatotoxicity due to MDMA, and also described the first cases of hyponatraemia. He has demonstrated, through clinical research, that vasopressin release is a pharmacological effect of MDMA.

Julie Holland, M.D. drholland.com
Dr. Holland is a physician in the psychiatric emergency room at Bellevue Hospital, with a private practice in New York City. She has been researching, writing, and speaking about the therapeutic potential of MDMA since 1985. She received the 1994 National Institute of Mental Health Outstanding Resident Award for her clinical research on schizophrenia. Dr. Holland also serves as a Clinical Assistant Professor of Psychiatry for the New York Univeristy School of Medicine.

Karl Jansen, M.D., Ph.D. K@BTInternet.com
Dr. Jansen is a medical doctor and consultant psychiatrist who was engaged in full-time study of the human brain for 6 years. He also has a Ph.D. in clinical pharmacology and is a member of the Royal College of Psychiatrists. He has made a special study of persons who use very large quantities of MDMA and ketamine.

Andrew M. Kleiman, M.D.
Dr. Kleiman is a fourth year resident in psychiatry at New York University Medical Center, Bellevue Hospital, in New York City. He is interested in clinical psychiatric research and is planning on establishing a private practice in psychiatry.

Matthias Emanuel Liechti, M.D. mliechti@bli.unizh.ch
Dr. Liechti is a medical doctor at the University Hospital of Psychiatry, Zurich, Switzerland, working in internal medicine and psychiatry. As a postdoctoral fellow and researcher he specialized in neuropsychopharmacology and elucidated the neuropharmacological mechanisms of MDMA's effects in humans.

Jessica E. Malberg, Ph.D. jessica.malberg@yale.edu
Dr. Malberg is a postdoctoral associate in the Department of Psychiatry at Yale University. She published the first papers investigating the interaction of environmental temperature, core body temperature and MDMA-induced neurotoxicity in the rat.

John Mendelson M.D. jemmd@itsa.ucsf.edu
Dr. Mendelson serves as Associate Clinical Professor of Psychiatry and Medicine for the Drug Dependence Research Center, University of California at San Francisco and is an internist interested in the human pharmacology of abused drugs. He is among the first to study the effects of controlled doses of MDMA on cardiovascular function and to investigate the pharmacokinetics of MDMA in humans.

Ralph Metzner, Ph.D. rmetzner@svn.net
Dr. Metzner, Professor of Psychology, California Institute of Integral Studies, is a consciousness researcher and psychotherapist who worked with MDMA in psychotherapy prior to its prohibition. He is the pseudonymous editor of *Through the Gateway of the Heart*, a compilation of experiential accounts of MDMA assisted therapy and meditation. He is also the co-author of *The Psychedelic Experience* with Timothy Leary, and the editor of *Ayahuasca—Human Consciousness and the Spirits of Nature*.

Michael Montagne, R.Ph., Ph.D. mmontagne@mcp.edu
Dr. Montagne has researched and taught on the social-cultural aspects of psychedelic drugs and their use for twenty–five years. His research also has focused on the role of meaning, symbolism, and metaphors in depression and the use of anti-depressant medications. He is currently the Rombult Distinguished Professor of Pharmacy, Massachusetts College of Pharmacy & Health Science.

Claudio Naranjo, M.D. hermesalud@euskalnet.net
Dr. Naranjo was originally trained in psychiatry and psychoanalytic therapy, and became one of the three successors to Fritz Perls at Esalen Institute. He later became known as an author, an educator, and an integrator between the world of psychotherapy and that of the spiritual traditions. He was the first to observe the characteristic effects of MDA and to point out the usefulness of MDA in psychotherapy. He was also the first to point out the characteristic effects of the "feeling enhancers" (now called empathogens) and to conduct clinical research with them.

Dave Nichols, Ph.D.
Dr. Nichols, Professor of Medicinal Chemistry and Molecular Pharmacology, Purdue University, has published more than 200 scientific research articles on various aspects of the medicinal chemistry and neuropharmacology of drugs that act in the brain. His laboratory carried out the first studies to establish the pharmacological mechanism of action of MDMA, and it was he who coined the term "entactogens" as a name for the novel pharmacological class of which MDMA is the prototype.

Joseph G. Rella, M.D.
After training in emergency medicine and completing a fellowship in medical toxicology at Bellevue Hospital, Dr. Rella collected data regarding MDMA toxicity in patients who were reported to the New York City poison center for seven years. He is well-acquainted with the acute toxicity of MDMA and is continuing research into its physiologic effects. He currently serves as Assistant Professor of Emergency Medicine, University of Medicine and Dentistry of New Jersey at Newark.

June Riedlinger, Pharm.D.
Dr. Riedlinger is Assistant Professor of Clinical Pharmacy and Director, Center for Integrative Therapies in Pharmaceutical Care, Massachusetts College of Pharmacy and Health Sciences. She took the witness stand to testify about the therapeutic effects of MDMA in 1985 and subsequently authored and co-authored several articles on MDMA and presented at the Drug Policy Foundation international conferences. Dr. Riedlinger is currently working in the Complementary and Alternative Medicine field through which she has been able to offer educational programs that include topics relating to psychedelic drugs and MDMA.

Douglas Rushkoff, Ph.D. www.rushkoff.com
Professor Douglas Rushkoff is the author of seven best-selling books on culture and
technology, including *Coercion, Media Virus, Cyberia, Playing the Future,* and the novels
Ecstasy Club and *Exit Strategy.* He writes a column for the New York Times Syndicate,
delivers commentaries on National Public Radio, and makes documentaries for PBS
Frontline. He is currently Professor of Virtual Culture at New York University's
Interactive Telecommunication Program. He has been studying psychedelic subcultures
since he became friends with Timothy Leary in 1988.

Rabbi Zalman Schachter
Rabbi Schachter, Professor of Religious Studies at Naropa University, is an ordained
Lubavitch-trained rabbi whose belief in the universality of spiritual truth led him to
study with Sufi Masters, Buddhist teachers, Native American elders, Catholic monks,
and humanistic and transpersonal psychologists. As such he also experienced
psychedelics and wrote about his experience in *The Ecstatic Adventure.* He is also the
author of *Spiritual Intimacy* and *Paradigm Shift,* and co-author with Ronald Miller of
From Age-ing to Sage-ing.

Emanuel Sferios emanuel@dancesafe.org
Mr. Sferios is the founder and current executive director of DanceSafe, a nonprofit
harm reduction organization that promotes health and safety within the rave and
nightclub community.

Alexander "Sasha" Shulgin, Ph.D.
Dr. Shulgin's academic background has been in chemistry and in biochemistry, with
post-doctorate studies at the University of California San Francisco Medical School.
His research work for the last forty years has been the design, synthesis, and evaluation
of new psychoactive drugs, with special concentration on the psychedelic drugs. His
early work with MDMA led to his co-authoring the first human studies describing its
action.

Ann Shulgin ashulgin@atdial.net
Ms. Shulgin worked for three years as a lay therapist, using MDMA, before it was made
illegal. Since many of the therapists who discovered the virtues of MDMA before it was
scheduled are still using it underground, they cannot appear in public or in publications
to speak about its use in therapy. She, on the other hand, stopped doing MDMA
therapy in the mid-1980's and can talk and write openly about it.

Harry Sumnall spun@liv.ac.uk
Mr. Sumnall is a Ph.D. candidate at the Department of Psychology, University of
Liverpool, UK. He is currently writing his thesis on the behavioral consequences of
exposure to a neurotoxic regime of MDMA. He is the co-author of several scientific
articles awaiting publication concerning the cognitive and psychopathological effects of
Ecstasy and other "dance drugs."

Franz X. Vollenweider, M.D., P.D. vollen@bli.unizh.ch
Dr. Vollenweider is a psychiatrist, research scientist and lecturer at the Psychiatric
University Hospital of Zurich. He is actively involved in both clinical and basic
research on the neurobiology of psychoses and affective disorders. Since 1987 he has
focused on basic research addressing the behavioral and neurobiological effects of

indoleamine hallucinogens, dissociative anesthetics and psychostimulants using Positron Emission Tomography (PET), Electroencephalography (EEG), and measures of information processing such as the prepulse inhibition paradigm of the acoustic startle reflex.

Andrew Weil, M.D. drweil.com
Dr. Weil is the director of the Program in Integrative Medicine of the College of Medicine, University of Arizona. He has a general practice in Tucson, focusing on natural and preventive medicine and diagnosis. Dr. Weil is also the founder of the National Integrative Medicine Council in Tucson and the author of eight books including the international bestsellers, *Spontaneous Healing, Eight Weeks to Optimum Health* and *Eating Well for Optimum Health.*

Further contact information can be found at drholland.com

INDEX